Women, Power, and Therapy: Issues for Women

Women, Power, and Therapy: Issues for Women

Marjorie Braude
Editor

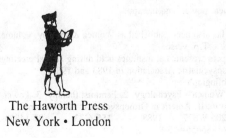

The Haworth Press
New York • London

Women, Power, and Therapy: Issues for Women has also been published as *Women & Therapy*, Volume 6, Numbers 1/2, Spring/Summer 1987.

The Haworth Press, Inc., 12 West 32 Street, New York, NY 10001
EUROSPAN/Haworth, 3 Henrietta Street, London WC2E 8LU England

Library of Congress Cataloging-in Publication Data

Women, power, and therapy.

"Has also been published as Women & therapy, volume 6, numbers 1/2, spring/summer 1987"—T.p. verso.
Papers presented at institutes held during annual meetings of the American Orthopsychiatric Association in 1983 and 1984.
Bibliography: p.
1. Women—Psychology. 2. Feminist therapy. 3. Power (Social sciences) I. Braude, Marjorie. II. American Orthopsychiatric Association.
HQ1206.W877   1988   155.6'33   87-14873
ISBN 0-86656-653-8

To my daughters:

Ann, who introduced me
to women's history
and Liza, who says it with
art, music, and poetry.
May your voices be loud and clear.

—MB

Women, Power, and Therapy:
Issues for Women

Women & Therapy
Volume 6, Numbers 1/2

CONTENTS

run psychotherapy groups for women. My newest interest is in co-leading education groups for adult daughters from alcoholic families. I have a background in history and literature and have taught and written in these areas.

R. LORRAINE COLLINS, PhD: I received my PhD from Rutgers University in 1980 after which I completed a two-year research post doc at the University of Washington. I am currently at SUNY Buffalo where I am a Research Scientist III, at the Research Institute on Alcoholism. I am also interested in commonalities across addictive behaviors and in the role of alcohol in aggression against women (physical and sexual abuse).

VIRGINIA DONOVAN, PhD: I have a PhD in psychology and am a psychotherapist. Since 1971 I have been a member of the Women's Mental Health Collective, a not-for-profit clinic in Somerville, MA. Our approach to psychotherapy has been informed by our awareness that individual, couple, and family problems can only be understood in the context of broader social issues. My particular area of interest is understanding the implications of emerging feminist psychological theories of development for the practice of therapy.

IRIS FODOR, PhD: Received a PhD in Clinical Psychology at Boston University, 1965. Training in child and adult clinical; Chair: NYU (SEHNAP) Women's Studies Commission (1984-85), Professor and trainer of Psychologists for the Schools; Clinical supervisor. Writer, lecturer and practitioner of Cognitive Behavior Therapy, Women's Issues and Mental Health, Assertiveness, the integration of CBT and Gestalt Therapy.

VIOLET FRANKS, PhD: I am a behaviorally oriented, non-sexist therapist particularly interested in problems which affect women. I have a private practice and also am employed in an inpatient psychiatric hospital. I edit a series for Springer Press entitled "Focus on Women."

MIRIAM GREENSPAN, MEd: I have been a feminist therapist in private practice in the Boston area for the past eleven years. I work primarily with women and couples—both heterosexual and homosexual—between the ages of 20 and 50. I also enjoy working with men. I have been involved in teaching, supervising and consulting as well as giving talks on the subject of women and therapy throughout the United States. In the past few years I have extended my consultation services to include workshops on gender relations in high tech industry. My first book *A New Approach to Women and Therapy*, was published by McGraw-Hill in 1983.

JUDITH HERMAN, MD: I received my MD degree from Harvard Medical School and my training in general and community psychiatry at Boston University Medical Center. For the past 14 years I have been a member of the Women's Mental Health Collective, together with Virginia Donovan and Michelle Clark. I am also Assistant Clinical Professor of Psychiatry at Harvard Medical School. My first book, *Father-Daughter Incest*, was published by Harvard University Press in 1981. Both my writing and my clinical work continue to focus on issues of violence in sexual and domestic life.

MARCIA HILL, EdD: My training at Rutgers focused mainly on children and systems, but my work as a psychologist has included a little of everything, from consulting in a variety of settings to therapy and teaching. From this range, I've gradually chosen clinical work, which

I continue to find absorbing and endlessly instructive. I now work primarily with women as a feminist therapist in a full time private practice. I am also involved with a local shelter for battered women. My professional interests include the political aspects of therapy, experiential therapy, violence against women, and the nature of the change process.

SHERE D. HITE, MA, is author/researcher of *The Hite Reports*, published 1976 (MacMillan) and 1981 (Knopf), and the forthcoming final Hite Report, to be published October, 1987 by Knopf. She has been published in 17 countries, and lectured in universities in the U.S. and around the world on women's sexuality and the place of women in history. She has addressed many academic societies, including keynote speeches, to the American Assn. of Sex Educators, Counselors and Therapists, the American Psychological Association, the American Historical Association, the World Congress of Sexology, and others.

MARGARET A. KINGDON, PhD: I earned my PhD in 1974 from the University of Maryland. Currently, I am a feminist psychotherapist in private practice in the Washington, D.C. area where I work with adult women who have a wide variety of concerns including depression, sexuality issues, separation and divorce, sexual abuse, and career and life-style changes. I am also a training consultant and conduct workshops and seminars in areas such as communication skills, women in management, stress management, time management, and career development.

JEAN LATHROP, MA: The first seven years of my adulthood were spent at home trying to be the perfect wife and mother and regarding other women as only competition for the goodies of a patriarchal society. When this life approach failed to work, I went to work, back to school, began co-counseling and joined a women's group. From then on my work (paid and unpaid) became increasingly centered on working with women in educational, therapeutic, and political settings. Currently I teach (women's studies) and counsel in an adult degree program whose primary population is women in transition and am chair of the university status of women committee.

BARBARA MILLER, PhD: Born and grew up in New York City. Went to Sarah Lawrence College and then earned a PhD from Columbia University in 1961. Have had an individual psychology practice for approximately 23 years in the New York area as well as Denver, Colorado, Washington, D.C., and currently Burlington. Specialty areas include: women's self-esteem and coping, adolescence and ethnic minority concerns and stress. Married with 3 children.

JEAN BAKER MILLER, MD, is Clinical Professor of Psychiatry at Boston University School of Medicine and Scholar-in-Residence at the Stone Center, Wellesley College. A recipient of the Rockefeller Foundation Humanities Fellowship, she has written *Toward a New Psychology of Women* (1976) and edited *Psychoanalysis and Women* (1973), as well as numerous articles on depression, dreams and the psychology of women. Fellow of American Psychiatric Association, American Orthopsychiatric Association, American Academy of Psychoanalysis, and have been a member of the board of trustees of the last two. Member, consultant to, and teacher of several womens' groups.

NICOLA MORRIS, MA: I am a teacher and advisor at Goddard College, a small progressive school in Central Vermont. I teach Feminist Studies, Literature, and writing. Many of my students are women who are studying and questioning their own lives and placing their experiences in a political context. I work with women who are seeking to develop a strong sense of self, women who want to find and develop their own power. I have an abiding interest in the barriers that women have to overcome in order to write.

PATRICIA A. RESICK, PhD: I earned my PhD in 1976 at the University of Georgia. After graduating I took a position as an Assistant Professor at the University of South Dakota. In 1980 I was promoted to Associate Professor. After a year as a visiting Associate Professor at the Medical University of South Carolina, I took a position as an Associate Professor at the University of Missouri-St. Louis. My area of research is reactions to victimization, and trauma and therapy of victims.

JILL V. RICHARD, MSW, MA, is currently a Psychiatric Social Worker for a public school system, south of Boston. She provides family, individual and couples therapy, as well as parent education to the families of pre-school and school-aged children. Her background includes administrative and supervisory experience. In addition she has spoken and written on topics related to women and psychology.

MARGIE RIPPER, BA: Currently a faculty member in Sociology at Flinders University in South Australia. Doctoral student in Medical Sociology, with research in the area of the social construction of femininity and illness. Previous research interests include women's health — particularly menstrual cycle effects, feminist theory, self-help, and medical education. Teaching experience includes Women's Studies, Sociology & Community Health.

MARYLIN SAFIR, PhD, moved to Israel in 1968, where she taught the first course on Behavior Therapy, helped to found the Israel Behavior Therapy Association of which she was the first President. She is currently a Senior Lecturer in the Psychology Department and directs the Women's Studies Department at the University of Haifa. She recently co-edited *Sexual Equality: The Israeli Kibbutz Tests the Theories* (Norwood Press, 1983) and *Women's Worlds – From the New Scholarship* (Praeger Publications, 1985). Her current research interests focus on Sex Roles and Sex Stereotypes as they relate to sexuality, to sex differences in intellectual functioning, and to socialization practices in city and kibbutz, in addition to feminist therapy.

LINDA T. SANFORD is a licensed psychotherapist and the Coordinator of the Sex Abuse Treatment Unit at Coastal Community Counseling Center in Braintree, Mass. She is the author of *The Silent Children: A Parent's Guide to the Prevention of Child Sexual Abuse* (McGraw-Hill, 1982) and she and Mary Ellen Donovan co-authored *Women and Self-Esteem: Understanding and Improving the Ways We Feel about Ourselves* (forthcoming Viking-Penguin paperback, September 1985). In the past 11 years, she has worked with over 600 sexually victimized women and children and also provides training and consultation on a national basis.

JILL MATTUCK TARULE, PhD, is an Associate Professor at Lesley College in Cambridge, Massachusetts where she teaches and directs the Lesley College Weekend Learning Community, an interdisciplinary program for returning adult students. A developmental psychologist, she is completing a collaborative research project and a resulting book: *The Other Side of Silence, The Development of Women's Ways of Knowing* (Basic Books, forthcoming). Her other research, teaching, administration and publications are in adult development with a particular emphasis on higher education as a support for personal and intellectual development. Her undergraduate degree is from Goddard College, her doctorate is Counseling Psychology from Harvard Graduate School of Education. She lives in Plymouth, Massachusetts with a husband, daughter, two dogs, a cat and, unfortunately, a nuclear power plant.

LENORE TIEFER, PhD, BOOK REVIEW EDITOR: Born a New York Jew in 1944, the daughter of a high school teacher and X-ray technician. Given an excellent public education, including the renowned all-girls' high school, Hunter. BA in 1965, and PhD in 1969 from University of California at Berkeley — and imagine the effect of Berkeley in the 60s! First job, because I got my degree before the movement hit, teaching psychology at Colorado State University in Fort Collins. Discovered feminism in 1972. Moved to New York, clinical work, medical center life and the joys of a patchwork career in 1977.

ANN VODA, PhD, is a menopause and menstrual cycle researcher. She was educated initially as a nurse and received advanced graduate training in physiology specializing in reproductive physiology. She has published widely in scientific journals, presented papers at national and international meetings. Her research and writings reflect a feminist perspective with regard to the medicalization of events related to women's menstrual cycle physiology. She is also a member of the Women's Studies coordinating committee at the University of Utah.

SUSAN WOOLEY, PhD: Received BA in Philosophy, Antioch College, 1964; PhD in clinical psychology, University of Illinois, 1969. Since then on faculty of Psychiatry Dept., Univ. of Cincinnati Medical College. Along with husband and collaborator, Wayne Wooley, involved for many years in study of food intake/weight regulation; founded Eating Disorders Clinic in 1974. Major interests have included the prejudices against fatness; physiological bases of overweight and eating disorders; women and body image; experiential, feminist treatment techniques.

Foreword

This volume consists primarily of papers that were originally presented at the 1983 and 1984 Women's Institute, sponsored by the American Orthopsychiatric Association. Marjorie Braude, who co-chaired the Institute in 1983 and chaired it in 1984, has done a wonderful job of selecting, from the widely diverse papers presented, a coherent series on the subject of women, power, and therapy. The resulting collection is a unified anthology with a central theme, not an assortment of topics such as one usually finds at a professional conference.

At the same time, the diversity of the authors' backgrounds is immediately apparent. Marjorie, who appears in this collection as both Guest Editor and author, is a psychiatrist. Other papers are written by nurses, psychologists, social workers, a gynecologist, psychiatrists, and counselors—a reminder once again of the importance and productivity of communication across the disciplines.

Cross-discipline dialogue is particularly important right now, when many of us in the mental health field must attend to the struggle for professional recognition—from our states, insurance companies, national organizations, and even our peers. The increasing emphasis on legislation for licensure and certification can promote inclusion and exclusion tensions. These separate and divide us, provoking jealousy and distrust of one group for another. In times like these it is crucial to keep focused on our central commitment to the improvement of conditions for women. We can all too easily lose sight of our common struggles and our shared visions. Here is a volume that brings us together.

Ellen Cole
Esther D. Rothblum

The author wishes to thank Catherine Royer for her assistance with the manuscript of this book.

Preface

. . . Power is the capacity to produce a change.

Jean Baker Miller

The past twenty years have produced an explosion of women's studies which has created a rapidly expanding body of knowledge. This volume is intended to be on the cutting edge of that expansion and therefore describes new and frequently controversial ideas and programs.

This knowledge enables us to change the way in which we assume power and deal with existing power in every part of our lives. This volume contains insights and models for assuming power over our relationships, minds, bodies, and positions in society. It deals with issues of power over the intimacies of our bodies and our psyches, as well as power in the workplace, professional societies and the courts. We who work in mental health deal in all of these arenas. In order to understand these issues more fully, this volume describes some of the historical and social contexts in which we have not had power.

This volume contains woman-created models for programs that provide services and resolve problems in new ways and that empower others to do so. These programs form a series of models that demonstrate how we women can implement our conceptions and that serve as starting points for other women to create other programs.

Women have always had visions for change that we have expressed in our organizations, meetings and affiliations. These visions have often not been generally known because they have occurred on a separate track, relegated to the women's page or magazine, and women did not have the political power to implement them. They were not considered to be scientific or serious effort worthy of the mainstream of knowledge. Women's meetings have been islands where women can experience a wholeness and female consciousness in an atmosphere temporarily free of the dominant male culture.

In recent years we women have also attempted to assume more power in academic, scientific, and political arenas. Some of this has been done in separate women's organizations, but more of it in sections or sub-groups of larger "mainstream" organizations.

One such group has been the annual two-day women's institute sponsored by the American Orthopsychiatric Association, an interdisciplinary organization of mental health workers. A group of women, starting with the leadership of Jean Baker Miller, formed a planning collective which put together a feminist experimental program, which included radical delineations and approaches to problems as well as thoughtful academic approaches, to make an exciting gathering place for women who seldom obtained a hearing in academic circles. A deliberate decision was made to extend the presentations to health and social arenas since these so often play a major role in defining mental health. Each year a different woman was elected to leadership and another woman assisted her. Volunteers formed a planning committee at the meeting. A theme was chosen, a call for papers was issued, a reviewing process was formed to decide which papers were accepted, and an institute was created.

This volume consists primarily of papers from the presentations of the 1983 and 1984 institutes. I was co-chairperson in 1983 and the chairperson in 1984.

There are common themes that emerge in these papers. One is the theme of equality both between people who work together to give treatment and between treater and client in situations where in the past they have related as superior and inferior, dominant and subordinate.

Another is the self-in-relationship theme, in which the manifestation of power in oneself is expressed through the relationship with and the empowerment of others. Relationships are given prime value. Some papers give a new and revolutionary vision of relationships, and others stress their relationship to the past.

Another theme is that accessible and reliable information about ourselves is power.

Another is respect for the individual life styles of other human beings.

Another is the assumption of power in important situations where women have traditionally or historically experienced lack of power. These papers offer many examples. Here technology and the knowledge of how to use it play an ever expanding role.

Some women have been able to assume power by implementing new values and programs in existing institutions, others by participating in separate programs that maintain a tie with existing institutions, and others by approaching problems in new ways and setting up new and separate structures and models. Which method works best is a matter of the philosophy of the organizers and the amount of resources and technology involved. An inpatient psychiatric service or complete woman's health services require a level of resources, technology, and expertise beyond those required by an information and referral service.

The authors range from established scholars and administrators to women who have formed collectives. Conflicts in philosophy and practice are inevitable. Some women perceive power as the product of rising in our existing system; some women want to develop alternative systems. As women develop more power and rise to leadership in health and mental health questions arise: will we take on the existing values which we feminists wish to change, or will we use those positions of power to implement feminist values and programs? That is, will we use new power to join the establishment or will we change it?

In order to understand the importance of our struggles and our models, it is necessary to understand women's roles in the past. In the year 1900, men ran the lives of women and children on a dominance-submission model. Only men could vote, own property, or sign contracts. A wife was the chattel of her husband. He had the legal right to enforce this with physical chastisement. The suffrage movement was the determined attempt to change this. Women did not have the right to vote until 1920.

The health and mental health practices not only reflected this dominance submission model but aided in its enforcement. The male medical establishment was very closely allied with the anti-suffrage leadership of ministers and politicians. These doctors opined that for health reasons women were not equipped to be educated or to hold responsible and demanding positions of leadership. Rather women should stay home to protect their reproductive capacities and be obedient wives and domestics. The roles of doctor and midwife were taken over by male physicians who barred women from medical schools, medical societies, and hospital staffs on the grounds that women were physically and emotionally incompetent, especially during their menses. Women were permitted only to be nurses or social workers who carried out the orders of the male physicians, including psychiatrists. At the same time, these male physicians declared women to be physically and emotionally inferior, and described as diseased normal aspects of female physiology such as menstruation, child-birth and menopause. Our tradition of gynecological and psychiatric care comes out of this history, and past and present oppressive practices can only be understood in its light.

Our values and mental health as women are so intertwined with our female reproductive physiology and practices which have evolved around it that separation becomes artificial. In fact, the separation of our functioning into a number of medical and psychological disciplines keeps us from perceiving the whole and helps to keep oppressive attitudes and practices in place. Witness the current arguments about menstruation. Attention is focused on the premenstrual phase. There is no common definition of what is normal, what is abnormal, what is emotional, and what is physiological. A woman who experiences premenstrual difficulty could have her problem defined as psychological or physiological. She could be treated with hormones, diuretics, vitamin B12, a low carbohydrate diet, antidepressant medication, or guided imagery depending on the type of practitioner she consults. Or she could, with the help of a feminist therapist, come to view the anger and depression that she feels as an appropriate response to her situation. It is only by unified thought that we will stop being the butt of the latest treatment fad and be able to plan intelligently for our own needs.

There are other major divisions and arguments in psychiatry: for example, there is a current argument over the relative roles of biology and social context in depression. Gretchen Grinnell and other writers in this volume describe the interpersonal and social contexts of depression. They are in stark contrast to some psychiatrists who are so impressed with advances in knowledge about the chemistry of the nervous system and the improvement of some depressed persons with medication that they consider depression to be an inherited physiological condition to be treated primarily by medications. Some of them do not consider psychotherapy or interpersonal changes to be necessary or even relevant. It can be enormously disempowering to the patient to be informed that only medication, and not her own insights and changes can benefit her, especially at times when the medications are not effective. This is in powerful contradiction to the contributions of feminist writers and researchers.

A similar division exists concerning anxiety and panic experiences. As researchers learn more about the physiological aspects of anxiety and panic and the specific effects of medications in counteracting the physical responses of panic, some psychiatrists regard anxiety and panic as primarily biological disorders to be treated by medication. This again is ignoring the information of cognitive, behavioral and interpersonal approaches to panic as described by Iris Fodor in her paper on agoraphobia.

Power has many faces, many dimensions and many forms. We can produce change with new ideas, new evaluations of social and psychological issues, or the assumption of physical, legal, economic and personal power over one's own life. We can take leadership in existing organizations and change them, or we can form new structures, networks and alliances. We can perform an action or empower others to do it. Each of us must make a personal decision as to where to take a stand and where and how to place our energies. The essays in this volume will give each reader new ideas and a new vision of the powers possible for herself and for society. I dedicate this book to the effective, joyful, creative, and constructive exercise of that new found power.

Marjorie Braude

SECTION I

Extending Perceptions —
Contributions to Theory

Each of the papers in this section presents perceptions and theoretical insights into an important area of our psychological knowledge and our experience as women.

Jean Baker Miller has used her own definition of power, "the capacity to produce a change." She has clearly, simply, and decisively enunciated principles of the psychology of women. Since 1984 she has been director of the Stone Center for Developmental Studies at Wellesley College where she has worked with women devoted to the study of the psychology of women. She delineates and speaks out on the forefront of women's psychological issues. In her paper she defines power in female terms and discusses our internal barriers to fully experiencing and achieving it.

Alexandra Kaplan discusses the role of gender differences in therapy, and demonstrates why the values and qualities which we present as women are those upon which successful therapy depends. These qualities enable female therapists to perform better than males in research studies on the outcome of therapy.

A number of the writers extend the traditional definition of countertransference from an individual to a social focus, to include reactions experienced by a gender, race, or class.

Teresa Bernardez focuses on gender issues in countertransference. Whether the therapist reinforces traditional female roles or permits or encourages change is profoundly related to the therapist's responses to a woman's expression of anger and grief, and to

xxvii

whether the therapist responds positively to behaviors which are active and experimental or to behaviors which are passive, submissive and compliant.

Gretchen Grinnell makes a powerful statement about the aggressive and disordered aspects of the male model of society in which we live. She makes the equally powerful statement that depression is a reasonable response to this model, and outlines a framework for treating depression by enabling a woman to experience and acknowledge her own signals, language, ideas, and reality.

Charlotte Krouse Prozan describes her ability to use the insights from her feminist evolution while maintaining her relationship with her psychoanalytic past. She selects out those psychoanalytic concepts and methods which continue to have integrity and validity to her when utilized with feminist concepts and goals.

Frances Newman, in her paper on distressed adolescent females, provides a feminist model for research. She describes the kinds of unresolved countertransference issues which can make investigation of a particular group unreliable and unethical, and proposes a model for ethical and reliable research with those who appear different from ourselves.

Margo Okazawa-Rey, Tracy Robinson and Janie Victoria Ward take us on a journey from the oppressions and stereotypes of black women to the enjoyment of each woman's strength and individuality. They discuss the role of the intersection of race and gender.

Iris Fodor is a writer in transition. She describes the cognitive behavioral model of agoraphobia, and discusses its problems. She then brings in psychodynamic and family perspectives, as she evolves her own model for therapy.

Rachel Josefowitz Siegel discusses her growth as a heterosexual therapist as she works with lesbian clients. She describes how both her clients and a greater social understanding of their situation have contributed to understanding her own countertransference issues. Another view, that lesbian therapists can be more effective with lesbian clients than heterosexual therapists, is well described by Nanette Gartrell (1984).

REFERENCE

Gartrell, N. (1984). Combating Homophobia in the Psychotherapy of Lesbians. *Women & Therapy, 3*(1).

Women and Power

Jean Baker Miller

In recent conversations people have told me stories that raise interesting questions.

For example, a woman came up to me after a meeting and told me that she was supervisor of a large number of sales workers. She asked, "Can you tell me what to do with these women?" Then she went on to say that her company has a big meeting once a month in which all the leading sales workers are recognized individually and asked to say a few words. In the past year or so, quite a few women have been among the sales people who are recognized. The women get up and say things like, "Well, I really don't know how it happened. I guess I was just lucky this time," or "This must have been a good month." By contrast, the men say, "Well, first I analyzed the national sales situation; I broke that down into regional components and figured out the trends in buying. Then I analyzed the consumer groups, and . . . I worked very hard—overtime three-fourths of the nights this month—and . . . " The point is, of course, that the women were doing something like that too—or something in their own style which was just as effective.

Another kind of example came my way when a woman was describing a project she initiated. She said as she starts to work, she thinks (and colleagues and friends have told her) this work might be genuinely significant and good. "Maybe I'm really onto something here," she tells herself. And immediately, almost in the same second, she says, "This is nothing," or "Everybody knows it anyhow."

Those two examples, I think, point to the question of women and power. In recent years there have emerged some writings about women and power (Janeway, 1980), and some meetings to consider

---

The author is a psychiatrist who is Director of Education of the Stone Center for Developmental Services and Studies, Wellesley College. She is also a clinical professor of psychiatry at Boston University School of Medicine.

1

women and power (Janeway, 1980), and some meetings to consider it from several viewpoints and disciplines. But if we are really going to build the kinds of institutions and personal lives that allow women to grow and flourish, I believe that we must invest much more conscious, concerted, direct attention to women and power. At the same time I believe that most of us women still have a great deal of trouble with the whole area. The only hope, it seems to me, is to keep trying to examine it together.

I am not implying that men don't have trouble with power (just look around the world!), but their troubles are different from those of women at this point in history. As with other major topics, I believe women's examination of power not only can illuminate issues which are important to ourselves, but also can bring new understanding to the whole concept of power. It can shed light on the traps and problems of men, perhaps illuminating those things most difficult for men themselves to discover.

I shall begin this initial consideration by reviewing some fairly common occurrences for women — analyzing them from a psychological perspective derived from clinical work.

DEFINING POWER

There have been many definitions of power, each reflecting the historical tradition out of which it comes; also, various disciplines of study have devised their own definitions (McClelland, 1979). An example given in one dictionary says power is "the faculty of doing or performing anything: force; strength; energy; ability; influence . . ." and then a long string of words leading to "dominion, authority, a ruler . . ." then more words culminating in ". . . military force." I think the list reflects accurately the idea that most of us automatically have about power. We probably have linked the concept with the ability to augment one's own force, authority, or influence, and also to control and limit others — that is, to exercise dominion or to dominate.

My own working definition of power is *the capacity to produce a change* — that is, to move anything from point A or state A to point B or state B. This can include even moving one's own thoughts or emotions, sometimes a very powerful act. It also can include acting to create movement in an interpersonal field as well as acting in larger realms such as economic, social, or political arenas.

Obviously, that broad definition has to be further differentiated.

For example, one may be somewhat powerful psychologically or personally but have virtually no legitimate socially granted power to determine one's own fate economically, socially, or politically. Also there's the question, "Power for what?" One may think in terms of gaining power for oneself, or one may seek influence for some general good or some collective entity.

WOMEN'S VIEW OF POWER

While more precise delineations are necessary, I think it is probably accurate to say that generally in our culture and in several others, we have maintained the myth that women do not and should not have power on any dimension. Further, we hold the notion that women do not need power. Usually, without openly talking about it, we women have been most comfortable using our powers if we believe we are using them in the service of others. Acting under those general beliefs, and typically not making any of this explicit, women have been effective in many ways. One instance is in women's traditional roles, where they have used their powers to foster the growth of others—certainly children, but also many other people. This might be called using one's power to empower another—increasing the other's resources, capabilities, effectiveness, and ability to act. For example, in "caretaking" or "nurturing," one major component is acting and interacting to foster the growth of another on many levels—emotionally, psychologically, and intellectually. I believe this is a very powerful thing to do, and women have been doing it all the time, but no one is accustomed to including such effective action within the notions of power. It's certainly not the kind of power we tend to think of; it involves a different content, mode of action, and goal. The one who exerts such power recognizes that she or he cannot possibly have total influence or control but has to find ways to interact with the other person's constantly changing forces or powers. And all must be done with appropriate timing, phasing, and shifting of skills so that one helps to advance the movement of the less powerful person in a positive, stronger direction.

As a result of this vast body of experience within the family as well as in the workplace and other organizations, I think most women would be most comfortable in a world in which we feel we are not limiting, but are enhancing the power of other people while simultaneously increasing our own power. Consider that statement more closely: The part about enhancing other people's power is difficult for the world to comprehend, for it is not how the "real world" has defined power. Nonetheless, I contend that women would function much more comfortably within such a context. The part about enhancing one's own powers is extremely difficult for women. When women even contemplate acting powerful, they fear the possibility of limiting or putting down another person. They also fear recognizing or admitting the need, and especially the desire, to increase their own powers.

Frankly, I think women are absolutely right to fear the use of power as it has been generally conceptualized and used. The very fact that this is often said to be a defensive or neurotic fear is, I believe, a more telling commentary on the state of our culture than it is on women. For example, in current times one can read that women are not being strong enough or tough enough. Such statements overlook the incredible strengths that women have demonstrated all through history, and they usually refer to some comparison with men's operations in our institutions. I believe they tend to overlook a valid tendency in women—that is, the desire to enhance others' resources—and to know, from actual practice and real experience, that it is an extremely valuable and gratifying life activity. On the other side of the picture, however, such statements reflect part of a truth—that women do fear admitting that they want or need power. Yet without power or something like it (which may eventually be described by another term) on both the personal and political level, women cannot effectively bring about anything.

WHEN WOMEN CONFRONT POWER

Now I'd like to focus on women's fears in confronting power, using individual examples which will further illustrate what may have been going on in the women I described briefly at the beginning of my remarks. I will highlight some women's inner, or intrapsychic, experiences.

Power and Selfishness

Abby was a low-paid worker in the health field who sought therapy primarily because of her depression. She had spent much of her adult life enhancing her husband's and her two children's development—using her powers to increase their powers. She then started work and did an excellent job, largely because she approached her patients with the basic attitude of helping them to increase their own comfort and abilities and to use their own powers.

After much exploration, Abby recognized that she tended to become depressed not when things were clearly bad, but when she realized that she could *do* something more—for example, better understand and effectively act on a situation. She felt this especially when she wanted to act for herself. For example, she knew that she was actually better at some procedures than the doctors were—not just technically better, but *totally* better, for she helped patients to feel more relaxed, more in control, and more powerful. She began to feel that she should get to do more of the interesting work, get higher pay, recognition, etc. She also realized that almost at the same moment she felt this way she became blocked by fear, then self-criticism and self-blame. This seemed to be a complex internal replica of the external conditions. The external conditions clearly blocked her advancement; she was a woman who worked in the lowest rank of the health care hierarchy. But the internalized forces created even more complex bondage. Initially, for Abby, as for many women, there was the big fear of being seen as wanting to be powerful. This provoked notions of disapproval, but more than that, at a deeper level, evoked fears of attack and ultimate abandonment by all women and men.

Further exploration unearthed several more sticking points: One was that the prospect of acting on her own interest and motivation kept leading to the notion that she would be selfish. While she could not bear the thought that others would see her as selfish, it was even more critical that she could not bear this conception of herself. I find this theme to be extraordinarily common in women—often women in surprisingly high positions and places—and, by contrast, a rare theme in men. With this theme for Abby there usually would come the notion that she was inadequate anyhow. She felt she should be grateful that anyone would put up with her at all, and she should best forget about the whole thing.

Eventually, this inadequacy theme gave way to yet another state in which she felt that she indeed did have powers and could use them, but doing so meant, inescapably, that she was being destructive. For Abby, this stage was illustrated by thoughts, fantasies, and dreams indicating destructiveness.

Power and Destructiveness

Another woman, Ellen, was at a different point in dealing with the same problem. She felt able to work and to think well so long as she worked on her ideas and plans in her own house. She could not bring them into the work setting. As she used to put it, "If only I could bring my inside self outside." Eventually, she said that this fear seemed to stem from the experience that as she went into the outside world or to work, immediately she became attuned to the new context, readily picking up its structures and demands. She felt she couldn't help but respond to that context and those demands.

Again, this kind of feeling is common in women, and again it reflects a very valuable quality. Historically, a woman's being attuned to and responding to her context and to the needs of everybody in it has been part and parcel of helping other people to grow and helping a family to function. Women can bring a special set of abilities to many situations because they *are* able to attune themselves to the complex realities that are operating. (This perhaps is the essence of what mental health researchers have tried to describe in characterizing mother's contributions to infant development — Winnicott, 1971.)

But consider the other side: Ellen felt that she could not get her own perceptions, evaluations, and judgments moving from inside her to the outside, although she had important contributions to make. To bring her ideas and actions into the outside context she had to overcome her ready tendency to be only responsive.

But that wasn't all. She felt to do so would disrupt the whole scene. In other words, she would be destructive — and that was not a way she felt she should operate.

In each person such a theme forges its specific expression from the individual's history, but the basic theme occurs regularly in many women: To act out of one's own interest and motivation is experienced as the psychic equivalent of being a destructively aggressive person. This is a self-image which few women can bear. In other words, for many women it is more comfortable to feel inadequate. Terrible as that can be, it is still better than to feel powerful, if power makes you feel destructive.

Let me emphasize this thesis: Any person can entertain the prospect of using her or his own life forces and power — individually motivated, in a self-determined direction. In theories about mental health, this is said to bring satisfaction and effectiveness. But for many women it is perceived as the equivalent of being destructive. On the one hand this sets up a life-destroying, controlling psychological condition. On the other hand it makes sense if one sees that women have lived as subordinates, and, as subordinates, have been led by the culture to believe that their own, self-determined action is wrong and evil. Many women have incorporated deeply the inner notion that such action must be destructive. The fact that women have survived at all, I believe, is explained by the fact that women do use power all the time but generally must see it as used for the benefits of others.

Don't misunderstand me: Using one's abilities and powers for others is not bad by any means. It does become problematic for women and for men, however, when such activity is prescribed for one sex only, along with the mandate that one must not act on one's own motivation and according to one's own determinations. In most institutions it is still true that if women do act from their own perceptions and motivations, directly and honestly, they indeed may be disrupting a context which has not been built out of women's experience. Thus, one is confronted with feeling like one must do something very powerful that also feels destructive.

Power and Abandonment

Another woman, Connie, illustrated this dramatically: She had difficulty finishing her work. But she discovered that she would become "blocked" not when she was really stuck, but when she was working well, streaming ahead, getting her thoughts in order, and making something happen. At those times she would get up from her desk, start walking around, become involved in some diversion, talk to someone, and generally get off the productive trajectory. Further exploration of why this happened led eventually to her saying that if she let herself go on when she was working well, "I'd be too powerful and then where would I be . . . I wouldn't need anyone else." For Connie, the prospect was that she would be out in some scary place. She said she would feel like some unrecognizable creature, some non-woman. She spoke of the prospect as if it signified the loss of a central sense of identity. Her sense of identity, like that of so many women, was so bound up with being a person who *needs* that the prospect of *not needing* felt like, first of all, a loss of the known and familiar self.

On the other hand, it was an unnecessary fear. On the other hand,

Connie touched on a sense that is present in many women — namely, that the use of our powers with some efficacy and, even worse, with freedom, zest, and joy, feels as if it will destroy a core sense of identity. One feature of that identity, as reflected by Connie's statement, demonstrates how deeply women have incorporated the notion, "I exist only as I need." Again, I think women are reflecting a truth which men have been encouraged to deny — that is, all of us exist only as we need others for that existence — but cultural conditions have led women to incorporate this in an extreme form. Along with it we women have incorporated the troubling notion that, as much as we need others, we also have powers and the motivation to use those powers, but, if we use them, we will destroy the relationships we need for our existence.

The Troublesome Equations

With these examples I have outlined some of the inner experiences women have related to me as they confronted the issue of power. They include:

A woman's using self-determined power for herself is equivalent to *selfishness*, for she is not enhancing the power of others.

A woman's using self-determined power for herself is equivalent to *destructiveness*, for such power inevitably will be excessive and will totally disrupt an entire surrounding context.

The equation of power with destructiveness and selfishness seems impossible to reconcile with a sense of feminine identity.

A woman's use of power may precipitate attack and *abandonment*; consequently, a woman's use of power threatens a central part of her identity, which is a feeling that she needs others.

It is important to emphasize again the many sides of all of this: On the one hand, most women are keenly aware of an essential truth that we all need others, need to live in the framework of relationships, and also need to increase the powers of others through our activities. On the other hand, most women have been encouraged to experience these needs as a predominant, central, almost total definition of their personalities. And their experience tells them that change can occur only at the cost of destroying one's place in the world and one's chance for living within a context of relationships. I believe this reflects accurately the historic and cultural place, and the definition of women.

The Challenges Ahead

The examples I have cited not only tell about individual neuroses but also reflect characteristics of many women. Right now I think it is important for women to recognize that we do need to use our powers. Many times, I think, women have done things which eventually proved to be destructive, often without being fully aware, because we actually felt so much pain and reluctance even to think about the topic.

Also, we need to help each other in several important ways: First, we can give sympathetic understanding to ourselves if we recognize the weight of the historic conditions which have made power such a difficult concept for most of us. Second, we can consider seriously the proposition that there is enormous validity in women's *not* wanting to use power as it is presently conceived and used. Rather, women may want to be powerful in ways that simultaneously enhance, rather than diminish, the power of others. This is a radical turn—a very different motivation than the concept of power upon which this world has operated.

Out of this, we can see that women already may have a strong motivation to approach the concept of power with a different, critical, and creative stance. Once admitting a desire and a need for power, women can seek new ways of negotiating power with others in personal life, work, and other institutions. Certainly this is a large and difficult prospect. It can appear naive or unreal even to talk that way. But the fact that it sounds unreal must not stop us! Once we recognize the undeniable truth that the world has been explained so far without the close observation of women's experience, it is easier to consider that seemingly "unreal" possibilities can become real.

Bear in mind these truths that have not been taken into account:

—Women's experience is usually not what it has been said to be.
—It is not men's experience. It does not necessarily operate on

the same bases, same motivations, or the same organization of personality.

— What we find when we study women are parts of the total human potential that have not been fully seen, recognized, or valued. These are parts that have not therefore flourished, and perhaps they are precisely the ingredients that we must bring into action in the conduct of all human affairs.

— Certainly these emerging notions must be used for the benefit of women, which is reason enough to pursue them, but they must be used also for the ultimate benefit of others.

REFERENCES

Janeway, E. (1980). *Powers of the weak.* New York: Knopf.
McClellan, D. C. (1979). *The inner experience.* New York: Irvington.
Winnicott, D. W. (1971). *Playing and reality.* New York: Basic Books.

Reflections on Gender
and Psychotherapy

Alexandra G. Kaplan

This paper will touch on many topics: psychotherapy outcome research, psychological development in women and men, the nature of the psychotherapy relationship, psyche and society, the interplay of cultural norms and treatment, psychotherapy training, and sex role socialization. Clearly not all of these topics will be covered in depth. Rather, what I would like to do is weave a theme through them to make the following argument: (1) that there is sufficient research to make some general statements about the factors associated with positive change in therapy, (2) that these factors are related in complex ways to major distinctions in the psychologies of women and men, (3) that our field, as a whole, has paid scant attention to how normative characteristics of women and men bear on their work as therapists, and, (4) that we need to examine how we all can enhance our work as clinicians by an examination of how gender-based factors affect the process and outcome of therapy.

In making this argument, I am suggesting that we think about therapy in a way that we are not accustomed to doing—to think about patients and therapists as being gendered, women or men. This is not to say that there is a direct, one-to-one correspondence between gender and personality. Clearly not all men are alike, nor are all women. But we do live in a highly gendered society, with strong norms about appropriate modes of being for men and women. However, regardless of the extent to which we consciously accept or reject these norms, we act in some relation to them and are experienced by others in relation to them. Thus, we will first look at

The author is a psychologist. She is a research associate and co-director of Counseling Services at the Stone Center, Wellesley College.

therapy outcome studies, and then examine the extent to which gender-related factors may be involved.

THERAPY OUTCOME RESEARCH

When we turn to the issue of therapy outcome research, we are entering an area of inconsistent results, wide variations in the ways success is measured, and differences in the vantage point by which data are gathered (e.g., the therapist, the patient, a non-participant observer). Fortunately, however, there are some excellent reviews of this literature, and from these reviews clear trends are evident. I am referring to reviews by Dent (1978), Gurman (1977), Orlinsky and Howard (1978), and Strupp, Wallach and Wogan (1964). Despite the range of perspectives represented by these authors, a common theme emerges in all of these writings. That theme is that the cutting edge of success in therapy lies in the nature of the relationship between patient and therapist. In the words of Howard and Orlinsky, the positive quality of the *relational bond*, as exemplified in the reciprocal interpersonal behavior of the participants, is more clearly related to patient improvement than are any of the particular treatment techniques used by the therapist.

But a thorough exploration of the nature of the patient-therapist relationship has been ignored in most clinical training almost as much as have gender influences. For most of us, training has centered on cognitive formulations. In terms of patients, curricula emphasize diagnosis, psychodynamic conflict or behavioral deficits, and in terms of therapists' responses, the stress is on interpretations and techniques of intervention. These components are of course necessary and important elements of training. But they are not sufficient, in that they stop at the point of translation into a way of being with the client that will best foster their natural connection. This situation is only partially remedied in supervision, which also tends to focus on cognitive formulations rather than on the quality of contact during the therapy hour. Indeed, an entire supervisory hour can be spent elucidating the client's history, identifying key dynamics, and evolving diagnostic formulations without ever exploring the clinical process of listening and responding. Again, diagnosis and dynamics are important, but they are not the entire process, in addition, such emphasis can work against the therapists' attentiveness to the client. Too much focus on "formulating an intervention" can draw the therapist's attention away from direct affective contact with the client and sensitivity to the nuances of her or his experiences.

It can be argued additionally that in clinical training there is a subtle *devaluing* of the client-therapist relationship. To the extent that relational issues are discussed in supervision, it is often in terms of their negative impact. Much more seems to be known about how a therapist can relate poorly than how a therapist can relate well. For example, there are the "problems" of overinvolvement, fostering dependency, or being manipulated. All of these can and do occur in therapy, and they warrant attention and correction. But in the absence of knowing more beneficial modes of relating, the temptation may be to compensate by greater distance rather than by better relationship. This greater distance may go unrecognized because it is often "masked" by accepted techniques such as silence, or *intra-psychic* interpretation. If there are "problems" in the client-therapist relationship, if the relational bond is not promoting the work, it is reasonable to assume that the difficulty lies within the relationship, not simply within the psyche of one of the participants. It is noteworthy that there are no commonly used parallel terms to denote insufficient relationship, such as fostering disconnectedness, underinvolvement, or not responding to the client's needs.

The second component of the relational bond, empathy, requires some careful definition, because I am not using it here as it is commonly conveyed in teaching programs. Specifically, as Jordan (1984) has described, empathy is typically considered as a "mysterious, contagion-like, and primitive phenomenon, or has been dismissed as a vague and unknowable state." Especially when discussed in terms of "maternal empathy" as in the writings of Winnicott and others, empathy becomes linked with such primitive states as merger and fusion. Empathy, then, often is described as mysterious and/or regressive, something that "just happens." In Jordan's perspective, however, empathy instead is recognized as a highly developed cognitive and affective process. It requires a high level of development—the capacity to take in the experience and affect of the other without being overwhelmed by it on the one hand, or defensively blocking it out on the other hand. For a therapist, this means that one needs to surrender oneself to the affect of another, while at the same time cognitively structuring that experience so as to comprehend its meaning in terms of other aspects of the client's psyche, its relationship to current dynamics in the therapy relationship, and the mode of response that will best convey this experience to the client. It requires that one be comfortable and familiar with the worlds of affect and the nature of connections between people.

GENDER AND THE RELATIONAL BOND

If the relational bond, consisting basically of understanding and empathy, is the key to successful psychotherapy, then we can ask the question: How is this relational bond affected by the sex of client and therapist? From the therapist's side, there has long been a recognition, within analytically-oriented therapies, of the importance of counter-transference. However, counter-transference is typically considered an individual, gender-neutral area of exploration, which exists as a function of the individual's historical, unconscious conflicts. By contrast, I am suggesting that we need to look at the therapist's contribution to what Stone (1981) calls the "here and now": her or his attitudes, values, style, presentation as they are experienced by the patient. Recent writings by Gill (1979), Langs (1973), and Stone have highlighted the importance of attention to this area, but again on an *individual* basis. I am adding that for each therapist we do not need to begin from "scratch." Instead (while I am not suggesting that all women and all men will behave alike), there are certain socially constructed, expectable, normative modes of being that constitute the "proper" stance of women and men, and that influence how women and men behave and how they are seen by their patients. Knowledge of these basic gender-linked trends provides an essential context for then exploring each individual's particular rendition of this.

Similarly for clients, there are few guidelines for understanding in a systematic way, what particular symptom patterns, key conflicts, behavioral styles, or ways of relating to the therapist might mean given that the client is a man or a woman. If, for example, one is working with a depressed woman, there is no widely accepted, comprehensive theory that addresses symptomatology or the experience of depression in light of women's normative roles and internalized self-concept, even though depression is overwhelmingly a women's problem. In other words, in the major prevailing theories of depression (or phobias, or eating disorders or borderline personalities — all primarily diagnoses received by women), gender con-figurations are not attended to in a theoretically coherent, system-atic and viable way — except by women or, more accurately, feminist therapists (e.g., Rawlings and Carter).

There are several conditions that have strongly influenced the absence of gender considerations in therapy as generally taught. The first pertains to the absence of virtually any exposure, in gradu-ate school or post-doctoral training, to the now vast literature on the psychology of women, especially as a required course. The prob-lem, of course, is circular: without a concern for gender influences, there is no need for courses on the psychology of women, hence no basis for identifying gender issues, etc. And yet, going back to the *understanding* component of the relational bond, knowledge about *women's* psychology, given that women make up the vast majority of our caseloads, seems critical. Without attempting to summarize the voluminous research findings in this field, several major areas of understanding can be highlighted. Observable sex differences in behavior are but the end point of a chain of contextual factors, and in some ways the least important. More central to the fullest under-standing of the meaning of behavior are the situational factors which ultimately shape these differences. Several examples illus-trate this point. There are clear *norms* about what is considered appropriate for each sex, which affect how behavior is understood and evaluated. There are differential *attributions* made by each sex about the reasons for their own behavioral outcomes (e.g., men tend to attribute their successes to their innate ability, while women tend to attribute their successes to luck). *Role determinants* play a factor in determining how one's behavior is seen. That is, women may behave in certain self-effacing ways that are more a function of their being in a subordinate role than they are a function of their being female. And finally, perceptions of the *value* of behaviors are influ-enced by the gender of the actor. Products or stances tend to be valued more highly if they are associated with a man than if they are associated with a woman. In terms of understanding women, then, if such contextual variables are not considered, individual problems tend to be seen in therapy as the result of individual failings alone, rather than a product of the interaction between culture and psyche. This, of course, can be a powerful impediment to conveying to the woman client that her reality has been given "just due," and thus promoting the understanding that facilitates growth in therapy.

While knowledge of the social sciences study of the psychology of women is of great benefit to clinical work, research studies per se are at best only the raw material out of which clinical understanding emerges. Even more central to our work are the theories of psychological development which inform our perceptions of normal and pathological behavior. Here we face a quandary different from that of the research literature on the psychology of women, which is available in abundance but lacking in exposure in clinical training programs (Kaplan, 1984). By contrast, as Miller (1984) has stressed, the developmental theories that are most frequently adhered to—Freud, Sullivan, Erikson, and Mahler—do not describe women's psychological experience. Common to all these traditional theories is a sequence of developmental stages in which each stage is a milestone over the preceding one and a prerequisite to the subsequent one. This sequence moves from a state of presumed enmeshment, or symbiosis, or merger, toward increasing levels of self-identity, independence, or autonomy. Ego strength and cognitive capacities are said to increase as one becomes an increasingly separate and bounded self. Elements of earlier stages, especially as they suggest relational needs (read: dependency) are frequently suspect. While all theories contain some adult phase of "heterosexual, genital attachment" there is little in them that explains how one evolves toward this form of intimacy, and even less on the continuing evolution of other forms of connection including that between members of the same sex, between parent and child, and so on. As is clearest with Freud, Sullivan, and Erikson, their theories were explicitly designed with men in mind, although Miller (1984) has suggested that these theories better describe the male *ideal* in Western society than the male reality. Because women are assessed in terms of theories that were not designed on the basis of their experience, not surprisingly women are found to be deficient, either lacking something they should have—such as a penis or an identity prior to intimacy, or a fully developed super-ego—or having something that they shouldn't have, which is usually some form of striving for connection. As a further result, elements of personality that particularly pertain to women's psychology are seen as inferior, or pathological, or irrelevant.

Both of these trends, women as deficient because they lack what they should have, and women as inferior because what they do have is not correct, can be found in the social science research literature as well as in developmental theory. Social scientists are equally at fault for evaluating people on dimensions that pertain to the male experience, and then finding women to be lacking. If we take for example some of the major paradigms that have been isolated for study in social psychology they invariably reflect some aspect of autonomy, or separation, or self-enhancement outside of connection. Thus, again, we have major paradigms of achievement motivation, or locus of control, or field dependence/independence, or cognitive dissonance, or attribution theory. Further, in those cases where direct gender comparisons are made such as with locus of control or field dependence/independence, it is always "better" to be centered in the self — to have an internal locus of control, to be field independent. And, inevitably, since these dimensions flow from the male paradigm, men not surprisingly fit the "better side" and women are found to be lacking.

Fortunately, in the last ten years, fields of the psychology and sociology of women have emerged and made major strides in correcting these imbalances. More recently, women clinicians and theorists have been turning their attention to the specific topic of women's psychological development. Three very influential books have become the cornerstone of this work — the writings of Miller (1976), Chodorow (1978) and Gilligan (1982). All of these works have in common an in-depth careful examination of women's psychological experience viewed from a perspective which places women in their own reality, not the reality as understood from an examination of the male perspective. Thus, they permit the acknowledgement and exploration of women's strengths (Miller, 1976) and a focus on dimensions of development that had heretofore been relegated to second-class status.

By far the most central dimension to emerge from these works is that of the nature, meaning and place of connection, or self as a relational being, in women's psychological experience. Chodorow and Gilligan have highlighted some specific aspects of this phenomenon. Building on the work of Miller (1976), scholars at the Stone Center have begun a detailed examination of the development of women's relational core self-structure (e.g., Miller, 1984; Jordan, 1984; Kaplan, 1984; Stiver, 1985; and Surrey, 1985). From these and other papers contained in the Stone Center Work in Progress series, a description is emerging of the relational pathway of women's psychological development. Only a brief synopsis can be given here; further elaboration can be found in the above papers.

The Stone Center relational model is structured around the *continuities* in the developmental process, not the discrete changes that are highlighted in the stage theories of most other models of development. What we have identified in women's development is the continuity throughout the life span of a core relational self-structure that evolves around increasingly complex and situationally grounded capacities for empathic attunement, and growth through active participation in mutually based relational processes. What is central for the developing woman is action within relationship; participating in the kind of relationship which enhances self and others, meaning that it is built around mutual empathic attunement. Such connections, as Miller (1986) has recently described, result in a greater feeling of energy and zest, a greater sense of empowerment and capacity for action, greater knowledge of self and other, an increased sense of self-worth, and motivation for further connection through which this process will continue. Relationship, in this model, is seen as a synergistic process, containing properties that evolve from the flow of mutual understandings and mutual connections.

While most prevailing developmental theories, especially those of the object relations school, highlight relationship as a key component of development, a closer examination of these theories suggests that for them relationship is often synonymous with "supply-giver" — the object rather than the subject of a relational process (Surrey, 1985). Emotional or material support from the other enhances the development of the self through a process of internalization. The quality of support from the external caregiver in turn strongly influences the emotional well-being of the individual recipient. By contrast, the Stone Center model emphasizes not a one-way dimension of giver and receiver but an interactive *process* in which the flow of connection becomes the arena through which growth occurs. In studying relational development, our interest lies in the evolution of mutual relational action, including how this form of action fuels or empowers other forms of action and specifically how increasingly mutual and empathic processes of connection emerge.

We trace the early stages of this relational process to the nature of relational connections, including but not limited to the early mother-daughter relationship. If we look for the most general, cross-cultural phenomena that can account for the virtual universality of women's relational core self-structure, what emerges is that in virtually all societies, young babies are raised by women. From this, two basic processes emerge. First, the daughter has a same-gender person with whom to begin a process of connection, including connection around the empathic and caretaking aspects of the maternal role (Surrey, 1985). This process can contain some rudimentary qualities of mutuality, in that the mother may more easily encourage her daughter to be like her and to respond to her. Boys, by contrast, are exposed from early in life to forces which encourage dis-identification from maternal qualities such as caretaking and affective expression, and increasing distance from the mother herself. Further, there is seldom a regularly present, actively engaged father with whom to form these early connections, but more likely an idealized, minimally present image. Thus, girls begin with a closer connection to an adult who engages the daughter in caretaking and affective closeness and encourages sameness. Second, because for daughters mothers encourage self-enhancement based on and in relationship, girls learn that self-knowledge and emotional growth occur best by moving into connection with others. By contrast, boys are encouraged to learn that self-knowledge and enhancement come from movement away from connection; that closeness may be a threat to the developing core self-structure. As Miller has stated, there is an implicit "amazing" notion in the developmental literature that development, especially for boys, is development away from connection with mother (or more generally, women). This fundamental psychological gender imbalance is further discussed in Chodorow (1978) and illustrated in Gilligan's (1982) TAT findings that women evidence greatest anxiety in the face of isolation, and men in the face of intimacy.

Miller (1984) has described in depth key aspects of women's relational self from early childhood through adolescence, including a comparison between our model and those of such theorists as Erikson and Freud. At every stage, what she highlights is the evolution of a continuous and growing relational process that maturational change makes possible, but which is excluded or minimized by other theories. This theme can be applied to the developmental moments that characterize the major theoretical approaches. Thus, the "rapprochement" phase of the object relations school would be propelled not by sufficient distance and separateness from mother, but centrally by the security of attachment with mother that makes cognitive, behavioral, and relational strides possible. Similarly, Freud's "Oedipal" years are marked not by rejection of the mother, but by an expansion of the girl's relational network to include greater emotional connection with the father. The latency years, in turn, are marked not by the absence of sexuality (which may not be the case at all), but rather by the intense and growth-promoting relations that develop between same-sex peers. Similarly, though adolescence is often characterized by conflict with parents, this conflict may well represent not a struggle for separation but a demand to be recognized and heard by parents even as the adolescent changes in ways that might run counter to parental values and expectations.

IMPLICATIONS FOR THERAPY

We can now begin to consider whether these different developmental pathways have any implication for the outcome of therapy depending on whether the therapist is a woman or a man. To assess this, we need to turn to the literature that discusses the relationship between gender and outcome, and look closely at those processes that are thought to affect outcome. Here again, there are ways in which the study of gender differences in outcome has led to inconsistent results, confusion in the definitions of such basic terms as "success," and inconsistent conclusions even given similar findings. Despite these inconsistencies, certain general trends have begun to emerge. Mogul (1982) has pointed out that within this literature " . . . there appear to be some demonstrable trends, under certain circumstances, toward greater patient satisfaction or benefit from psychotherapy with female therapists and no studies showing such trends with male therapists." This situation does not apply equally to all male and all female therapists. Specifically, as Howard and Orlinsky illustrate (1979), a gender effect is less evident with experienced than with non experienced therapists. Based on multiple ratings of the outcome of therapy with a group of female and male therapists working with female patients, the authors grouped each therapist into one of the following categories: (1) those for whom at least 50% of their clients were considerably improved with the rest improved and none worse than before therapy; (2) those for whom at least 33% were considerably improved and fewer than 10% were improved, and (3) those for whom fewer than 50% were improved and more than 10% were worse. Using these distinctions, no differences in therapist "quality ratings" were found between moderately experienced (2-6 years) and very experiienced (over 7 years) women therapists, both of whom were equally as good as the very experienced male therapists. These three groups had average rates of 4% worse, and 41% considerably improved. In contrast to these three groups were the moderately experienced male therapists, who had at least twice the others' rate of worse and unchanged patients and half the others' rate of considerably improved patients.

Howard and Orlinsky end their paper by asking: "On whom are the male therapists to practice until they become highly experienced?" While this is certainly a question which needs to be pondered, there is another question to be asked, concerning those clinical qualities which will improve their work: What do male therapists gain by their experience in therapy that seems to be in place for only moderately experienced women therapists? The answer to this question should be apparent by now, based on the nature of women's developmental pathway as just described. Given that the primary avenue for change in therapy occurs within the relational bond, what experienced male therapists must gain from their clinical experience is precisely that: experience in a process of growth-through-relationship. Clearly this experience enhances therapy, but there is some evidence that experience alone is not sufficient. Howard and Orlinsky, in the same paper shed light on some difficulties experienced more by the women patients with male than with female therapists. Specifically, when the authors compared the patients' self reports of therapy according to sex of therapist, they found that

> those seeing male therapists reported more eroticized affection, anger, inhibition and depression than those seeing female therapists. After therapy, the women with male therapists saw themselves as less self-possessed, less open, and more self-critical than did the women with female therapists. The male therapists were described by their patients as more demanding, less encouraging, and less expansive than were their female counterparts.

It seems a reasonable conclusion from the bodies of literature reviewed that the greater capacity of women therapists especially in their early years of training is linked to women's relational developmental pathway. Those qualities which allow greater avenues for change in therapy overlap and complement the nature of growth-enhancing experiences for women: active, empathically-based participation in relational processes. This is certainly not to say that all women make good therapists, or that there is a group of therapists who need only minimal training. But it is to suggest that attention to the process of connection in therapy is one that needs far greater emphasis, possibly for some therapists more than others.

A CHALLENGE FOR FUTURE TRAINING

Differences in the psychological realities of women and men have created obstacles to learning about women's lives through women's own reports, and to empathy with women's affective experiences. The work of both women and men therapists can suffer from these obstacles, but we can now identify them more systematically for members of each sex. That the obstacles exist is not surprising. Traditional psychological theory and the cultural mores within which therapy is embedded strongly support and affirm the male reality. Men have little encouragement in their professional lives to consider the limitations of their own experience, to "suspend" their reality, and to be receptive to and validate the "other" as it is reflected by their women clients. Many women therapists have been encouraged to give greater credence to current theory and the values in which it is embedded than to their own experience, and therefore have been too ready to "suspend" their reality in the face of ideas that contradict their experience.

Yet, increasingly, women are demanding to be heard. This has implications for family and work life and social structure. Male therapists may need to ponder those areas in which they have limited understanding and turn to writings by women and the women in their own lives for guidance and information. But such a stance typically is not encouraged in men. In part, it calls for a measure of humility, recognizing that one has much to learn from others, and that new learning might threaten what one already "knows." In part, it means developing receptivity to the experience of another along with a suspension of one's own preconceptions. Some argue that this goes against the basic structure of our culture's historical models of thinking. If so, it poses a formidable challenge.

The risk for men is that, as part of the majority culture, they will respond in a defensive, invalidating way to those whose experiences are different and directly challenge their own. There is some evidence that this pattern does occur with male therapists and female clients, to the detriment of the women's satisfaction with their treatment. The challenge presented to male therapists is great, but the potential gains in personal and professional growth are even greater.

Many women, therapists or not, are not yet accustomed to helping others and giving information openly. Certainly the culture has not fostered such characteristics. Where theory conflicted with their own intense emotional experience, some women therapists have opted for theory and seeming "safety," attempting to resolve conflict in a way that ultimately is detrimental to themselves as well as their clients. Nonetheless, the research I have cited suggests that in the privacy of their offices some of the basic relational values come through — in spite of socialization and professional training.

Full and open discussion of these issues in all therapy training would constitute a major stride toward growth among therapists of both sexes. Such discussions would be initiated ideally at the very beginning of therapy training and continue throughout its course. Such training would validate self-exploration and lay the groundwork for continued work toward genuine understanding of differences in women's and men's experience. Until such concerns are addressed as a matter of course in major training facilities, it is unlikely that individual practitioners will have the impetus or support to undertake this important and difficult work by themselves.

REFERENCES

Chodorow, N. (1978). *The Reproduction of Mothering*. Berkeley: University of California Press.

Dent, J. K. (1978). *Exploring the psychosocial therapies through the personalities of effective therapists*. DHEW Publication No. (ADM) 77-527. National Institute of Mental Health.

Gill, M. M. (1979). The analysis of the transference. *Journal of the American Psychoanalytic Association, 27*, 263-88.

Gilligan, C. (1982). *In a Different Voice*. Cambridge, MA: Harvard University Press.

Gurman, A. (1977). The patient's perception of the therapeutic relationship. In A. Gurman and A. Razin (eds.), *Effective Psychotherapy: A Handbook of Research*. New York: Pergamon Press.

Howard, K. & Orlinsky, D. (August, 1979). What effect does therapist gender have on outcome for women in psychotherapy? Presented at the American Psychological Association, New York.

Jordan, J. (1984). Empathy and self boundaries. Wellesley College: Stone Center, *Work in Progress*, Wellesley, MA.

Kaplan, A. G. (1984). The "Self-in Relation": Implications for depression in women. Wellesley College: Stone Center, *Work in Progress*, Wellesley, MA.

Langs, R. (1973). *The Technique of Psychoanalytic Psychotherapy, Vol. I. The Initial Contact*. New York, Jason Aronson.

Miller, J. B. (1976). *Toward a New Psychology of Women*. Boston: Beacon Press.

Miller, J. B. (1984). The development of women's sense of self. Wellesley College: Stone Center, *Work in Progress*, Wellesley, MA.

Miller J. B. (1986). What do we mean by relationship? Wellesley College: Stone Center, *Work in Progress*, Wellesley, MA.

Mogul, K. (1982). Overview: The sex of the therapist. *American Journal of Psychiatry, 139*, 1-11.

Orlinsky, D. & Howard, K. (1978). The relation of process to outcome in psychotherapy. In S. Garfield and A. Bergin (eds.), *Handbook of Psychotherapy and Behavior Change*. New York: Wiley Press.

Rawlings, E. & Carter (1977). *Psychotherapy for Women*. Springfield, IL: Charles C Thomas.

Stiver. I. (1985). The meaning of care. Wellesley College: Stone Center, *Work in Progress*, Wellesley, MA.

Stone, L. (1981). Some thoughts on the "Here and Now" in psychoanalytic technique. *Psychoanalytic Quarterly, 50*, 709-31.

Strupp, H., Wallach, M. & Wogan, M. (1964). The psychotherapy experience in retrospect. *Psychological Monographs, 78*, Whole No. 586.

Surrey, J. (1985). The "Self-in-Relation": Clinical implications. Wellesley College: Stone Center, *Work in Progress*, Wellesley, MA.

Gender Based Countertransference
of Female Therapists
in the Psychotherapy of Women

Teresa Bernardez

The issue of a gender role bias in psychotherapy has been investigated in recent years but the findings are inconsistent (Abramowitz, Abramowitz, Tittler & Weitz, 1976a). A major obstacle is the absence of projects in which the process is investigated in its depth and richness over time. Until then, the observation of clinicians, particularly those whose responsibilities in teaching and training psychotherapists put them in contact with a good number of colleagues, are a valuable source of material.

Although the term countertransference has been used for characteristic patterns of reactions in therapists to gender role behaviors (Abramowitz, Abramowitz, Roback, Corney & McKee, 1976b) the term is only proper at its most general conception. My objection to this designation is that the psychoanalytic term does not incorporate culturally-determined reactions and that the specificity of the reactions and of the underlying determinants I am to describe are not the product of individually or family specific conflicts in the persons involved in the therapeutic endeavor.

From the start, I want to underline that these reactions that therapists manifest in the treatment of women are the product of our socialization and have become observable because of our increasing awareness of biased assumptions about gender role behavior and recent insistence that gender issues be examined in the therapeutic and supervisory relationships (Alonso & Rutan, 1978; Beiser, 1977; Benedek, 1973; Bernardez, 1976; Kaplan, 1979).

The author is a professor of psychiatry at Michigan State University, Lansing, Michigan.

Since our socialization about gender starts in the family, the therapists' responses may be mixed with diverse components of more classically termed transferences and countertransferences but can be set apart because they are culture-specific and they have unconscious determinants shared in commonality with a large and "average" group. These are reflections of prevailing mores, prejudices or preferences which have the capacity to be considered normative at times. We are blind to them because so many others share them (including our patients and colleagues) and they are resistive to examination and change because they are for the most part out of our awareness and because they are continuously reinforced in our daily lives.

In my first presentation of the subject (Bernardez, 1976) I placed emphasis on three specific reactions of therapists to the women they saw in psychotherapy. They were:

1. the discouragement and disapproval of behaviors that did not conform with traditional role prescriptions for the female, e.g., rejection of motherhood, role reversal in marriage, lesbianism and/or rejection of heterosexuality.
2. the disparagement and inhibition of expression of anger and other "negative" affects as well as a whole spectrum of aggressive behaviors not expected of women and;
3. the absence of confrontation, interpretation and exploration of passive-submissive and compliant behavior in the patient within or without the therapeutic situation.

All of these reactions from therapists constitute errors of commission or omission in therapeutic conduct that have as a common denominator shared beliefs about what is expected of a female in this society. Some of the expectations have changed in recent years. Increasing flexibility and awareness of the constrictions of gender roles in our society have permitted therapists to explore the patient's choices without dictating or expecting conformity to sexual stereotypes. Evidence of this has been gathered by authors replicating the original Broverman study (Zedlow, 1978). However, many of these studies use paper and pencil tests which do not capture the more irrational, emotional reactions evoked by the live contact with patients over time. In theory most therapists genuinely desire to offer freer choices and more flexible and creative lives for their patients but in practice this desire is often limited by fears, dreads and prohibitions stimulated (and shared) by patients and supported, albeit ambivalently, by the social milieu. This is particularly true of long term treatment situations in which unconsciously determined reactions on patients evoke equally unconscious responses in therapists that maintain the status quo. Although the dynamic, insight-oriented therapies have as a safeguard the identification and study of the phenomenon of countertransference, these reactions are culture-syntonic and have not been identified as the result of prejudicial beliefs. In other instances, these reactions have been isolated as if they are only encountered in a particular female patient-therapist dyad. It has been due to the attention showered on these issues by feminist scholars and clinicians that we are beginning to realize the universality of certain reactions on the part of therapists that keep their female patients from exploring, understanding and resolving conflicts that have large social determinants.

In what follows I will take up the most common reactions to female patients by female therapists that betray affectively charged beliefs and conflictual themes regarding women. I will explore the possible determinants of these conflicting beliefs and I hope to clarify the effects that the resolution of these reactions have on the process and outcome of psychotherapy.

Findings of no differences in the outcome of therapy by women and men appear to be contradicted by Abramowitz (1976) and others' (Hoffman, 1977) findings of female therapists showing greater empathy and ability to facilitate self-disclosure than males (Hill, 1975). Abramowitz et al. (1976b) find that male counselors and testers prolong testing sessions and therapy length and the research suggests that voyeurism and sexual curiosity may account for this.

Such propensities in male counselors may be compounded by the tendency of women patients to establish dependent bonds with therapists due in part to their socialization towards affiliation and away from autonomy, resulting in possibly longer treatment of female patients with male therapists.

Other factors increase this risk: one is the erotization of the transference that takes place not infrequently in female patients/male therapists dyads. Another is the socialization of the male for dominance. The male therapists may be more inclined to reproduce the dominant-subordinate position by unconscious encouragement of the female's compliance, submissiveness and passivity. These difficulties are much less frequently encountered with female therapists, although they are possible in the male-identified female.

A problem for therapists of both sexes is the strong gender role prohibition against female anger, criticism, rebellion or domination. The reactions of the therapist to the female patient's aggressive behavior are the most pervasive, the most crucial, if resolved, to permit the therapist's helpfulness to the female patient. They are so frequently encountered, ignored or justified by therapists and supervisors that they are neither properly identified as obstacles nor explored and resolved within the therapist.

There is considerable confusion in the minds of therapists of both genders as to what constitutes healthy aggressiveness, particularly for the female. Anger is often equated with hatred, destructiveness, or with the outcome of its thwarted expression —bitterness and resentment. The expression of anger when it is direct and uncontaminated with indictments and judgments is an important conquest for the female patient, who is usually confined to the indirect expression of negative feelings or to devious ways to communicate dissatisfaction by manipulation, passive-aggressive behaviors, subtle retaliation of depression (Bernardez, 1978). It is precisely the exploration of feelings of bitterness, resentment and dejection that can lead her to the sources of dissatisfaction and eventually to more assertive action to resolve those dissatisfactions. The energy required for realistic protest and creative action has been blocked by prohibitions and discharged through indirect and self-defeating channels that only foster an increasing sense of helplessness. Therapists of both genders have difficulties with a whole array of aggressive behaviors in their women patients. I will take up examination of these problems in the female therapist. They are manifested by intolerance to the patient's expression of negative feelings: dislike, disapproval or rejection of the content and attitudes in the patient that explicitly or implicitly convey criticism, competition, exercise of power or domination over others. It is the incapacity of the therapist to maintain a benevolent neutrality toward the patient at those times that alerts us to the existence of strong feelings about them. The therapist may respond verbally or non-verbally to these behaviors of women. The response may be to ignore, discard, interrupt, discourage the communication or to become directive and implicitly disapproving. A more subtle and at times more dangerous therapist's response is to interpret the "aggressive behavior" of the female patient in ways that increase guilt and arouse self-criticism without allowing exploration and understanding of underlying dynamics. In essence, the interventions of the therapist (including her silence) have the direct or indirect aim of suppressing, discouraging and inhibiting those communications and attitudes.

When the therapist has an opportunity to explore her reaction she tends to use adjectives that reflect a negative view of the patient and a condemnation of her behavior sometimes in moralistic terms. Although women therapists tend to use less derogatory terms than male therapists to give vent to the disapproval felt, they communicate their distaste for the patient's behavior. The negative reaction of the therapist has the purpose of protecting the therapist from similar feelings in her of which she disapproves. In the fantasies of therapists the stereotype of the vengeful and omnipotent female is aroused. This stereotype has the characteristics of an unloving woman. In the female ideal, her loving traits, her benevolence and her consistent nurturance of others are the salient characteristics that disappear in the negative stereotype. In every woman, the image of the idealized mother lies barely beneath the surface. As are others in our culture, therapists are also subject to expectations about females that betray the necessity to hold onto an idealized maternal image. In her paper, "The Fantasy of the Perfect Mother," Chodorow (1982) testifies to the pervasiveness of this expectation of females whether they be mothers or not. Mothering is seen not as a role, task or occupation but rather as a set of intrinsic characteristics and dispositions that we inadvertently come to expect of all females. The betrayal of that unconscious wish calls upon very dreaded images of equally irrational proportions: the vengeful mother. I will not go into further detail here about the origins and meanings of these early images of mother that every woman may at one time arouse. Suffice it to say that the prohibitions about female anger have been corroborated by other clinicians (Kaplan, 1976) and researchers (Brodsky & Hare-Musin, 1980; Bernardez, 1976) in recent years. Dinnerstein (1977) has drawn a compelling picture of the profound impact of the mother-of-early-childhood in men's and women's fantasies about their roles and of their influence of patterns of heterosexual interaction.

The female therapist needs to be free of the dread of "female destructiveness" and of the compulsion to expect in all women nurturing and maternal characteristics.

Particularly in the case of the hostile, domineering and openly aggressive female patients this situation is vital. For the patient is often complaining about a real injustice in her life but doing it in such a way that it can be dismissed or not heard. At times, these

patients utilize this stance as a defense against awareness of other
feelings that are often intolerable unless the patient has been reas-
sured by the therapist that she has acknowledged her desire for inde-
pendency, autonomy, sense of mastery and control of her own life.
The feelings that are warded off often have opposite valence: helplessness, passivity, longings for nurturance and sometimes depressive feelings and self-deprecatory attitudes. Because these patients
are unaware of the importance and validity of their grievances they
collude in having others dismiss them. The therapist here is well
advised in hearing out and helping the patient make her criticism
and dissatisfaction more explicit. The aim would be to help the
patient become more successful in expressing her dissatisfaction,
more competent in identifying and asserting her needs. Once these
concerns have been dealt with we can be successful in interpreting
the anger as a defense against "forbidden" affects.

This aspect is not so different from its counterpart in the male
patient. Males often defend against passive longings and dependent
wishes with an anger experienced in comfortable syntonicity
(Bernardez, 1982). In male patients those aspects that are warded
off are also negatively valued by the culture. Female patients, on
the other hand, are more likely to be devalued by their angry or
dominant attitudes. Defiant or aggressive behavior is thus deviant
for females while gender-syntonic for males. This is a fundamental
difference, and it requires that the therapist not be distracted in her
therapy of these women patients by the apparent and yet false sense
of power that the behavior may superficially convey.

Paradoxically, it is this patient who most needs the therapist's
assurance that she will neither control nor dismiss her and that she
can expect her help in addressing her grievances. But the element of
self-centeredness often required of patients to engage their resources to help themselves is regarded with ambivalence by our
culture when it is exercised by women. The tendency to expect
other-directed, altruistic behavior of women may be reflected in
therapists' reluctance to encourage women patients in self-serving
behaviors no matter how appropriate to their development and how
desirable an improvement.

The female patient then, because of long held collective expectations about her role in society coupled with the therapist's own affectively charged notions of unconsciously dreaded female stereotypes is in serious danger of not examining and resolving in her
psychotherapy the very complicity with the role prescriptions that

prevents her growth. I am here speaking of the capacity to develop autonomy and independence, self-sufficiency and competence, self-esteem and assertiveness and freedom to express a whole range of emotions including anger, criticism or disapproval. It is within the therapeutic situation that such premises need to be examined, tested and changed and new behaviors tried. If a therapist cannot tolerate criticism from the female patient, how is she to become competent to use discriminating judgement, to express her opinion with authority and comfort, to trust and express her dislikes? Indeed, how is she to learn to discriminate resentment and bitterness from a wholesome expression of dissatisfaction, to differentiate and choose direct rather than indirect and devious ways of expressing anger, to exchange forceful and honest self-disclosures rather than manipulative or passive-aggressive communications? The integration of loving and critical aspects in the self, of both aggressive and erotic components can not be achieved in women if only one aspect is encouraged and explored. The present grievances of women have a lot to do with this sense of having been exploited, used for the service of others and praised only when selfless and altruistic. Women's other realms of experience need to be integrated and for that eventual outcome plenty of room for exploration, resolution and change has to be allowed. To permit this freedom, therapists need to be aware of their own gender role biases, their own views of their own gender restrictions and their own relationships to their mothers. In this way, therapists do not become a party to the patient's domination or control or usurp control themselves.

Throughout all of this difficult and hazardous search, the therapist's ability to maintain equanimity and compassion for the patient is just as crucial. It is more difficult to have the required understanding if the therapist has not had the opportunity to have her own complaints about the restrictions of her gender addressed, heard and transformed or if the therapist has not had her own therapy to resolve her own grievances about women in her past. Supervision offers the possibility of examining and working through these dilemmas if the supervisor exhibits the same attitudes and awareness that she wants to promote in the therapist (Benedek, 1973). If the supervisor is tolerant and nonjudgmental of the negative behavior in the supervisee but inquiries about the reasons and sensitivities for such reactions with interest and empathy she can uncover them and be able to support the therapist.

In the occasions in which I was called as a consultant to resolve protracted problems in the psychotherapy of women patients I was able to address the therapist's own socialization to help her understand the situation of her patient. The problem that is most often encountered with women patients is that of prolonged depression. The richest avenue for understanding of the therapeutic impasse is the therapist-patient relationship. Often the therapist needs relief from her anxiety and guilt over the potential criticism of the patient, understanding of her role in subverting desirable critical behaviors in her female patient and a hearing of her own dissatisfaction and anger about the patient's inability to change. Unfortunately, it is the therapist who does not seek consultation or who has no access to supervision who is most at risk. These situations often result in the patient abandoning treatment or getting worse and having the treatment terminated by the therapist. But in some cases, the danger is precisely in the compliance of the patient in adapting to the therapist's unconscious biases and improving in a way confined to feminine role prescriptions.

CONFLICTS WITH ANGER
AND THE FEMALE THERAPIST

Female therapists appear to have greater flexibility than their male colleagues in supporting choices of women that do not fit the traditional model (Hoffman, 1977). In regard to anger and negative feelings, however, they seem to share with male colleagues similar assumptions and prohibitions. Unlike men, their conflicts reflect similar origins to those found in their patients. The female therapist has a strong bond with the patient because, often, she has been socialized in a similar way. She has, as potential advantages, experiences in education and professional work for which a certain degree of competitiveness and aggressiveness is required (Carter, 1971).

One of the dilemmas of women in professions is that they may be required to identify with men and masculine styles and assumptions to survive or succeed in predominantly masculine environments. In these situations an increasing alienation from females may result and a problematic derogation of feminine qualities with concurrent idealization of masculine traits that leads to behavior with female patients not very different from that of male therapists. These therapists, may tend to devalue their own feminine identification and wish not to be differentiated from male professionals. Paradoxically, they may react negatively to characteristics in the woman patient that they display themselves; they are power-conscious with interest in having control and authority over others; they are more openly aggressive and competitive, and they reveal counterdependent traits of toughness and exaggerated autonomy. They also tend to show disapproval of more traditionally "feminine" conduct such as dependency, self-deprecation, submissiveness, this derogation being linked to female models that they have rejected. The underlying dislike of women has its origins in disappointment with these female role models and their wish to escape the negative fate of females. At the same time these conflicts have not been sufficiently resolved to permit a positive female identification and a sense of commonality with other women.

Another common problem with female therapists lies in the opposite tendency: to respond to the requests or demands for nurturance, support and dependency without the freedom to deny and frustrate these needs when appropriate. Kaplan (1979) has emphasized how women therapists may be culturally handicapped in taking on their own authority while being quite able to be empathic. The anger of the patient when criticizing the therapist for her ungivingness may evoke guilt in the therapist and attempts at placation. These may result in the inability to draw firm enough limits so that the female patient can test the boundaries vigorously, become aware of her back log of anger in the past, particularly towards women and feel free of guilt herself when not meeting inappropriate expectations of her.

A different reaction is observed often times if the angry behavior of the female is directed towards a male. This behavior often produces an awareness of conflict and discomfort in the therapist followed by a variety of interactions that signal disapproval or encourage deflection. In this situation the female therapist reacts out of concordant views with the female patient about forbidden role reversal in male-female relations. Dominance over the male is a social taboo for the female, and the fear of female dominance as well as the belief of male vulnerability to female aggression replicate similar unconscious dreads in male therapists.

Although the fears are similar, the underlying dynamics are different. The female therapist fears the arousal of her own anger and of forbidden aggressive impulses towards the male and this in turn, threatens the dissolution of dependent bonds with men and of loving affiliations with them. The whole architecture of heterosexual arrangements is threatened when assumptions about the nurturance and motherliness of women are challenged. In the public sphere we find a similar dread and prejudice. The assumption is often made that the freedom of women to have greater choices and more flexible, integrated roles would destroy the family and the community. That is in part due to the fact that male roles are not correspondingly examined and questioned. It also betrays a belief in the unequal and excessive responsibility assigned to the female in matters that should deeply concern both genders.

Whatever the impact of this collective expectation of responsibility, the female therapist is not immune to it and may inadvertently react in accordance with societal expectations. This may lead her to dismiss the charges her patients express toward men in their lives or to react in a critical and moralistic manner not unlike her male colleagues. But unlike them, female therapists experience discomfort similar to their patients in the expression of their own anger. They have a similar difficulty in differentiating anger, hatred, resentment and rivalrous feelings. In the experience of conducting experiential workshops for women therapists I have noticed the exquisite sensitivity women show about the potential to hurt others and the strong inhibitions of competitive and aggressive impulses in female groups.

This observation is in contrast to the popular fantasy that such groups would encourage angry expressions and deprecation of males. Females have an unusual difficulty in externalizing their anger at men and feel often guilty if their behavior betrays such feelings. There are instances, however, when the female therapist identifies with the female victim and she herself voices her indictment of males. That is often the case therapists dealing with rape victims. The therapist finds herself enraged while the patient expresses no affect or she speaks predominantly of her depression and her devastation. In these instances, the female therapist takes up the role of the patient's expression of rage because the patient may find it so overwhelming or destructive that she blocks it altogether. These are dramatic and extreme examples of occurrences that are otherwise frequent in the therapy of the female. I am speaking of the tendency in the female patient to split-off the anger onto the other and speak about the depressive and hurtful feelings. Such occurrences are also common in the process of describing a family or personal situation when the patient makes perfectly clear that she is being exploited or mistreated by a man but voices no anger, defiance or criticism. The therapist becomes the recipient of the split-off anger of the patient and may often act out by voicing it. Clearly the patient may receive confirmation and satisfaction from it but she is not helped in acknowledging, exploring and expressing her own negative feelings as the situation demands. On the other hand, the female therapist, having become the depository of the hostile feelings toward the male that the patient disacknowledges, may defend against them by identifying with the patient in her sadness and grief, becoming powerless to help the patient.

THE THEME OF BEING "CHEATED" IN THE BACKGROUND OF FEMALES

Females often voice resentment at their mothers for depriving them of love and self-esteem. Repeatedly the complaint of not having been valued and respected as a female child is voiced. Either a male sibling has been favored or the expectations about her capacities and development have been seen as limited in comparison to males. Equally painful is the disappointment of the girl in the mother's behavior, position and aspirations. Many females criticize their mothers without recognition of the subordinate role and limited choices their mothers had. The mother is perceived as the person responsible for the second class status of the girl and for the indoctrination into obedience and compliance in the role of woman. This aspect of the conflict may lead to defensive identifications with males. If this conflict is not resolved the female continues to hold a devalued picture of her herself as a woman and since she is forbidden to take cognizance of her subordinate position in the social world, her complaints about her mother and maternal objects become the focus of the resentment. On the other hand, the desire for mother's special attention, for being valued and for being taken seriously, for being regarded with joy and hopefulness about the future persist and appear in the transference reactions of women patients to female therapists. The "identificatory hunger" with female role models and supervisors that have been observed in female therapists in the process of professionalism attest to these absences in their background.

REACTIONS TO THE GRIEF, LOSS, AND SORROW IN THE FEMALE PATIENT'S LIFE

If the therapists' reactions to anger in women patients are frequently responsible for therapeutic impasses, the troubled reactions in the therapists to the expressions of deep grief and sorrow in the woman patient's life contribute to an incomplete and inaccurate picture of the patient's dilemmas. I am referring to the persistent discouragement and inhibition of the emergence of deep grief and the active ignoring of the cues that the patient gives in signaling the existence of these troubling feelings.

A tentative explanation for the therapists' reactions, is that the strong affective impact of the patient's grief tends to overwhelm the therapist. This observation has been found true of experienced and competent therapists as well. They ward off and avoid these manifestations in their patients in such subtle and consistent ways that it can only be interpreted as the therapist unconsciously selecting what is being avoided.

I have found it extraordinarily frequent to have women patients from all walks of life and diverse ages seem unable to restrain a compelling desire to weep that frightens them in their intensity and unexpectedness. The capacity to express sadness and to cry is not discouraged in women as it is in men (Filene, 1974). It is clear, however, that it is not only the intensity of the individual's expression that may be forbidden for its impact on patient and therapist but that it is the origins and circumstances of the grief which make so clear the collective fate of women that the social determinants cannot be denied. Depression being a prevalent disorder of women it is common to find in women patients the disposition to speak about their sadness. But what is different is the occurrence of uncontrollable weeping surprising in its intensity and which patients have described as a "dam broken loose." This charged communication that usually evokes a strong empathic response and leads to a positive and rapidly developing therapeutic alliance, produces in many therapists an avoidance reaction characterized by anxiety and fears of being "drowned" in the patients grief. Both men and women alike veer away from a strong empathic response.

Although the female therapists are less inhibited in their empathic contact with the female patient than the male therapists they often comment on experiencing "unbearable" pain. The patient moves them very deeply and places them in contact with their own grief.

Similar experiences of disappointments, betrayals and losses in their own lives and the awareness of the aloneness the woman bears in the midst of it are awakened. It is my impression that the capacity to let go of the restraints with which many women control the expression of sadness is in direct connection with the therapist's readiness to hear, acknowledge and empathically contain both the content and the affect of this important communication. The patient has longed for the opportunity to do so and in yielding to that need she becomes instantly aware of how alone she has felt and how divorced from her own internal states.

It is not difficult to assume that the therapist's clinical experience is a crucial factor in allowing these developments due course. Another important factor, however, is the affective readiness, openness and flexibility of the therapist. That affective receptiveness in the therapist is again gender-role related. In hearing the stories of the women patients, one after another, it becomes apparent that many women suffer similar fates. It is difficult, therefore, not to conclude that the same sources of unhappiness repeat themselves whether it is women abused or exploited or women mourning the loss of the self. The poignancy of the individual's story makes only more painful the awareness that a great source of women's sorrow is the result of the way their lives are conceived by the culture and their own cooperation with it. The awakening of the woman patient to the realization that the sacrifices made in the expectation of being compensated or valued for them have been useless and that the supposed gains are illusory is a common and painful experience. The female therapist confronted with this realization has to examine her life as a female and just as often the life of her own mother.

Both male and female therapists, for different reasons, tend to stifle, inhibit or prevent in the female patient the intense grief expression for fear of "hearing" the implications of the patient's sorrow. The inability to hear the complaint of "womankind" in the individual woman's grievances is due to a cultural prohibition, which we obey unconsciously. This *cultural countertransference* stands in the way of permitting the female patient to hear and explore the extent, intensity and origin of her complaints and thus effectively deal with them. It is as if the therapist was afraid to experience the guilt and powerlessness that comes with the awareness of social injustice. But hearing it in our patients demands that we explore as well implications for our own lives. The complicity of therapists with cultural prejudice defends them from the awareness of conflicts with established notions of equality in heterosexual relations and the necessity to examine and change their own behavior in profound ways.

The female therapist, by allowing herself to acknowledge the deep mutilation that social expectations create for women and by mourning these losses, often fears devastation by what appears to be a universal "hatred of the female." Her own dissatisfaction with her gender, in whatever measure present in her own dislike of femaleness, internalized notions of her own inferiority, only compound the shock of awareness of what is seemingly an ubiquitous malevolence. The other reaction is equally frightening to the female. Anger of great intensity can be aroused by the acknowledgement of the many ways in which our patients and ourselves have been maimed and restricted.

It is this fear of a paranoid position toward the world, of a grave disappointment with and distrust of men, of a feared loss of relations of loving nature with men and of an equally feared rage against women for their complicity, helplessness, and victimization, that the acknowledgement of the devastating effects on women of their socialization and compliance with their victimization cannot be allowed in consciousness except in small degrees and at controlled intervals. This defense against overwhelming despair or disorganizing rage is tampered with when the woman patient's deep sorrow is allowed to emerge.

For the patient, however, the experience of integrating these losses into a pattern of awareness of the social determinants of suffering and inequality in women is deeply healing. It stands to reason that the therapist should be responsible for increasing her awareness of her own cultural countertransference and dealing with her own grief and anger in her situation in the world so that she can permit maximum growth in the female patient.

REFERENCES

Abramowitz, C. Z., Abramowitz, F. I., Tittler, B. & Weitz, L. J. (1976a). Sex related effects on clinicians attributions of parental responsibility for child psychopathology. *Journal of Abnormal Child Psychology, 4*, 129-138.

Abramowitz, F. I., Abramowitz, C. Z., Roback, H. B., Corney, R. & McKee, E. (1976b). Sex-role related countertransference in psychotherapy. *Archives of General Psychiatry, 33*, 71-73.

Alonso, A. & Rutan, S. (1978). Cross sex supervision for cross sex therapy. *Am. J. Psychiatry, 135*(8), 928-931.

Beiser, H. (1977). The woman psychiatrist as supervisor of women. *Psychiatric Annals, 7*(4), 15-23, April, 1977.

Benedek, E. (1973). Training the woman resident to be a psychiatrist. *Am. J. Psychiatry, 130*, 1131-1135.

Bernardez, T. (1978). Women and anger: Conflicts with aggression in contemporary women. *JAMWA, 33*(5), 215-219.

Bernardez, T. (1976). Psychotherapists' biases towards women overt manifestations and un-conscious determinants. *North Carolina Journal of Mental Health, VII*, Number 5.

Bernardez, T. (1982). The female therapist in relation to the male role. In Solomon and Levy (eds.), *Men in Transition: Theories and Therapies for Psychological Health*. New York: Plenum Pub.

Brodsky, A. & Hare-Musin, R. (1980). *Women and psychotherapy: An assessment of re-search and practice*. New York: The Gineford Press.

Carter, C. A. (1971). Advantages of being a woman therapist. *Psychotherapy: Theory, Re-search and practice, 8*, 297-300.

Chodorow, N. (1982). The fantasy of the perfect mother. In Barrie Thorne & Marilyn Yalom (eds.), *Rethinking the family: Some feminist questions*. New York: Longman.

Dinnerstein, D. (1977). *The Mermaid and the Minotaur. Sexual arrangements and human malaise*. New York: Harper Colophon Books.

Filene, P. G. (1974). *Him/Her/Self: Sex roles in Modern America*. New York: Harcourt Brace Jovanovich, Inc.

Hill, C. E. (1975). Sex of client and sex and experience level of counselor. *Journal of Counseling Psychology, 22*, 6-11.

Hoffman, M. (1977). Sex differences in Empathy and Related Behavior. *Psychological Bul-letin, 84*, 712-722.

Kaplan, A. G. (1979). Toward an Analysis of sex role related issues in the therapeutic rela-tionship. *Psychiatry, 42*(2), 112-120.

Kaplan, A. G. (1976). Androgyny as a model of mental health for women: From theory to therapy. *Beyond Sex-Role Stereotypes*. Little Brown, pp. 353-363.

Zedlow, P. B. (1978). Sex differences in psychiatric evaluation and treatment: An empirical review. *Archives of General Psychiatry, 35*, 89-93.

Women, Depression and the Global Folie: A New Framework for Therapists

Gretchen Grinnell

Folie

Mania; craziness; folly: "a costly undertaking having an absurd or ruinous outcome . . . Archaic French: evil; 'In place of folly there can be sanity and purpose' (Norman Cousins)."

American Heritage Dictionary: 1973

Folie a deux

A rare syndrome characterized by the simultaneous occurrence of psychosis in two people who have a close relationship — i.e., they live together.

In such cases, one of the two (the inductor) is usually suffering from paranoia or some other paranoid.

The inductee — generally a woman or a passive male — seems to accept the delusional attitudes of the dominant person and often is his spouse or child.

When the passive person is separated from the domination of the inductor, her psychosis is likely to disappear, while the inductor retains his abnormal symptoms.

Encyclopedia Britannica 15th Edition 1974

The author is a psychotherapist in private practice in Toronto, Canada.

Presented to the American Orthopsychiatric Association Women's Institute April, 1984. Toronto, Canada.

Folie a doute

Abnormal doubts about ordinary acts and beliefs; inability to decide upon a definite course of action or conduct.

Taber's Medical Dictionary 14th Edition 1981

Paranoia

A chronic psychotic entity characterized by fixed but ever expanding systematized delusions of persecution.

General characteristics are sensitiveness, suspiciousness, jealousy, brooding, excessive self consciousness, fixed ideas developed into well systematized logical delusions, megalomania, . . . and inability to make concessions.

Taber's Medical Dictionary 14th Edition 1981

THE GLOBAL FOLIE

This essay examines and analyzes feminine depression based on my clinical work with individuals, pairs and families who have presented with the usual problems and perplexities one would find in any middle-class counselling practice.

The people who come to see me are not abnormal per se, but are, by virtue of various crises, in trouble emotionally. The women I see are depressed, anxious, self-doubting or have psychosomatic complaints. I am a drugless practitioner and often counsel those who have been through psychiatric treatment but have given up because they have experienced little or no change in their anxiety levels, sometimes with high doses of medication. I also see men, mostly those who fear they are about to lose their wives or girlfriends and feel puzzled and upset about why things are going wrong in the relationship. These men all have a unified theme: "There is something wrong with her; please fix it and then our relationship will be saved." Their partners agree.

My observations have led me to re-frame and re-name certain concepts and attitudes re: depression and to examine the roots of male and female depression. I now contextualize depression as a natural result of a paranoid masculine dominated system based on a

Testosterone Imperative which creates a Global Folie hitherto unnoticed and undiagnosed as a sociological phenomenon.

The premise of this paper is that we are indoctrinated into a mild form of the Folie a deux and that depression is a natural response to this, as is its companion, the folie a doute. Therefore I have reframed depression as a "resting potential" rather than a disease. Depressed people are not "sick." Rather, they are mistaken in believing that they themselves are malfunctioning while those who dominate them are "well." The opposite is often true — depression is a correct reaction to a disordered surround.

I want at the outset to emphasize that in folie the inductor lives in a hierarchical system and indoctrinates dependents into this system as well. He persuades them to rely on his better judgement; to believe his transcendent dogmas and philosophy; to assimilate his history and ascend to his "higher" values. His goals and doctrines are to be taken as "truth" and "reality" whether or not these require a suspension of disbelief. In a Folie it is forbidden to have a tendency to argue, to be atheist to his gods, as it were, or to think in opposition to his premises. His methodology must be utilized and one's personal experience and perceptions all must filter through his belief system. All must be compared with it and eclipsed if they do not fit his reality.

Psychologist Jerome Bruner notes that in control of thought one must both "seduce and coerce by shaping the conception of the world" in which we live. This is done through "monopolistic preemption . . . of the sources of information to which an individual is exposed, and control over the order in which this information is encountered" (Bruner, 1971).

And sociologist Dorothy Smith describes how our reality is manufactured sociologically as we adopt patterns of thought which are in fact not "truth" but elaborated fabrications or mythic variations of it. We are thus impelled to mistrust our perceptions as each is systematically preempted by a socially accepted "norm" which is not fact, but an embroidered fantasy of fact. Under the indoctrination of the Folie we have been led to believe that male supremacy and rationales of competition are "natural" tendencies. This gives excuse for going to war on a religious basis or pretext of self defense while committing political aggression.

These are not natural tendencies as ethnologists and animal watchers would have us believe. Darwin himself noted his observations through the lens of the hierarchy of masculine values. His experience of his own world led him to see what he was familiar with: male supremacy. Upon further examination with a different lens, one could intuit that this might not have been necessarily the case despite his monumental contribution to the evolution of animal species knowledge (Darwin, 1909; Suzuki, 1985).

One can also intuit that delusional beliefs and biases are given credence because authorities believe them to be true. When a credentialed person says something is "true" we have been taught to believe it, even though eminent rationales may be emerging from disturbed, mythic or delusional social constructs. In the Global Folie male constructs are given greater credence than female ones, unless these aid and abet masculine experience.

In the Folie our perceptions, memories, imagination and conceptions of the world are "cathexed" — taken in and internalized to be our own — much as a fabric soaks up dye and becomes the color to please the eye of the artist. In his book *Ten Philosophical Mistakes*, philosopher Mortimer Adler lists ten concepts which form the ground for cathexis. These are: Our consciousness and its "objects"; the intellect and the senses; words and meanings; knowledge and opinion; moral values; freedom of choice; human nature and human society; human existence; happiness; and contentment (Adler, 1985).

Immediately I note that these constructs differ greatly for men and women. In mental and experiential living, "objects" and "objectivity" are masculine modalities. I believe feminine modalities are more subjective. We experience ourselves intuitively and know that we are in some way connected — part of a whole — earthy. We are indeed also seen as "objects" — love objects and sex objects — but this is often denied. Under the doctrines of the Folie, we are required to be objective rather than subjective, and to be rational rather than intuitive. Although females are passionate, their passion is considered to be irrational and is disallowed unless it is serving masculine needs. God forbid that this passion should be used on our own behalf.

In courtrooms, in the church, in medical practice, and in education, the masculine conceptions of competition and lack of emotion (which demote care-giving and fairness) are the norm. When we hear the statements "That's human nature," and, "It's just human nature to be greedy/competitive/warlike," we are hearing masculine constructs. Female passion in this construct has been subsumed into masculine nature. Women's psychology is only now being separated out from male nature. Much as anthropologists take artifacts and carefully piece them together, we are now naming what has previously been unnamed and piecing together subliminal feminine essences which are embedded in the primary system of masculine thought and experience (Gilligan, 1982; Miller, 1976; Schaef, 1981).

As Thomas Kuhn (1970) has described, it is the interloper who notices flaws in an established paradigm and points these out to incumbents who are established authorities. These see the interloper as an uncredentialed upstart who is misinformed, crazy, heretical or sick. Interlopers are Agents of Change and fundamentally serve to reorder "reality" and create the ground for a paradigm shift in knowledge as new information infiltrates and gradually replaces the old. Galileo, Semmelweiss and Pasteur were interlopers. As agents of change each opened a new paradigm which forever altered "truth" as it was known in his time. None could rescind this knowledge.

We are interlopers naming a new truth: Women's reality is separate from men's reality. We are heretics gathered together to review and to rename what we discover are flaws in prevalent beliefs about the nature of woman. In the search for truth, feminists are creating a paradigm shift which is the harbinger of a paradigm change. I believe this is a natural process in the evolution of our species and is not, after all, extraordinary. If this succeeds, our reality as we know it will alter in regard to authentic human development as opposed to the gender indoctrination which is now the prevailing pattern. It is natural for established doctrines, like the seasons, to change.

HIERARCHY AND THE TESTOSTERONE IMPERATIVE

The premise of this paper is that we are living under the terms of a global paradigm based on a pattern similar to the Folie a deux and its companion, the Folie a doute. This pattern is neither rare, nor is it unusual in its milder forms. It emerges from, and is embedded in, what I call the Testosterone Imperative.

This is a tacit, socially accepted contract which overtly forbids but covertly winks at the masculine appetite for unbridled rut and the glory of fighting. By virtue of their hormones, males at large in this contract, are excused from a fundamental responsibility for hostile aggression and sexual imperialism. This is because it is supposedly "natural" for males to react crudely when provoked or sexually aroused. Men are therefore able to remain primitive and animalistic under a thin veneer of civility because the Testosterone Imperative (first experienced at puberty as an almost uncontrollable hunger for sexual contact) implicitly orders them to remain captive to their adolescent appetites.

It seems that neither moral suasion, religious dogma nor the promptings of healers have made inroads into its pernicious existence. This is because males simply refuse to render it socially unacceptable among themselves but rather celebrate it and glory in it. Therefore it is women who have, by necessity, to put up with it and subconsciously to co-operate as their sons and daughters become initiated into its secret permissiveness.

Under the aegis of this Testosterone Imperative, we are indoctrinated into a state akin to the folie in which girls are induced to contain and to repress their own considerable erotic and aggressive urges (unless these serve masculine interests), and adopt false feminine behavior repertoires which are not natural to them. Boys (who are the tenderest of creatures until adult males get hold of them), are trained to withhold their natural altruism and are required to anesthetize their capacities for open empathy toward other men and to become instead homophobic and fearful of one another.

This Imperative enforces gender-appropriate behavior and forms the basis of indoctrination under the terms of a Global Folie. People are induced to become willing and able to deny their true nature, and to become paranoid about their ability to conform to masculine or feminine roles which are invented for them. With this in mind I believe that boys, like girls, can be socialized away from the false premises of the Imperative once it is revealed for what it is: a pseudo reality practiced assiduously throughout the world.

Under principles of the Global Folie indoctrination into The Testosterone Imperative begins at birth as newborns are coded in pink or blue to permit gender identifications. Training begins then: boys are meant to become competitive, tough and crude with one another, and girls to become gentle, compliant and sexually attractive (NOVA, 1980). I believe this renders males into mild sociopathic syndromes as they are taught to fear connection and vulnerability and encouraged to sexualize emotionality rather than to express it. Joan Sutton has described a form of masculine behavior which she calls a "Compulsive Male Personality" (Sutton, 1981). I believe this is condoned as a norm in many males who secretly believe it is true masculinity.

Girls and women, on the other hand, supposedly by virtue of an Estrogen Response — the theory that "biology is destiny" — are persuaded to depress themselves. Their identity and sense of individuality goes down to fit the doctrines of the Imperative. This is then seen as:

A strong female tendency to be whatever (society) demands at the time. The rewards for women who grow and become strong decrease, while the rewards for women who present themselves as young, sexy and vulnerable increase. (Bat-Ada, 1980)

I paraphrase Bat-Ada by adding that there is equal demand on males which results in a strong tendency to be whatever (masculine society) demands at the time. The rewards for boys and men who grow toward empathy and vulnerability to one another decrease, and the rewards for those who become sexually dominant, powerful and invulnerable, increase. Males are considered "abnormal" while women are called "sick, stupid, crazy, ugly or unfeminine" if they do not comply (Schaef, 1981).

This lays the groundwork for a pathological doctrine which forces each gender to compete: boys to fight with each other and girls to be mistrustful of their own and others' "assets." Herein are the roots of paranoia leading to "sensitiveness, suspiciousness, jealousy, brooding and excessive self consciousness" which renders adults captive to continued damage to the personality. These depress and stunt true growth in adult life and, I believe, are "fixed ideas developed into well systematized delusions." In this pathology, getting to the top in the assessments of others as "most beautiful" or "most powerful" becomes the underpinning of an anxious society.

The structure which creates Folie and permits the Testosterone Imperative is hierarchy — a vertical, upwardly-striving, goal-oriented modality where The Top wins — is "good" — and The Bottom loses — is disgraced. This is a success/failure paradigm and is the structure (that can be seen in any barnyard or zoo on a Sunday), which emerged from pre-history as we evolved from animal hierarchies. Early church and military rank-ordering sprang from this vertical monad in the ordination of kings, generals and priests with God above all.

In the hierarchy, winning denotes abundance and losing begets pity and contempt. One who has fallen in status has become lower – a lower animal – in the superior/inferior constructs inherent in these beliefs. Woman in this construct is seen as a "lower" being – a lower caste – an inferior. Men dread being "effeminate" or labelled inferior; it demotes them to a lower caste and bestows "loser" status upon them.

In hierarchy then, woman must bridle her own appetites and elevate masculine needs to conform to the demands of a Testosterone Imperative. In this Imperative there is also anxiety and a built-in paranoia about abundance and scarcity as well as dread of losing and contempt for things effeminate. In their writings of men and competition, both James Verser and Eugene Bianchi emphasize that "competition is based on a scarcity of resources" and it leads to violence in emphasizing winning and separateness (Verser, 1981). "Winning is all, even if it means trampling on one's fellow . . . a tough stance brings . . . material rewards. The place of woman . . . is essentially subordinate and derivative. She functions to bolster male toughness" (Bianchi & Ruether, 1976). Suffice it to say that hierarchy breeds paranoia – one must watch and be careful lest one be taken from behind.

Although we experience this underlying suspiciousness every day of our lives, we do not think of it as clinical in its implications. It has become a norm in the Folie of our living.

In fact, however, hierarchy is a construct, an invention, a convenient classification system which is legitimate when it is used to classify phenomena in botany, for instance, or biology. It is used to code and document elements from the most simple to the most complex and to explain in evolutionary terms how components relate to one another. But hierarchy is illegitimate when it is used to classify humans into "poor," "fair," or "excellent" in performance; or "good," "better," "best" as people. It is this false premise – the worship of hierarchy and the language of it – which permits the existence of the Global Folie.

I fear that in trying to gain more corporate power and political freedom, women are attempting to emulate the Testosterone Imperative; to become "as men" – tough; insensitive; learning to disobey their natural squeamishness about going in for the kill. Some are of necessity having to use similar emotional defenses to their male counterparts: rationalization, intellectualization, denial and worst of all isolation – separation of an idea from its associated feeling.

Women are now contemplating going to war to shoot other women's children at the behest of aging generals who refuse to do this for themselves. Female athletes are taking steroids and pumping iron to accommodate a male ideal and are playing at war games in the bush. These are "male cloning productions" in which inductees emulate the behavior of inductors (Harragan, 1977). Rather than insisting that feminine qualities expand ever outward until a false pattern is suffocated, some women are forced to enter the Testosterone Imperative if they are to gain a power-hold in the hierarchy of male dominants. The Boys-Will-Be-Boys Syndrome is spilling over and now Girls-Must-Be-Boys also in order to forestall sexual harassment and expectations that they will be unable to "cut the mustard" as independents in a male-ordered world. Actually woman has the ability to become quite ruthless when it comes to defense of her children, for instance. She can become murderous and coldly calculating on their behalf if she becomes enraged. But she does not march to war and use hostile aggression unless she is driven to it. Also some women are able to be properly astute in business without descending to the properties inherent in the Testosterone Imperative. However, some of these same women who single-handedly flourish and support whole families by themselves become Matriarchs. In this case we have an Estrogen Imperative akin to the Testosterone Imperative: absolute dominance over others becomes an echo of the masculine penchant for dominion and control. However I believe that the Matriarch is merely trying to serve and to save her family et al., rather than for the sake of having Power for Its Own Sake. The Testosterone Imperative is self-serving and egotistical whereas the Estrogen Imperative constitutes an attempt to regulate and to govern for the sake of others' welfare.

WOMEN AND DEPRESSION

A depression is "an area that is sunk below its surroundings, a hollow," says the dictionary. Under the terms of the Folie, women have been induced to push themselves down — to depress themselves — their identity and their authenticity. They have therefore to *be* depressed as part of their normal existence. They then become entrapped in a chronic subconscious sense that there is something wrong with them. There is a deep-down longing for sustenance. Coupled with this, there is a helpless wish for others to change and make things better. Should a crisis arise depression can become full-blown with profound physiological and emotional loss of energy.

In this paper I want to validate depression and the so-called psychoneurotic tendencies women seem to display. It has been ordained so far in the psychiatric literature, that depression is a disease — a bio-physiological imbalance in the body chemistry. This idea is simply and flatly erroneous. I believe that the terms "reactive" or endogenous depression are "blame-the-victim" statements. Though there may indeed be physiological symptoms, the condition of depression is sociological rather than medical. The cause is an enforced lifestyle of conflict and existence within the parameters of a "Double Bind" (Bateson, 1972). I spoke with Gregory Bateson when the first doubts began in my mind about depression as a medical disease. He agreed that depression emerges from a double-bind conflict. A double bind is a situation of intolerable pressure on the psyche when two simultaneous messages oppose one another but both must be obeyed. I believe depression (and its companion the Folie a doute) arises when entropy — "the measure of the capacity to undergo spontaneous change . . . specified by the relationship" — clashed with the command not to change because change threatens the relationship in which it occurs. Depression is due to a double-bind. This occurs because of entrapment in the command to serve others and the conflict to potentiate while enmeshed in the Folie where primary service is to males in relationships.

The victim must naturally react to all this with sub-clinical forms of humiliation and anger. But she is not allowed to show this. Therefore, the depressed state is appropriate as an opiate which dulls recognition of entrapment and postpones painful decisions which will go against becoming aggressive. Depression can be seen as a form of altruism: rather than hurt others by becoming enraged or deserting the home (for which she will be criticized), a woman turns against herself. This is duly ordained as masochism. In my opinion this demonstrates a heroic stance not, as we're led to believe, a psychiatric disorder. In fact if she does express rage openly, woman is labelled hostile, uncooperative and immature. Her "acting-out behavior" is diagnosed as maladaptive or unnatural. She is swiftly punished through chemical "uppers" or "downers" which render her once more obedient to the Testosterone Imperative.

It is no wonder then that she demonstrates mild or severe forms of the Folie a doute: self-negation, self doubt, "mental and emotional inability to decide on a definite course of action" which will protect her and free her at the same time.

The depressed woman is an anxious woman, one who is forbidden to take her power and must instead use herself as a psychological and personal source of nurturing. It may be good for a woman to do this with little children. But it is not natural for women to have to do this with, and for, grown-up males or other able-bodied adults. Joseph Pleck has named the major services women render to the male world which becomes covertly anxious if there is a threat of removal. The first is "expressive power" — the ability to express emotion. The second is "masculinity-validating power." Women must play a prescribed role of doing things that make men feel masculine. In these roles, women are seen as refuge from the war between males; they are symbols of success as well as mediators and serve also as an underclass representing the lowest status in the masculine hierarchy. He also quotes Elizabeth Janeway who points out that if women liberate themselves, men will not only risk falling to the lowest level (that of being woman) but that there will be "a new underclass composed of the 'weak' of both sexes" (Pleck, 1981).

It can be seen that the underpinning of relationship between the sexes is based on anxiety. The premise of this essay is that anxiety is not irrational. It is healthy. Anxiety signals that there is something wrong. However the difference between neurotic and sociopathic or psychopathic anxiety is the way anxiety is played out.

The psychopathic personality is anxious about getting needs met and is puzzled and annoyed if services are withheld. He thinks he is right, while those who disagree with him or complain to him are wrong. He is often unable to empathize with others who disagree with him. The sociopath is similar in that he fears deep connection; others might drain him or take away what he has in such small measure. He fears scarcity, and cannot experience the abundance which is possible in human relationships.

In the "normal" men who come to see me I suspect mild forms of disordered personality, reminiscent of sociopathy or mildly psychopathic responses. Under the terms of the Testosterone Imperative, I believe many normal men have been led to sociopathy and see themselves as healthy rather than antirelational, phobic and disordered. They cannot understand why some women seek help when they should find happiness and fulfillment in meeting the needs of their partners and family as is expected of them by "nature."

Neurotics on the other hand, know that there is something wrong. The dependencies which accompany neuroses are often a rich ground for change and transformation, particularly in depressed women. Anxious women are relationship-oriented and seek help and change — to get things to come right, as it were. But they are labelled infantile, overly dependent, manipulative and immature in pleading for rescue from the conflicts which immobilize and humiliate them. They are called "neurotic" if they display open anxiety or overfunction, while at the same time being held in contempt for their need to affiliate and to center around their relationships rather than centering on themselves as males have been taught to do. Women martyr themselves and are condemned for this as well. A martyr is one who will suffer torture for a cause. In the Global Folie women are indoctrinated into neurotic martyrdom while being blamed for driving others to distraction with their worrisome or "nagging" ideals. They are in existential double-bind as a lifestyle. No wonder they plead for help and for rescue from such a conflicted arena.

However people in double-binds often seek reassurance and approval from the very people who oppress them. They hope falsely for understanding from those who purport to love them. They are often blind to those who also secretly manipulate them to remain primarily obedient and dependent. These others may be lover, family members, good friends, business associates or parents, anyone whose domination is hidden behind a confident and expertly applied ongoing oppression in the name of love and concern for their welfare. Unfortunately this happens too often in the helping professions as well, particularly in psychiatry. Women are accused of "Learned Helplessness" (as if they deliberately caused this in themselves), then must add to their depressive repertoires the condition of iatrogenic malady brought on by the physician. Many physicians of both sexes who are traditional do not equate depression with social and relational oppression under the terms of a Global Folie.

I have learned that where there is depression and mild Folie a doute, to look immediately for an inductor. This person will seem to be well-meaning, self-confident, concerned, is often very worried about how "sick" the depressed woman is and wants her to "get better soon." In reality inductors are like hidden puppeteers who must at all times keep control and appear benign while doing so. I emphasize that dominants experience themselves as deeply sincere. They do not mean to harm by being helpful (controlling) while at the same time they cripple any movement toward autonomy in those they counsel using hidden agendas as stencils.

In marital, family and individual counseling, therapists and doctors often are themselves unaware of their own tendencies to indoctrinate or re-educate patients back into the Testosterone Imperative. They are led astray by the seeming health and logic of indoctrinators (who look calm, cool and concerned); they are distracted by the appearance of panic and craziness or deadness in the identified patient. The apparent robust health and power of the one is congratulated and given a clean bill of health, while the dilemma of the other goes unnoticed or is diagnosed as maladaptive.

The depressed person does not know that her love and loyalty to indoctrinators is, in reality, a fatal addictive tendency to ministrations which keep her captive. She finds it impossible to withdraw this loyalty because she has been led to believe domination is good for her, sexy, romantic, or denoting love and care. And yet if she is to grow, she must prepare herself to go through the pain of withdrawal from these same ministrations. It is impossible for her to come back to herself if she remains as a satellite revolving around the planet of her undoing.

The only remedy for a Folie is *separation from the source of indoctrination* (be this personal, cultural, religious or political in its framework). We cannot change hierarchy, nor its companion the Testosterone Imperative. Pleading for mercy from oppressors merely prolongs false hope and inaction. We must instead prepare to move away from hoping for change and reframe most of the constructs introduced by the Global Folie.

A NEW FRAMEWORK FOR THERAPISTS

How do we get out of pandering to the stencil of conformity which denigrates the effeminate and elevates "health" according to masculine values? Quite simple: we merely remove ourselves from the Barnyard Hierarchy (Harragan, 1977). We refuse to think or speak in terms of a pecking order and censor any further ideation based on ancient feudal elevator constructs. The hierarchy can be laid on its side and become instead a continuum — a horizon — a potential which is elastic rather than rigid. In this horizontal mode, depression can be seen as a "resting potential." Much as the heart rests between beats to preserve its strengths, the depressed person can be viewed as "resting" until she decides what she wants to do with her life.

Once it becomes clear that she has a choice, she can opt to stay in the relationship on a more voluntary basis. She will know what is happening and have more of an informed choice. The horizontal modality legitimates her decisions, because they are neither "higher" nor "lower" choices. She can move more into relationships or more into herself at the same time, as an expansion in both directions on the continuum.

Or she can decide to opt out by ending certain of her relationships. This may take months of preparation; woman's "neurosis" serves others. But it also makes her reluctant to reject others who oppress her.

With this new orientation in mind, I use five steps with depressed women which seem to be effective over time. First, I reframe her reality and explain the Folie to her: she is not at fault. Rather she acts obediently: she is a satellite revolving around dominants who have their own best interests rather than hers at heart. She usually recognizes immediately that this is indeed true and feels some relief once she realizes she is one of millions who are likewise ensnared. She also learns that many males are sub-clinically depressed but use sex, sports, technology and liquor to remain unconscious of their own pain and anxiety.

Second, I show her a model where vertical constructs give way to horizontal modes — she does not need to strive upward nor think in terms of success/failure. Instead she is on a continuum imagining what she wants and where she is going in her life. She will not be shown mercy from her benign oppressors but must herself start to plot a different course emphasizing that others do not intend either to help her or to change their own behavior. (Ironically, when she changes, they will change in response to her altered behavior — they cannot stay the same if she is different than before. But there will be pressure on her not to change — she will be sabotaged by family, friends and spouse or lover. I conspire with her, and we literally plot to predict where and when this will be applied.) If possible I quote or get her to read Gilligan's book on feminine morality in which her "self" is valued as much as "other," i.e., in self-service she is as deserving as others whom she serves. If she negates self, she is negating a member of the human race, even though the "member" in this case, is herself (Gilligan, 1982).

I validate her altruism toward herself as well as altruism toward others. Basically I believe we are all self-serving although women have been told they are not supposed to be "selfish." Depressed women negate the fact that humankind has self-service at the core of being. For instance why does a mother pick up a crying baby? Because its cry evokes anxiety in her and perhaps she also needs to empty her swollen breasts. (Incidentally the baby is well served in this; it is changed, fed, held and soothed as its cry is answered.) Nature has ordained that a certain tone in the mewling of younglings ensures that the parent's anxiety will bring swift attention to whatever is needed for the survival of offspring. Parenting is a "selfish" act when viewed in this way — a legally selfish act. I point out that if a person gives a gift it is either because one would feel guilty or foolish about not giving, or one gets pleasure out of watching the excitement of the recipient. In the same way she gives her gifts — talents, service, attention and self negation because it makes *her* feel good to do so. She is able to recognize that whatever she is doing is legitimately an attempt to save herself — to survive — even if she is told — pressured — that she is "hurting" others in doing whatever she needs to do on her own behalf. Taking her power back may beget verbal reprisals, and she needs to grasp the principles of ego-validation as a natural state in order to withstand the rejection she may have to endure. I conspire in therapy with clients about what I call "Altruistic Selfness."

Third, with this self-protectiveness in mind, we plot strategy in which she can take small gradual steps to get to where her needs call her: a walk around the block; going to a different corner store; typing one less letter a day; watching one different T.V. program; taking a bubble bath just for herself; putting on body lotion as if she was soothing another person rather than herself; anything to wake her to her own self-nurturing. She will not benefit from any strategy which scares her or is imposed on her. (One must not forget that her indoctrinators forbid her to become her own agent of change. She may have to be quite sneaky and quiet about what she is doing and some sessions must by necessity deal with her guilt and shame about this.)

Fourth, she is shown that she has become addicted to influence. She is encouraged to find surrogates to replace inductors — distant relatives perhaps; old long-lost friends, friendly neighbors; anyone who she is comfortable with but has been induced (by mate or mother) to give up because they were not considered to be "suitable."

Fifth, she can quickly learn to read and to honor her body signals. Her feelings are metaphors — inner signs and clues about who she is comfortable with (and with whom she is uneasy) — when she is "uptight" and when she feels expanded and more loose. She will notice which environments evoke relaxation and will be able to name at least two others in her life who neither thrill nor frighten her nor question her motives or values. These can be used to compare experiences and contrasts with dominant familiars. Little or no medication is needed once she gets the hang of "hanging out" so to speak, and her self-image takes on its proper perspective. She can be taught that all of her reactions are trustworthy once she has the courage to refuse to deny her internal inputs. When she begins to trust that her own intuitions are neither crazed nor false, she will trust her own judgement. Healthy animals take flight when threatened. If she is to be healthy, she too can learn to move away from situations or people who sabotage her personhood even if these same people tell her she is "off the wall" or "sick," "stupid," "crazy" or unfeminine. Unfortunately, some people will, and she must be warned of this. Being a psychological "quitter" is often the most intelligent act a person can commit if a moral, intellectual or psychological life (hers) is on the line. This may take several months of consistent validation from a therapist, who must in turn trust the client's ability to self-heal rather than thinking in terms of depressed women as "crippled" in some way. I find this very hard sometimes, and must myself seek validation when I become impatient with slow "progress" (the male model).

Eventually depressed people can pull out of the orbit of oppressive others who hold an emotional "gravity pull" over them. But anger is often slow to come and great mourning and sadness must be gone through first. I ask women in this state to take back the rituals of grieving which have become the property of church or state and create rituals of their own. One of these is to put on something black or to dress entirely in black. It is therapeutic, and it is proper to mourn an ending before one can begin a new beginning. This can be done entirely in private with no one the wiser.

In conclusion, I believe we can, in our own time, suffocate hierarchical constructs. We can think, speak and act closely aligned with nature by refusing vertical modalities. We can use language denoting a more powerful natural ordering of ideas: expansion/contraction; inward/outward; tides and wave forms; stopping and starting. Breathing in and out is the flow of life. In nature, activity is one of opening and closing; sexual tumescence and detumescence is not an "upward" phenomenon but rather one of increase, decrease, swelling and shrinking, excitement and calm. All of these are found at the heart of nature's pumping action and circulation. None of these is a hierarchical construct. We can ignore vertical thinking.

In the Horizontal Continuum and the New Language of Reframing, we can regenerate the feminine — name what has been unnamed or non-existent in dominant themes. The phallic term "consciousness-raising" gives way to "expanded (or contracted) awareness." We do not transcend, descend or ascend. Instead we can imagine ourselves stretching outward or pulling inward. Both are legitimate in reaching or shrinking from our potentials and entropic designs. Rather than striving, we can enlarge and embrace alternative modes of thinking creatively. I think it is vital to remember how vertical language creates a false reality, and the use of mechanical concepts manufactures isolation and separation of feelings from ideas.

I hope that as therapists, teachers, social workers and practitioners we will not pander to the DSM III — not try to readjust troubled people to their disordered surround. That breeds more field dependence and external locus of control. If practicing psychotherapy is itself indoctrination, let us be sure to "induce" men and women to be who they really are, not pseudo-men or male-ordered androids. We can safely leave that to robots.

As women treating women, I hope we can re-name and re-frame our reality away from hierarchy to direct energy, language and therapy toward active rejection of the Testosterone Imperative and The Global Folie.

REFERENCES

Adler, M. (1985). *Ten Philosophical Mistakes*. New York: Macmillan Publishing Co.

Bat-Ada, J. (1980). "Playboy isn't playing": An interview with Judith Bat-Ada. Laura Lederer. 121-133. *Take Back the Night: Women on Pornography*. New York: William Morrow & Co., Inc.

Bateson, G. (1972). *Steps to an Ecology of Mind*. New York: Chandler Publishing Co.

Bianchi, E. & Ruether, R. R. (1976). *From Machismo to Mutuality. Essays on Woman-Man Liberation*. New York/Toronto: Paulist Press.

Bruner, J. (1971). *On Knowing: Essays for the Left Hand*. New York: Atheneum Books, Harvard University Press.

Darwin, C. (1909). *Origin of Species*. New York: *The Harvard Classics*. P. F. Collier.

Gilligan, C. (1982). *In a Different Voice*. Cambridge, MA: Harvard University Press.

Harragan, B. (1977). *Games Mother Never Taught You*. New York: Warner Books.

Kuhn, T. S. (1970). *The Structure of Scientific Revolutions*. Chicago: University of Chicago Press, 2nd edition.

Miller, J. B. (1977). *Toward a New Psychology of Women*. Boston: Beacon Press.

NOVA. (September, 1980). *The Pinks and the Blues*. (Boston: PBS T.V.) WGBH Transcripts 125 Western Ave., Boston, MA 02134.

Pleck, J. H. (1981). Men's power with women, other men and society: A men's movement analysis. 234-244. *Men in Difficult Times*. Robert A. Lewis, Ed. Englewood Cliffs, NJ: Prentice-Hall, Inc.

Schaef, A. W. (1981). *Women's Reality*. Minneapolis: Winston Press, Inc.

Sutton, J. (1981). *All Men Are Not Alike*. Toronto: Seal Books McClelland & Steward.

Suzuki, D. (1985). *A Planet for the Taking*. (CBS T.V., Canada) Transcript: Canadian Broadcasting Corp. Box 500, Stn. A, Toronto, Ontario. M5W 1E6.

Verser, J. (1981). Strokes and strokes: Men and competition. 6-12. *Men in Difficult Times*. Robert A. Lewis, Ed. Englewood Cliffs, NJ: Prentice-Hall, Inc.

An Integration of Feminist and Psychoanalytic Theory

Charlotte Krause Prozan

This paper attempts to integrate feminist and psychoanalytic theory and to illustrate how this integration can be applied in clinical practice. I do not see the two as competitive theories of female psychology but rather see each as making valuable contributions to our understanding of women and treatment of our female patients. Special emphasis is placed on the feminist critique of the nuclear family as a patriarchal institution inherently oppressive to women and as incompatible with a life of independence and full development. I propose a way of looking at marriage and child rearing in the light of recent refinements in the recognition and treatment of the borderline syndrome and attempt a more optimistic view of marriage for women based on psychological theories of individuation and the value to women of work independent of the home.

I find it useful to distinguish between the two areas of contributions made by Freud: the developmental theory, and the technique of psychoanalytically oriented psychotherapy. I am very traditional when it comes to technique. I believe that the development and interpretation of the transference is our best tool for helping our patients uncover their fears and doubts, their anger and envy, and of course their need to be understood, appreciated and loved. By maintaining a professional distance and by not revealing our own lives and opinions, we facilitate the all-important projections which enable the therapist and patient to look inside and discover the sources of his/her misery.

The author is a psychotherapist in private practice in San Francisco, California. She has written and lectured on psychoanalytic theory and new developments in the psychology of women for UC Berkeley Extension and UC Berkeley Graduate School of Social Work.

59

Some feminist critics such as Chessler (1972) have accused the practitioners of this traditional mode of attempting to maintain a superior position to the patient, of using an authoritarian approach, and have accused therapy, therefore, of being another institution of oppression for women. This may well be true for some analysts and therapists; however, I don't believe that this is the real meaning of neutrality. I believe that it is to protect the patient. The atmosphere of neutrality is designed to discourage therapists from narcissistically using our patients to meet our own needs; to fulfill our thwarted ambitions, or to confirm our way of thinking and being in the world.

What we should not be neutral about is the health and welfare and progress of our patients. This means, for example, that we will not remain silent if a woman is reacting with passivity and masochism to a damaging relationship or to a life situation which threatens her self-respect and depresses her. A further criticism of traditional therapy, that it aims at getting the patient to conform and to adjust to an unjust society, cannot be countered by getting the patient to conform to what we as feminists or socialists or anti-nuclear activists hold out as our personal version of what is a just society. If we do, then we are making moral rather than psychological judgments.

Freud's theory of female development is based on very inadequate observation and limited research. Freud (1925) saw penis envy as the central issue in women's psychology and believed women had an inferior super-ego. Both of these ideas need substantial revision in order to incorporate the new research and theory developed since that time. For example, the Masters and Johnson (1970) research proved his theory of female orgasm incorrect. Gilligan's (1982) thesis, that the female super-ego is different than the male's, corrects Freud's assumption of "deficiency."

The two-volume work of Helene Deutsch (1944) which describes female psychology in terms of masochism, narcissism and passivity is fascinating and important but holds a number of assumptions about women with which I find much to disagree. What she calls masculine is what I call a healthy adult. What she calls feminine, such as her ideas about receptivity, sounds too much like an undifferentiated woman. Our theoretical understanding of what is normal and what is pathological for a woman is naturally going to have a significant effect on our work with her.

The image I hold is that women have the potential for being emotionally and physically strong, nurturant and creative, intelligent and competent and have the possibility for meaningful lives either within a family or in various individual pursuits or combining both. Feminists believe that women have been prevented from developing to their full potential by attitudes and mores of society, not by their anatomy, because society has narrowly confined them to the roles of wife and mother in a subordinate position to their husbands and dependent on them financially. Psychiatry is blamed for supporting and enforcing these stereotypes. The one good thing Freud is credited with is the recognition of women's strong sexual drive and the danger of repression of this drive which results in neurotic symptoms. Feminists recognize that anger is a natural and healthy reaction to the distorted view of women as weak, intellectually inferior, sexual objects, silly and so on, and feel sadness at how these beliefs are internalized by women, destroy self-esteem and then make women vulnerable to economic, political, social and sexual exploitation. The questions I ask and the comments and interpretations I make include a feminist analysis and integrates it into a traditional psychodynamic analysis thereby, I believe, broadening and enhancing both.

PENIS ENVY OR PRIVILEGE ENVY

As an example of this, let's focus on the concept of "penis envy." How might a feminist understand and use it to help women? In one sense I use it and call it privilege envy. This is very close to Lacan's definition of "a socially specific jealousy" (Turkle, 1981, p. 75). Of course, we all envy those who are privileged; the poor envy the middle-class, the middle-class envy the rich, blacks envy whites, the plain-looking the beautiful, women envy men, and in many cases men envy women. The little girl may have envied the boy for his penis, and her lack of it may have made her feel damaged and inferior. She has these feelings repeatedly reinforced by the actuality of women's inferior status in society and the promotion of her dependence on men. The little boy's envy of women can be more easily sublimated as society keeps reinforcing his ego by telling him that he is superior and promotes his independence. We can understand a woman's anger and accept her pain and frustration when faced with current prejudice or in recalling past injustice. We can work with her to channel her anger constructively by fighting arbitrary inequality.

CASE OF MS. A.

Ms. A., a divorced woman of 30, had been in therapy with me for about a year working on issues relating to her family of origin and to her dissatisfaction in her current love relationship. She is from a lower middle-class background and had not been sent to college in spite of what to me was clearly a superior mind. She felt ashamed and inferior because of not having gone to college and had worked as a secretary since high school. She recognized how important it was to her to please her boss and be a devoted and faithful employee for which she hoped to be rewarded by advancement and salary increases. In keeping with her wish to please, she worked very hard and put in extra hours without pay. In therapy she connected this with how she had tried to please her estranged father but never could. After some time passed and she did not get the longed-for recognition she became depressed and acted out her anger against herself in self-mutilating ways. My interpreting these symptoms as evidence of her anger at her boss resulted in her looking more clearly at her situation and recognizing that rather than being rewarded for her hard work and dedication, she was in fact being exploited. She approached her boss and asked to be compensated for her overtime work. When he refused, she refused to continue to work overtime. Once she was no longer trying to win his love and was able to work through her anxiety about losing her job by making her boss angry, she was able to go for legal advice and file suit against him to win her back pay. After months of effort she won her case and was awarded $1000. In the meantime she found another job. Her abilities were recognized and she was given specialized training with which she has been able to advance herself to a semi-professional capacity. In her personal life, she was able to leave the man she was living with who was cold and depressed and couldn't meet her emotional needs. Eventually she formed an attachment to a successful and much more giving man, whom she married.

WOMEN'S FEELING OF BEING DAMAGED

There is another way in which our understanding of the concept of penis envy can be used by therapists to help women and that is in relation to a feeling of being damaged, an irrational idea which can unconsciously represent a childhood idea of castration. I am always impressed with how many women feel there is something wrong with their bodies: too fat, too thin, hips too big, breasts too flat, breasts too big, legs too heavy, hair too curly, hair too straight and so on. Why have today's young women cooperated so willingly in the current fashion of being skinny — torturing themselves with diets, forced vomiting, laxatives and corseting themselves in tight pants? I have found it useful to ask some questions of women when the issue of their displeasure with their bodies comes up, especially in relation to shame at being seen naked by a man. I ask, "What do you think you're missing?", or "What is the secret that you think your clothes conceal?" They often are taken by surprise. I might say, "You do have breasts and female genitals, what would be disappointing about that to a man?" The feeling of something missing can also be displaced to the brain, with ideas about intellectual damage usually expressed as inadequacy or inferiority. Fortunately, this is less common than it used to be. However, a feeling of fraudulence occurs in some women when they become successful (Applegarth, 1977), and this can be related to the old idea of passivity as feminine and competence as reserved for men. Thus the feeling of being a fraud can be interpreted as the woman's fear that she is passing herself off as a man, as if only men have what it takes to be able, smart and successful.

If the brain were located in the penis, this fear would have some basis.

The anxiety about body image occurs once again at mid-life with the aging process, as women obsess about the appearance of wrinkles, grey hair and changes in skin texture. They spend billions of dollars on cosmetics in the hope of stemming the tide of this loss of youth. The key word here is *loss*: I had it — youth and beauty — but I'm losing it.

My idea is that women's autonomous development has been atrophied by cultural expectations which result in depression and psychosomatic symptoms. Freud defined mental health simply as being able to love and to work, yet traditionally a woman has been expected to love and to work for the objects of her love, her husband and children, thereby making her life's work intrinsically bound to her love life. In this way women have been dependent on men to fulfill them in both of these vital areas (Krause, 1971). We see midlife women in our clinical work who have never fully developed their identity nor completed individuation tasks. In their generation when adolescent boys asked the questions "Who am I?" and "What do I want to be?" the girls merely asked "Who will I marry?" Most went directly from high school or college to marriage without any period of independence or serious work. They lived vicariously through the lives of their husbands and children and neglected themselves. Women at mid-life are especially vulnerable to feelings of low self-esteem as signs of aging and loss of child-bearing capacity can make them feel worthless. Meaningful work can be especially crucial at this time so that the added skills and wisdom of her advanced years compensate for physical losses.

Feminists have raised our consciousness and understanding of many issues relating to women which have been very valuable to therapists. A few examples include rape (Brownmiller, 1976), abortion, pornography (Lederer, 1980), sexuality, menopause, hysterectomy, sex roles, father-daughter incest (Herman, 1981), mother-daughter relationships (Friday, 1977), battered wives, fat women (Chernin, 1981), third-world women.

SEXUAL ABUSE OF CHILDREN

These have influenced my work with patients. An example is that of the sexual abuse of young girls. As you all know, the traditional analytical theory held that stories of sexual abuse have in fact in many cases been fantasies that women patients have confused with reality. In 1977 an article appeared in the woman's journal *Chrysalis* (Rush, 1977) which questioned this interpretation. Florence Rush, a social worker on the staff of a home for delinquent girls, was impressed with the frequency and verifiability of such reports by these girls. She suggested that rather than viewing the reports as fantasy, perhaps it was necessary for the male analysts to view them as fantasy so as to protect the men involved, often men with whom they could identify as husbands, fathers and men of their own class. Current research indicates that 5.5 percent of male PhD psychologists (Nelson, 1982) and 5 percent of male psychiatrists admit to having intercourse with female patients. In a recent book Marie Balmary (1982) suggests that Freud's theory of focusing on the child's sexual impulses, rather than the parents', could have been an effort to defend his own father's reputation (Balmary, 1982). She points out that Freud's switch came a year after his father's death and suggests that Freud wished to conceal some facts about the sexual life of his thrice-married father, Jakob, and Freud's own illegitimate conception. In *The Assault on Truth: Freud's Suppression of the Seduction Theory* by Jeffrey Masson (1984), Dr. Masson makes a strong case for the truth of Freud's original theory that sexual attack in their girlhood by their fathers was the etiology of hysteria in his female patients. His retraction of this theory, according to Masson, was an effort to defend the reputation of his close friend Wilhem Fleiss. I talked with a number of friends about the *Chrysalis* article and was surprised that each one recalled sexual advances made by an adult man when she was a girl.

CAN MARRIAGE BE SAVED?

An issue of continuing debate is that of the effect on women of marriage and child rearing. Some feminists have seen the family as an instrument of capitalism and as the institution most deeply implicated in the oppression of women.

The question is, can we have both — closeness and independence, challenge and security, children and jobs? I believe that if we recognize the validity of the feminist critique of marriage as a patriarchal institution but also recognize the value of marriage as the institution which meets our needs for intimacy, security and child rearing, we can modernize marriage and make it viable for women by creating a new ideal for a relationship in which respect and autonomy are encouraged for both partners.

Nancy Chodorow's (1978) work emphasizing the lasting importance of the girl's primary identification with her mother as the internalized love object and the secondary nature of her attachment to her father would explain the feelings of loss many women experience during marriage since their primary needs for intimacy have been met by women and often cannot be met by their husbands. It also can explain the beneficial psychological effect of marriage for men who are, in marriage, reunited at last with the primary mother love object they had to reject in latency in order to identify with their fathers. This would explain the more severe reaction some men reportedly have to female rejection, to divorce and widowhood and their rapid re-marriage after divorce. Men often report never being able to attain the level of intimacy with male friends that their wives have with female friends and envy this in women. It is only with their wives or sometimes women friends that they can return to the bond of closeness, but remain ambivalent and fearful of the threat to their masculine identity if they feel too close.

Murray Bowen (1972) describes his differentiation of self scale. The greater the degree of undifferentiation the greater the emotional fusion into a common self with others. The basic self is a definite quantity illustrated by such "I" position stances as "These are my beliefs and convictions. This is what I am, and who I am and what I will do, or not do." The basic self is not negotiable in the relationship system, and is not changed by coercion or pressure to gain approval, as opposed to the "pseudo self" which is adaptive in order to enhance one's position in relationship to others. People choose spouses or close friends from those with equal levels of differentiation and the degree of fusion depends on that basic level before the marriage. One of the selves in the common self becomes dominant and the other submissive or adaptive, thus the dominant one gains a higher level of functional self and appears "stronger" at the expense of the adaptive one who gave up self and who is functionally "weaker." It doesn't take much imagination in studying Bowen's work to see how in a traditional marriage the dominant partner who would gain would be the husband and the submissive or adaptive partner who would regress would be the wife. It is with Chodorow's and Bowen's concepts in mind that I believe we can make sense out of the research on marriage that appeared in the 70s and identify quite precisely the danger of marriage to women, unless and until the woman rejects the role of wife as submissive and refuses to merge her identity with her husband and children. Of course similar dangers are inherent in marriage for a man who is passive and submissive, and we see men such as this in our practices as well. The difference is that the culture supports the fusion of the woman with the man, as illustrated by the practice of the wife taking the husband's name, whereas society is contemptuous of a man who adapts himself to his wife — he is referred to as henpecked. Lacan (Turkle, 1981) states that in the moment a young child realizes that his/her name is the name of the father (nom du pere), the entire patriarchal culture is transmitted to that child.

THE IMPORTANCE OF WORK
IN WOMEN'S LIVES

In Jessie Bernards's (1971) article, "The Paradox of the Happy Marriage," Bernard questions whether the qualities that are associated with marital happiness for women may not themselves be contrary to good mental health. Is it possible that many women are "happily married" she asks, because they have poor mental health?

She reported that more married than single women are passive, phobic and depressed. Using such factors as alcoholism, suicide attempts, medical complaints and reports of well-being, the group with the best mental health proved to be single women. The next healthiest was married men, married women following and the least healthy of all, single men. So much for our much-sung hero, the rambling man and his counterpart on the urban scene, the urbane bachelor, and also so much for our happy, contented married women.

Erik Erikson (1959) in his monograph "Identity and Life Cycle" has suggested that for women the resolution of their identity crises occurs after the choice of mate and the birth of children. D. J. Levinson's (1976) theory of stages of development focuses on the world of work which a man enters in his twenties and in which he matures through his thirties until becoming his own man at about forty. Neither of these authors related the role of work to identity formation in women. It has been so clear to male authors that work is of central importance to the self-esteem and maturational growth of men. Surely women mature as they take on the responsibilities of parenthood and running a house, but this would also apply to men. Women, just as men, need experience in the world outside the home to measure themselves, to test their skills, to feel competent and to interact with adults in exchanges or social and productive value to society. A woman who is totally dependent on her husband for financial support has a tough time feeling grown up, is more fearful of displeasing him and is thus more likely to compromise her autonomy in order to hold on to her husband's favor. In the extreme cases of battered women, they often state that they can't leave their husbands because they don't know how to support themselves.

Judith Birnbaum (1975) studied satisfaction and self-esteem at mid-life in comparable groups of married professionals with children, single professionals and homemakers. Both groups of professional women were more satisfied and had higher self-esteem than did the women who had lived out the traditional role pattern. In Sears and Barbee's (1977) analysis of Terman's sample of gifted women, married women were less satisfied with their life patterns than were women who were single, divorced or widowed. Satisfaction was highest among women who were both single and income producers. Of course the vast majority of working women, and men, do not work in professional jobs. However, we should not underestimate the psychological and social value that all people can get from work.

In a study in London (Brown, Bhrolchain & Harris, 1975) it was found that for women who were both under stress and unable to turn to a confidante, work served to prevent the development of psychiatric symptomatology; only 14 percent of such women who worked developed symptoms, compared with 79 percent of those who did not work. Walter Gove (1981) concluded that the higher rates of mental illness among women are largely due to societal and not to biological factors because they generally appear to be specific to particular societies at particular times and, most importantly, appear to be limited to married women, with never married, widowed and divorced women having comparable if not lower rates than men (Masters & Johnson, 1970).

Researchers Baruch, Barnett and Rivers (1983) report similar findings in a study of 300 women between ages 35 and 55. All groups of employed women rate significantly higher in mastery and lower in depression and anxiety. A woman's level of well-being could not be predicted by whether or not she had children. Married, employed mothers were the highest in well-being. This research supports my thesis that it is not marriage per se that is dangerous to mental health for women, but rather undifferentiation and dependency that is dangerous and which is less likely in a woman who works outside the home. Another important factor may be the opportunity to have close relationships with other women which is afforded by many job situations where women work. In factories, offices, stores or schools, women most often work around other women.

"EMPTY NEST" OR "NEGLECTED SELF"

The role that mothers play in the lives of their children has been studied for years in search of the causes of neurosis and schizophrenia. Feminists have studied the effects on women of having children and two reports focus on the so-called "empty nest syndrome." Pauline Bart (1971) in her work on Depression in Middle Aged Women, also titled "Portnoy's Mother's Complaint," studied depressed women at the time of first hospitalization in middle age, and concluded that role loss was the key factor in their depression. They all complained primarily of their children leaving home and how empty their lives were. She drew a connection between mid-life depression in women from ethnic groups that place the greatest importance for the woman on her role as mother, as compared to her role as a wife, and concluded that mental breakdown in middle age was more common among these ethnic groups. More recently, Lilian Rubin's (1971) research revealed a quite different attitude among working-class and middle-class women in the East Bay. Almost all of these women cautiously expressed relief that their children were leaving home so that their responsibilities were lessened and they could have time for themselves. Barbara Artson (1978) relabeled the empty nest syndrome the "neglected self" syndrome and feels mid-life women suffer from having lost themselves in the process of child rearing and experience an identity crisis when children leave.

In re-reading Bart's material, I was struck by the quotes of her women and concluded that rather than the problem of role loss, these were in fact women who had suffered from a borderline condition all their adult lives but had been able to maintain a non-psychotic defense system as long as their children were available to them to project upon and introject from. For example: "I didn't think of myself at all, I was just someone that was there to take care of the needs of my family" (Bart, 1971, p. 164). Another said, "My son is my husband and my husband is my son" (Bart, 1971, p. 179). One woman moved from Chicago to Los Angeles with her husband four months after her daughter, son-in-law and granddaughter did because "my daughter and only child moved here and it was lonesome for her, you know" (Bart, 1971, p. 171). She said she and her daughter were "inseparable." She thought the best time for a mother was from infancy till the child was 11 or 12 "because after that they become a little self-centered" (Bart, 1971, p. 172). We can now translate this to mean that they become independent, hopefully.

This material is important to us as therapists because it shows the inter-connections between a feminist analysis and a psychodynamic analysis. When Bart's work first appeared it was an important contribution as it pointed out the potential dangers to women in trying to get all their meaning in life from motherhood. Since then we have had the work of Kernberg (1975) and others defining clearly the borderline syndrome and we can now look back at these women patients and fill out the picture of the pre-psychotic personality: probably as severely obsessive and phobic, splitting off of anger so that they cannot experience anger at their children, a depressive-masochistic character, severe repression of sexuality which kept an

intimacy from developing with their husbands and, most importantly, a pathological boundary problem which merged them in a
symbiotic tie with their children and left them empty at their depar-
ture. The distinction here is between an appropriate sadness when
children leave home at one end of the scale and an empty woman at
the other end. In the middle are the majority of women, not borderline, but feeling frightened and alone because they never allowed
themselves to develop an autonomous identity apart from mother
and wife.

The external danger to women's autonomy and development has
been that society rewards with approval this pathological self-denial
as expressed through the so-called devoted mother, devoted daughter and devoted wife. The internal danger is the guilt and anxiety she
feels if she asserts herself, or in the case of more disturbed women,
the emptiness and panic they feel in trying to extricate themselves
from dependent relationships. Autonomy may unconsciously be
equated with destruction, abandonment and sadistic retaliation. I
believe that an integration of the best of feminist theory with the
best of psychoanalytic theory can combine to show us the way to
help women to live their own lives as healthy adults and at the same
time relate to husbands, children, bosses, lovers and parents as
whole people in reciprocally rewarding relationships without sacrificing their own or their children's mental health or destroying any-
body.

> You can't always change things . . .
> You're given so much to work with
> In a life and you have to do the best
> You can with what you got. That's what
> Piecing is. The material is passed on
> To you or is all you can afford to buy . . .
> That's just what's given to you. Your fate.
> But the way you put them together is
> Your business.

Quote from a quiltmaker.

REFERENCES

Applegarth, A. (1977). Some observations on work inhibitions in women. *Female Psychology*. P. Blum, ed. New York: Intl. Univ.'s. Press, Inc.
Artson, B. (1978). Mid-life women: Homemakers, volunteers, professionals. Unpublished
doctoral dissertation, California School of Professional Psychology.

Balmary, M. (1982). *Freud and the Hidden Fault of the Father*. Baltimore: Johns Hopkins Univ. Press, 1982.

Bart, P. (1971). Depression in middle-aged women. *Women in Sexist Society*. V. Gornick and B. Moran, eds. New York: Basic Books.

Baruch, G., Barnett R. & Rivers, C. (1983). *Life Prints: New Patterns of Love and Work for Today's Women*. New York: McGraw Hill.

Bernard, Jr. The paradox of the happy marriage. (1971). *Women in Sexist Society*. V. Gornick and B. Moran, eds. New York: Basic Books.

Birnbaum, J. (1975). Life patterns and self-esteem in gifted, family-oriented and career-committed women. *Women and Achievement: Social and Motivational Analysis*. M. Mednick, S. Tangri and L. W. Hoffman, eds. New York: Halstead-Wiley.

Bowen, M. (1972). Toward the differentiation of a self in one's own family. *Family Interaction: A Dialogue Between Family Researchers and Family Therapists*. Framo, ed. New York: Springer.

Brown, G. W., Bhrolchain, M. N. & Harris, T. (1975). Social class and psychiatric disturbance among women in an urban population. *Sociology, 9*, 225-254.

Brownmiller, S. (1976). Against our will. *Men, Women and Rape*. New York: Simon & Schuster.

Chernin, K. (1981). *The Obsession*. New York: Harper and Row.

Chessler, P. (1972). *Women and Madness*. New York: Doubleday.

Deutsch, H. (1944). *Psychology of Women* (vol. 1). New York: Grune and Stratton.

Erikson, E. H. (1959). Identity and life cycle. *Psychological Issues*, Vol. 1, No. 1 (Monograph No. 1).

Freud, S. (1925). Some psychical consequences of the anatomical distinction between the sexes. *CPW, 19*, 243-260.

Friday, N. (1977). *My Mother My Self*. New York: Delacorte Press.

Gilligan, C. (1982). *In a Different Voice*. Cambridge, MA: Harvard Univ. Press.

Gove, R. (1981). Mental illness and psychiatric treatment among women. *Female Psychology: The Emerging Self* (2nd ed.). S. Cox, ed. New York: St. Martin's Press.

Herman, J. (1981). *Father-Daughter Incest*. Cambridge, MA: Harvard Univ. Press.

Kernberg, O. (1975). *The Borderline Syndrome and Pathological Narcissism*. New York: Jason Aronson.

Krause, C. (1971). The femininity complex and female therapists. *Journal of Marriage and the Family, 33*, 476-482.

Lederer, L. (1980). *Take Back the Night*. New York: William Morrow.

Levinson, D. J. et al. (1976). Periods in the adult development of men: Ages 18-45. *The Counseling Psychologist, 6*, 21-25.

Masson, J. M. (1984). *The Assault on Truth: Freud's Suppression of the Seduction Theory*. New York: Farrar, Straus and Giroux.

Masters, W. H. & Johnson, V. D. (1970). *Human Sexual Inadequacy*. Boston: Little Brown and Co.

Nelson, B. (1982). Efforts to curb sexually abusive therapists gain. *New York Times*, November 23, 1982.

Rubin, L. (1971). *Women of a Certain Age*. New York: Harper and Row.

Rush, F. (1977). Freud and the sexual abuse of children. *Chrysalis 1*, 31-45.

Sears, P. S. & Barbee, A. H. (1977). Career and life satisfaction among Terman's gifted women. *The Gifted and the Creative: Fifty-Year Perspective*. J. Stanley, W. George, and C. Solano, eds. Baltimore: Johns Hopkins Univ. Press.

Turkle, S. (1981). *Psychoanalytic Politics: Freud's French Revolution*. Cambridge, MA: M.I.T. Press.

Working with Distressed Adolescent Females: Countertransference Issues

Frances Newman

In trying to help distressed adolescent females, a clear-sighted view of the nature of their experience is essential. When one gathers information through a research or clinical interview, major issues of countertransference can cloud one's vision. The usefulness of research rests upon the ability of the researcher to provide information that is, as far as possible, undistorted by error, bias or falsification on the part of either the inquirer or the responder. In short, how the information is gathered determines how accurate and useful it will be. This is particularly the case in research into the attitudes, psychological states and history of individuals, in which the interview is the principal method of data gathering. It is most particularly the case when the research is conducted with "clinical" or "at-risk" individuals who have learned to be suspicious of health professionals and who, because of their particular problems, are vulnerable to misunderstanding and even hostility and abuse by the very professionals who seek to treat and study them. This became clear to me when I began collecting data for my doctoral dissertation five years ago, for a study of ego development among a group of teenaged girls living in a hostel for indigent women.

First, I shall briefly describe the young women with whom I talked. Next, I shall briefly summarize theoretical issues about the formation of young women's identity—which was the focus of my

The author is a staff psychologist at Toronto General Hospital, Ontario, Canada. Her special interests include ego development, adolescence, women's issues and suicide.

Portions of this paper are based on the author's doctoral dissertation, Adolescent ego development in non-standard females: unfortunate life events and current function. Simon Fraser University, 1985.

73

work — and of the role that unfortunate life events can play in the identity formation process. Then, I shall describe the procedure I used and the countertransference issues that arose.

The young women I interviewed can be considered to be "non-standard," that is, not like those who are usually called "normal" adolescents, who live at home, go to school and generally avoid the attentions of social agencies. By contrast, the participants in my study were without family supports — some had been "kicked out" or had fled unpleasant and often intolerable family situations, some had been living in group or foster homes for a variety of reasons, they typically were not attending school regularly or had dropped out of school, and they had histories that included numerous contacts with the Children's Aid Societies, social welfare agencies, truant officers, parole officers and police.

EGO IDENTITY FORMATION THEORY

What I was attempting to investigate with the help of these young women was the adolescent psychosocial task of ego identity formation outside the standard context of home and school support. According to Erik Erikson (1954; 1956; 1963), by examining the ways in which the adolescent negotiates the pressures from within (developing psychological, psychosexual, and cognitive structures) and without (societal demands) it is possible to understand the formations of ego identity upon which the individual relies in coping with the demands of adulthood. The successful resolution of the major task of adolescence — ego identity formation — allows the young adult to take on the business of providing for herself by doing meaningful work; sharing herself in an intimate relationship with another; caring for and sharing herself with the next generation, and ultimately finding satisfaction in the way in which she has chosen to lead her life.

At the end of childhood, the individual has experienced a number of psychosocial crises in the context of a growing awareness and experience of a society of others. At each stage of development, Erikson tells us, the major criterion of ego strength is the quality of the resolution of the crisis at that stage. In the context of "an average expectable environment" (Erikson, 1956), where adults, the representatives of society, co-operate to guide and support the developing child, the resolution of each crisis provides the child with a firmer sense of herself and of her place in the society. In the average expectable environment the resolution of each crisis results in a favorable balance between alternative approaches to the world. That is, at the first stage, basic trust in the environment outweighs basic mistrust; at the second, autonomy dominates shame and doubt; at the third, initiative dominates guilt; at the fourth, industry outbalances inferiority. However, in a healthy individual some degree of mistrust, shame and doubt, guilt, and inferiority have also become integrated parts of the personality. At the end of childhood, a last crisis of ego development remains before adulthood begins: The structure of identity, the social aspect of ego, requires completion. "Identity" refers to many aspects of personality both conscious and unconscious, both personal and social. In order to complete this complex and essential structure and be ready for the tasks of adulthood, the adolescent must actively, though by no means always consciously, transform the experiences and identifications of childhood into a coherent self-system. This active transformation of childhood identification is perhaps the most obviously important stage in the entire process of identity formation, which begins " . . . in the baby's earliest exchange of smiles (in which) there is something of a *self-realization coupled with a mutual recognition*" (Erikson, 1956, p. 69). Identity formation continues throughout childhood, and indeed throughout the life span in the context of a supportive social milieu in which there exists a certain mutuality, or "cog-wheeling" of individual needs and abilities with societal needs and expectations. It is a strenuous task, and one which, if not accomplished, leaves society at a disadvantage, since society depends upon the cooperation of a collection of strong and flexible egos to carry on the care and maintenance of the next generation (Erikson, 1956; 1963). Even given a series of average expectable environments in which to develop, the young person faces a formidable task, crucial both for herself and for her society.

What of the adolescent who faces the identity crisis with few or defective supports from the individuals and institution appropriate for this "formidable task"? Unsupported by parents, without the structure of the school that provides the training and socialization necessary for adolescent work, the individual may be at a disadvantage, compared to those who do their work in an average expectable environment. These same adolescents, whose earlier experiences have been less than optimal, may also not have resolved important antecedent crises satisfactorily.

Identity Diffusion, the polar opposite of Identity Achievement, is the unfavorable outcome of the adolescent Identity crisis. According to Erikson (1956), a number of family and childhood factors are associated with the unfavorable outcome of the identity crisis. Among these are insecure attachments in childhood, absent or weak adult models with whom to form identifications, and severe physical trauma "either in the oedipal period or in early puberty associated with a separation from home" (Erikson, 1956, p. 92).

Empirical data regarding the state of identity in adolescence among young people who currently lack adequate social supports and who may also have experienced less than average expectable environments in the past would increase our understanding of the relationship between self and environment in the development of ego.

IDENTITY FORMATION AND UNFORTUNATE EVENTS

In addition to asking the question of how the adolescent crisis is dealt with by non-standard young women, I was also trying to discover the relationship between the form of the adolescent identity crisis and early unfortunate life events, including physical and sexual abuse; major separations from parents; loss of and death of parents; placements in foster and group homes; school failure. This necessitated my asking them about a large number of painful issues.

The young women with whom I worked had had many unfortunate experiences, including sexual abuse which would lead them to see themselves as deviant, unworthy, and as debased sexual objects whose limited choices might lead them to prostitution as an occupation and lifestyle (Newman & Caplan, 1982). Fewer than 10% of the young women had not experienced some form of serious sexual or non-sexual physical abuse by the time I interviewed them (at that time, their ages ranged from 16 years to 18 years, 11 months). In all but one case, the sexual abuse was inflicted by a male – a father or father surrogate, a brother, babysitter, boyfriend, pimp or male stranger, and this occurred in the lives of over half the young women interviewed. Non-sexual physical abuse occurred in the lives of 79% of the young women. From infancy to the time at which I interviewed them, almost 70% of the young women had experienced some form of major physical abuse by parents (mothers and fathers were equally likely to have inflicted this abuse) and 38%

had been abused by others. Over half the young women had been placed away from home in foster homes and group homes, at some time in their lives, and 75% of them had lost one or both parents through death or abandonment. Over 57% of the young women had failed one or more grades in primary and secondary school, over 85% had been out of school for one year or more, and none of them had completed high school. In adolescence, 14% were or had been actively engaged in prostitution, 19% had or were engaged in drug abuse, 19% had or were engaged in alcohol abuse, and 44% had appeared in court and been charged for a variety of charges, including property, violence, drug and status offenses.

MEASURES AND INTERVIEW

Ego development was assessed using two well-validated and widely-used sentence completion forms: The Ego Identity Incomplete Sentences Blank (Marcia, 1966; Wagner, 1976) and the Sentence Completion Test (Loevinger & Wessler, 1970; Loevinger, Wessler & Redmore, 1970). The unfortunate life events were assessed by means of a detailed, semi-structured history interview. Both of these forms of information or data gathering require the participant to share her view of herself and of the world with the inquirer. It is important to note that when inquiring into the life and self-structure of individuals, the researcher must be aware of and respect the constructed nature of reality from the point of view of the responder. There are no *facts* in this line of research, there is point of view. Beyond ascertainable, objective events that can be corroborated by agency reports, eye-witness reports, school reports and so on, the rest is the stuff of which the individual self consists. For this reason, and bearing in mind the need to provide unbiased, accurate and useful information, as outlined at the beginning of this paper, it is essential to take pains to encourage in the participant-responders a sense of trust and confidence in the interviewer-researcher.

I was aware at the outset that what would be data to me was in fact the very stuff of the lives of these young women and that my work must be at very least unintrusive and respectful, and at very best, useful to them. It became clear to me as I began to plan the research that the young women and I would become collaborators. In order to achieve my aims I would have to behave in a way that was worthy of the trust of my collaborators. In order to find out meaningful and useful information about the lives and self-constructions of these young women I would have to be willing to engage with them in a shared enterprise in which mutual respect would result in a product of value to them as well as to me. For in the very act of investigating their lives I was becoming a part of the social world of these young women. It is my belief that the way in which I entered their world determined, in part, the quality of the information I was offered.

PROCEDURE

Because the residents of the hostel where I conducted my research constituted a kind of at-risk population (many of their life situations included exploitation, neglect and abuse, and most had ongoing contacts with group homes, parole officers and a variety of social agencies), particular pains were taken to establish the ground rules for the study with them. I identified myself as a psychology student doing research for my doctorate and said I was interested in how young women without families to help them, cope with the problems of growing up. I explained that since their information would be valuable to me, they would be paid for their participation. The limits of confidentiality were also explained: It was guaranteed that the only personnel who would have access to participants' files would be me, my assistant (a mature female trained in sociology) and my supervisors. Only group data without identifying information would be reported in written or verbal reports of the study, and nothing any participant revealed about herself or her life would be repeated to a third person (including any hostel staff member) unless the matter had first been discussed with the participant herself. With this last provision I anticipated the possibility that a distressed young woman might reveal some problem that would properly become the concern of those responsible for her. In no case did a participant refuse her consent on these or any grounds: several young women asked explicitly that their parents not be informed of their participation in the study; one young woman asked to be allowed to use a pseudonym on the study forms and receipt (a list of pseudonyms had been prepared in advance) and three young women refused specific information during the course of the interview. (The information refused in each case concerned sexual history or history of sexual abuse.) One further point was made to each young woman before the signing of the consent form: I identified myself as one who had experience working with adolescents in clinical settings (a doctoral internship at a Family Court Clinic was referred to) and who was especially interested in and familiar with the problems of young people. At the same time, it was made clear that I was not available as a therapist (several young women had eagerly asked the hostel staff if it might be possible "to talk about my problems") but that I could, in consultation with the hostel staff, make referrals to appropriate social agencies for counselling or other help in dealing with personal concerns.

In only two cases was there sufficient cause for concern about interview information to cause me to suggest to a participant that the information should be shared with hostel staff; in each case the matter concerned expressions of depression and thoughts of self-harm. In these two cases, the participants agreed that the matter should be discussed with the staff and appropriate measures were taken by staff people to work with the participants and observe the behavior closely. In several cases, a participant and I agreed that talking to a staff person, a social worker, or case-worker already involved with the participant might be helpful. The concerns expressed included sexual and physical abuse (three cases), estrangement from a parent (two cases) and, in one very unusual case, the potential kidnapping, by her parents, of an Asian-born Canadian citizen back to her native country for an arranged marriage.

Appropriate referrals were discussed with staff, made to outside agencies and reported to my local supervisor. Follow-up discussions were held with the participant and staff. There were no unfortunate sequelae of these cases, and in no case was any participant noticed to be disturbed or alarmed by the interview process.

The above issues are dealt with here in some detail for three reasons. First, indigent young people whose histories include experience of abandonment, neglect, abuse and exploitation by parents and others, can be considered to be "at risk." Even a relatively benign interview and inquiry by a well-intentioned researcher can be a threatening situation for such young people. Care was taken to ensure that the research would be at least non-invasive and at best useful to these young women. Second, ethical considerations required that these young people and the agency temporarily responsible for them be fully informed about the purposes and procedures of the research. Third, as Baker (1983) has pointed out, much more

happens in interview research with young people than a simple giving and collecting of information. The interview is one kind of human interaction, a social encounter in which the interviewed and the
interviewer exchange information. For the adolescent, the adult interviewer provides information about adult thought and language
patterns and about adult values. The interview is an occasion for the
management of identity as the adolescent reflects on her experiences and values while formulating answers to questions about her
life. Modern role theory, according to Sarbin and Mancuso (1980),
offers yet another way to understand the importance of the interview. In order to locate oneself in the social ecology,

> a person makes use of an inferential process: on the basis of
> available cues and knowledge of the role system, the individ-
> ual infers the role of other(s) and concurrently of oneself. The
> process can be described as the efforts of an individual to find
> answers to the question *Who am I?* Ordinarily the answer is
> constructed from considering at the same time the reflexive
> question: *Who are you?* Finding one's place in the role system
> is a reciprocal event — answers to the question *Who am I?* are
> determined by the answers to the question *Who are you?* and
> vice versa. The totality of such answers defines a person's
> social identity. (Sarbin & Mancuso, 1980, p. 211)

Throughout the encounter with the interviewer, from the discussion of the consent form, to the interview, to the payment offered at
its conclusion, the experience is itself an instance of adolescent socialization. The vulnerable adolescents interviewed in this research
had had many experiences of less than optimal socialization with
adults; one of the aims of the research procedure itself was to provide an opportunity for a non-exploitive, useful exchange with an
adult. Sigel (1981) has pointed out the role of current social experience in cognitive development. According to him, inquiry, especially by teachers and other sensitive adults, activates representa-
tional thought and challenges established constructions; change is
thereby provoked.

At the beginning of the two-hour testing period the participant
was provided with a brief oral outline of the research, description of
the tests and the interview and a copy of the written consent form.
The consent form was discussed in detail, with emphasis on confidentiality and issues relating to the participant's right to terminate

participation at any time. I explained that the two sentence-completion forms would be completed before the interview. It was promised that the participant would be given the opportunity to discuss the tests and interview and to ask questions concerning any aspect of the process at the conclusion of the interview.

All testing and interviewing took place in a small staffroom; the participant was seated at a desk while she completed the two tests. Because of the possibility that a participant might find it uncomfortable to remain alone in a room while completing a school-like task, I remained in the room with her. The two sentence-completion forms were always presented first for two reasons: (1) so that material discussed in the interview would not influence responses to the tests, and (2) so that participants would have some opportunity to become familiar with the testing situation and the tester before answering personal questions about their lives.

After the participant had completed the EI-ISB and the SCT she was offered the opportunity to take a short break. When the participant was ready to begin the interview I reminded her that if she preferred not to answer any of the personal history questions she had only to ask to move on to another interview topic.

To begin with, demographic information was requested; the participant was then asked to give a brief history of how she came to be living at the hostel. Working back from this current history, the participant and I went through the interview schedule page by page while I took verbatim notes on the schedule itself. Whenever a participant indicated distress in recounting personal information I temporarily put aside the interview to focus on helping the participant to deal with her distress. Returning to the interview was determined by the participant's willingness and by my assessment of her ability to continue without further distress. In some cases, areas of questioning that caused distress were not returned to; however, no participant refused to continue with other areas of the interview.

When the interview was concluded, the participant was encouraged to ask questions about any areas of the testing and interview that were of interest or importance to her. In addition, I spent some time with each participant reviewing the history in such a way as to encourage the participant to regard the interview not as the recounting of a collection of unfortunate events but as a partial chronicle of her life, including fortunate as well as unfortunate events, personal strengths as well as weaknesses.

Each participant was thanked for her contribution to the research; she was further invited to address any additional questions about the research to me. I then paid the participant and received a signed receipt. All the participants spontaneously indicated that the interview had been not an unpleasant experience; many said that it had been "interesting" and some said that they would have been glad to take part "for nothing."

I do not include all this detail in order to hold myself and my research up as a model for other people to follow but to give some idea of the issues I faced when planning and carrying out my study. Indeed, I am aware now of some limitations of my study both from a scientific and from an ethical point of view. For example, my interview did not include sufficient questions about each individual's assessment of her strengths or of the protective relationships she had experienced. I therefore did not provide my participants with an adequate opportunity to reflect on the creative and positive aspects of their lives and therefore I failed to discover some of the very important information about how such young women understand and cope with their own experience. Erikson has formulated a very important distinction between the case history and the life history, a distinction that ought to be important to us when we undertake to investigate the stuff that lives are made of.

> A genuine case history gives an account of what went wrong with a person and of why the person fell apart or stopped developing; it attempts to assign to the particular malfunctioning a diagnosis in line with the observer's psychodynamic views; and it arrives at therapeutic suggestions as to what could or can be done to reactivate a sounder development in this and in similar cases. A life history, in contrast, describes how a person managed to keep together and to maintain a significant function in the lives of others. (Erikson, 1974, p. 13)

I am aware that it is not appropriate to write *life* histories of young women aged 16 to 19. On the other hand, I think it is important to include in such investigations the life history perspective as well as the case history perspective. And included in this life history perspective must be an awareness of cultural assumptions, biases and prejudices and the ways in which these have implications for the lives we investigate.

There is, currently, growing interest in the ways in which traditional theorists of personality, cognitive and social development regard *female* development as an aberrant or deviant from of male development. As Carol Gilligan has said: "What some psychological theories take to be women's deficiencies are in fact mere differences from men" (Gilligan, 1982). Among these theories are those about moral development (Kohlberg, 1964) identity construction (Erikson, 1963; 1968) and personality development (Freud, 1953; 1961). Much work has recently been done to demonstrate that female development in these areas is different rather than deficient or deviant. With respect to identity development and moral development, Carol Gilligan in *In A Different Voice* (1982) has pointed out that, because of gender-linked differences in cultural expectations and child-rearing practices, girls are encouraged to maintain connections forged in infancy and childhood, compared to boys, whose early development consists of relinquishing early attachments and connections. This difference has implications for both identity development and moral reasoning and makes females more likely than males (1) to establish identities based on personal relationships *and* achievement and (2) to resolve moral dilemmas by negotiating individual needs rather than by invoking moral principles. Paula Caplan in *The Myth of Women's Masochism* (1985) has argued that because girls are raised and educated to consider the needs of others before their own and to be nurturant, they are more likely, as women, to be willing in everyday life to behave in unselfish and self-sacrificing ways than are men.

In order to contribute something to this current reexamination of traditional views of women, I chose to investigate the ways in which these particularly disadvantages, one might say deviant, females have gone about the business of making some sense of their lives in order to make something of themselves.

COUNTERTRANSFERENCE ISSUES

It is not only in psychological theories that faulty assumptions about females are likely to lead to faulty conclusions. Commonly-held views about females may inform the ways in which the very investigations designed to gather objective information are carried out. Even more so are young street girls likely to be the recipients of the prejudices and biases of the people who work with them.

As detailed in a review (Newman et al., 1985) of the four major views of prostitution in the twentieth century, prostitutes may be seen as (1) victims of bad genes; (2) targets for the social reformer's zeal; (3) objects of academic study; or (4) the results of psycho-dynamics gone wrong. In each of these views, the person as an active creator of her own life is relatively ignored.

Young street girls, "bad" girls, who fail to conform to social expectations by living apart from home and school, can be the targets of the prejudices, biases and unexamined motives of those who choose to work with them. These countertransference issues must be confronted and attended to if we are to (1) be of use to the young women themselves and (2) be successful in obtaining valid and worthwhile information about their lives. These are issues not only for the researcher but also for the educator, the clinician and the front-line worker.

Among the most common unexamined reasons for working with distressed young women are (1) because we want to reform or save these "victims"; (2) because we are angry, having been the recipients of some of the prejudices and biases women often experience; (3) because we have a need to work through our own unresolved adolescent conflicts.

In the case of #1, the wish to reform or save "victims," we may, in our zeal, forget that each of the young women is an individual with her own history, her own internalization of this experience, and her own strivings to construct an identity and to make a life. If we think of these individuals as victims we deny them the respect and considerations we would accord to those we consider in control of their lives, and thus we perpetuate the very prejudices and myths we might wish to change. In addition, we might be tempted to implement inappropriate remedies and solutions for their distress. Adolescents who have suffered abuse at the hands of uncaring adults are not likely to respond well to programs offered by judgmental and moralizing adults. Nor are "reform" programs likely to be tailored to the needs of young women whose early experience has left them developmentally scarred: teenagers whose early dependency needs have not been met and who often seek to avoid depression by engaging in frantic and often self-harming behavior require consistent experience with adults who value them and accept them as they are. The development of trust in an accepting adult must come before any attempts at change; an adult who sees in the young distressed street girl a flawed or bad person will not be trusted.

In the case of #2, our own anger at the unfair treatment that women in general and these young women in particular have received, we must be careful to understand how we have responded to this treatment ourselves. If we have experienced discrimination and unfair treatment because of gender-based myths and prejudices, (1) we may have accepted these ideas unconsciously and thus feel badly about ourselves and tend to see women in general as unworthy and deficient; (2) we may have rejected these false ideas completely and thus be blind to their effects on the lives of those we work with; or (3) we may have become so angry that we are motivated to right wrongs, to the exclusion of listening and responding appropriately to individuals and their individual concerns and needs.

In the case of #3, the need to work through our own unresolved adolescent conflicts, we are most subject to problems. As women we have all experienced the adolescent process of rebelling against adult authority, and many of us have, in that rebellion, behaved in ways that may continue to make us feel ashamed or unworthy. It is important not to use the young women we work with as vehicles for the resolution of these feelings, as the objects of our own need either to punish or to reward rebellious behavior.

All of the countertransference issues mentioned above must be confronted and examined before we begin our work with distressed adolescent females, whether we are researchers, clinicians or educators. Unless we understand our own motives and learn to separate them from the experiences and needs of the young women we will not be useful or ethical in our work.

As outlined in Newman and Caplan's paper (1982) the current perspective in the study of young street girls is to view them as active, creative human beings who are striving to construct their lives and identities. Unless we separate our own motives and unresolved conflicts from theirs we will not be able to experience their uniqueness and individuality. And unless we confront our own unresolved conflicts about adolescence and the experience of being women who are often the targets of prejudices and unfair treatment we will not be able to make use of our own feelings to understand the feelings of the very young women we wish to help.

ETHICAL CONSIDERATIONS IN SCIENCE

In scientific research, the traditional view regarding ethics is that work is not ethical if it is not scientific. Thus, if procedures and measures have no scientific validity, i.e., can not be demonstrated to be valid and reliable and appropriate to the subject under investigation, then the research is deemed unethical. The underlying assumption is that what is scientifically rigorous and valid, is likely to be ethical. I would like to propose the opposite. If procedures, methods, measures, and even the very questions themselves are not ethical then the entire investigation is unscientific. If we do not take into account the point of view, needs, concerns and individuality of those we work with then our interactions with them will be distorted by our own often unexamined biases and prejudices. The result of distorted interactions — whether clinical, educational or investigative — can only result in a product that has little value for the participants and the larger community of which we are a part. As women working within women we must be especially aware of the myths, stereotypes and prejudices that operate against women, lest we ourselves unwittingly participate in their perpetuation.

REFERENCES

Baker, C. (1983). A "second look" at interview with adolescents. *Journal of Youth and Adolescence, 12,* 501-519.

Caplan, P. J. (1985). *The myth of women's masochism.* New York, E. P. Dutton.

Erikson, E. H. (1954). On the sense of inner identity. In R. Knight and C. Friedman (Eds.), *Psychoanalytic Psychiatry and Psychology.* New York: International University Press.

Erikson, E. H. (1956). The problem of ego identity. *Journal of the American Psychoanalytic Association, 4,* 56-121.

Erikson, E. H. (1963). *Childhood and society.* New York: W. W. Norton.

Erikson, E. H. (1968). *Identity: Youth and Crisis.* New York: W. W. Norton.

Erikson, E. H. (1974). *Dimensions of a new identity: the 1973 Jefferson lectures in the humanities.* New York: W. W. Norton.

Freud, S. (1953). Three essays on sexuality. In J. Strachey (Ed. and Trans.). *The standard edition of the complete psychological works of Sigmund Freud* (Vol. 7). London: Hogarth Press.

Freud, S. (1961). Female sexuality. In J. Strachey (Ed. and Trans.). *The standard edition of the complete psychological works of Sigmund Freud* (Vol. 21). London: Hogarth Press.

Gilligan, C. (1982). *In a different voice.* Cambridge, MA: Harvard University Press.

Kohlberg, L. (1964). Development of moral character and moral ideology. In M. Hoffman and L. W. Hoffman (Eds.), *Review of Child Development Research.* Vol. I. New York: Russel Sage Foundation.

Loevinger, J. & Wessler, R. (1970). *Measuring ego development,* Vol. I. San Francisco: Jossey-Bass.

Loevinger, J., Wessler, R. & Redmore, C. *Measuring ego development, Vol. II. Scoring manual.* San Francisco: Jossey-Bass.

Marcia, J. E. (1966). Development and validation of ego-identity status. *Journal of Personality and Social Psychology, 3,* 551-558.

Newman, F. & Caplan, P. (1982). Juvenile female prostitution as gender consistent response to early deprivation. *International Journal of Women's Studies, 5,* 128-137.

Newman, F., Cohen, E., Toban, P. & MacPherson, G. (1985). Historical perspectives on the study of female prostitution. *International Journal of Women's Studies, 8,* 80-86.

Sarbin, T. & Mancuso, J. (1980). *Schizophrenia: Medical diagnosis or moral verdict?* New York: Pergamon Press.

Sigel, I. (1981). Social experience in the development of thought: Distancing theory. In: I. Sigel, D. Brodzinsky & R. Golinkoff (Eds.). *New directions in Piagetian theory and practice*. Hillsdale: Lawrence Erlbaum Assoc. Publishers.

Wagner, J. (1976). A study of the relationship between formal operations and ego identity in adolescence. Unpublished doctoral dissertation, State University of New York at Buffalo.

Black Women and the Politics
of Skin Color and Hair

Margo Okazawa-Rey
Tracy Robinson
Janie Victoria Ward

Since 1853, when William Wells Brown, the first published black novelist was published, black women have been depicted as white, if not whiter than her caucasian counterpart; beautiful black women had long, flowing hair cascading down their backs, clear, light eyes, and finely-cut, well-molded features. This image of black female beauty appeared repeatedly in novels such as *Clotel* (Brown, 1969), *Iola Leroy* (Harper, 1971), and *The Chinaberry Tree* (Fauset, 1969). Over the decades, color-specific portraits of black women continued in literature, in the theater, and in films. Later novelists explored the fate of the woman who did not meet this standard of beauty. In Wallace Thurman's *The Blacker the Berry* (1970), the protagonist learned the horror that her dark color evoked. As the story ends, we learn that the tragically dark-skinned girl could never overcome the lessons learned in childhood: envy those lighter and despise those darker than herself. In "If You're Light and Have Long Hair," Gwendolyn Brooks (1974) wove a story of a black man who, neurotically attracted to a light-skinned woman, abandoned a darker woman for what he considered a more desirable catch.

Nowhere were the differences in life experiences of dark-skinned and light-skinned black women illuminated more clearly than in

Margo Okazawa-Rey is an assistant professor of social work at the University of Alaska in Fairbanks. Tracy Robinson is a doctoral candidate at the Harvard Graduate School of Education. Janie Victoria Ward is a developmental psychologist working in the Boston area.

This article appears in slightly different form in the *Women's Studies Quarterly* 1986: 1 & 2 Special Issue—"Teaching Women, Race, and Culture," published by The Feminist Press at the City University of New York.

Toni Morrison's novel, *The Bluest Eye* (1970). Maureen Peal, the pretty, "high-yellow dream child," was elevated above everyone else because of her light skin, light eyes, and long brown hair. Little Maureen was always treated favorably, and had a qualitatively different experience as a black child due to the advantages bestowed upon her.

> She enchanted the whole school. When teachers called on her, they smiled encouragingly. Black boys didn't trip her in the halls; white boys didn't stone her, white girls didn't suck their teeth when she was assigned to be their work partners; black girls stepped aside when she wanted to use the sink in the girls' toilet, and their eyes genuflected under sliding lids. (p. 53)

Zora Neale Hurston interjected the painful truth into the prevailing depictions of black womanhood in an insightful piece entitled "My People, My People" (Hurston, 1984).

> If it was so honorable and glorious to be black, why was it the yellow-skinned people among us who have so much prestige? Even a child in the first grade could see that this was so from what happened in the classroom and on school programs. The light skinned children were always the angels, fairies and queens of school plays. The lighter the girl, the more money and prestige she was apt, and expected, to marry. Was it really honorable to be black?

Literature, of course, reflects life, and within the lives of black women, stereotypic attributions and pre-judgments based on skin color have led to a variety of intra-group rivalries. Often it is within the family, where a variety of skin colors may be represented among individual members, that black children first learn the values attributed to differences in skin color. When the child enters the larger social world, she carries these color-conscious attitudes beyond the confines of the home, and, in turn, those attitudes are reinforced by that world. Many black women can recall from childhood verbal and physical attacks provoked by color envy or dislike. The school experiences of many black women confirm the painful differences of black female socialization depicted in Toni Morrison's novel. For example, darker girls remember beating up the resented lighter-skinned girls, and conversely, lighter-skinned girls recall how they spitefully excluded their darker classmates from various social activities.

As members of this American society, a woman's self-concept develops, in part, from observing and internalizing what others think about her. Consequently, the attributes society assigns to the "attractive" and "unattractive" black female have profound implications for her psychosocial development.

While many light-skinned black women have been psychologically comfortable with their color, some have not. Too often in the Black community, lighter-skinned women have been considered more desirable. Subsequently, the lighter-skinned woman has felt misunderstood by darker blacks who have failed to understand the pain and conflict associated with what is a biological occurrence. Understand the dilemma of the light-skinned girl who during childhood was told repeatedly that, because of her color, she is among the prettier and the best. Is it any surprise then that in adolescence she may find herself wondering whether the boys, in choosing her, can see beyond her physical characteristics and view her as more than just a pretty face.

If we carry this argument further, and consider the pathological effects of racism which has affected some black men (their attraction to light skin), it is not outrageous to imagine a scenario in which a light-skinned black woman finds herself chosen by a man who, she later discovers, is acting out some subconscious desire to possess the unobtainable white woman. In such an instance, the black woman may feel she is being settled for as the next best thing to a white woman.

On the other hand, if a dark-skinned young girl is constantly told that she is ugly, and experiences treatment that supports these views, she may begin to feel as such. This is particularly true when the treatment she receives within her community of origin, the black community, is consistent with the negative and self-deprecating messages doled out by the larger society. Throughout her development she hears both implicit and explicit messages stating that due to her color she is considered undesirable. For a dark-skinned black girl who is aware of these negative pronouncements against her physical appearance, there can be a driving motivation to compensate for her devaluation either through education or some other activity in which she may excel and redeem her sense of worth. In these two extreme but frequent cases, it is easy to see how one's self-esteem can be undercut by a societal definition of woman's worth that subordinates all of her other qualities to a fundamentally immutable characteristic such as skin color.

Although our illustrations focus upon childhood and adolescent experiences, similar assumptions and judgments based on skin color repeat themselves across the life span of black women. For example, relationships between black men and women are often tinged with the issue of skin color preference. Color often enters into the choices black people make of whom to date and whom to marry. In the presence of a newborn, one can still hear passed down folklore which predicts the baby's future skin color and hair texture. Though oblivious to these concerns, the young black infant must learn to function in a society in which the shade of one's skin functions as a status determining characteristic.

HISTORICAL OVERVIEW

Color-consciousness is rooted in the social, political, and economic conditions that existed during the centuries of slavery in the U.S. As a result, skin color has held a unique significance in the Black community. In the American south, Blacks were subjected to enforced segregation, while white men were allowed to victimize enslaved and defenseless black women. The biracial offsprings were called "mulattoes": light-skinned, straight-haired children born of interracial parentage. Social advantages were often granted to these children by their fathers who offered them a better quality of life than that available to other blacks. Concrete benefits were gained, such as release from field work, better housing, education (formal or informal), clothing and, even on some occasions, emancipation, despite the mother's continued enslavement. In this way, the free Negro population was enlarged in the years prior to the Civil war.

Although liberated before the masses of other black slaves, many mulattoes lived a marginal existence, and although they were not recognized as equals by whites, they often chose to disassociate themselves from other blacks. Fleeing persecution and discrimination in the South, the mulattoes came North, bringing lighter skin color and its elitist affectations with them. Many held disdain towards their darker brothers and sisters, preferring instead the supposed gentility and culture of the white race. Following The Emancipation, the mulattoes quickly discovered that their lighter color functioned as a valuable social resource. Successful social and economic integration of blacks into the closed white society was afforded to a scant and select few. Education was a primary vehicle for entrance, and, due to the preferential treatment afforded light-skinned blacks in the mission schools and black colleges established after the Civil War, skin color served as a foundation for the emerging black middle class. Sociologist E. Franklin Frazier (1957) explained how even within black educational institutions, many lighter blacks had been socialized to differentiate themselves from the black masses by conforming to white puritanical standards and avoiding the ungrammatical speech and dialect of the sons and daughters of slaves. On the other hand, history also informs us of several incidents where cleverly skillful light-skinned black men and women posed as white in order to gain admission to segregated white colleges and universities, and later upon completion of their degrees, reclaimed their racial identity. In many urban areas, other major social institutions such as the black church also divided along color and class lines: middle-class, usually lighter-skinned congregations sought to dissociate themselves from the overt religiosity of the common black people.

Color-consciousness in the black community was supported by the larger society, where racism entrenched in America's institutions, upheld notions of white superiority. Many white psychologists believed that the more white blood found within a person, the better (morally, physically and mentally) that person was. Beginning as early as 1912, psychological studies (usually utilizing IQ tests) were undertaken attempting to prove opposing hypotheses about mulattoes: that persons of racially mixed ancestry were inferior to those of pure (unmixed) backgrounds: or, that racially mixed persons were superior to pure backgrounds (Guthrie, 1976). Whether the field of psychology paved the way for racism to flourish, or whether psychologists were merely reflecting the attitudes and perceptions of the day is an intriguing topic for debate. Whatever the case, clearly the larger American institutions supported and endorsed this value of "whiteness as rightness" and in its wake, the black community fell victim to its twisted perception of social status and human worth.

World War II initiated a period of increased social and physical mobility for the black masses and inaugurated a new stage in the evolution of the Negro middle class. Family background and color snobbishness were slowly being supplanted by education and occupation as the essential ingredients for social class membership. Darker skinned blacks were found to be making increased progress up the social class ladder. However, attitudes were hard to change. For example, many black people, particularly women, (since they were the ones most often affected), can still recollect the proliferation of numerous fraternities and sororities in which the correct skin hue and hair texture were essential. Widely acknowledged were the exclusivity of certain "blue vein" social clubs, in which membership required a skin color light enough for ones blood veins to be seen; or, similarly other associations which instituted a hair comb test, where the more easily a comb could flow through the hair, the higher one's chances of gaining club admission.

Recently, a study of eminent blacks determined that the inheritance of light skin color (generally from the mother, who is twice as likely to have been lighter skinned than the father), as well as the mother's education, occupational attainment, and income, served to increase a family's social position over time (Mullins & Sites, 1984). It is little wonder then that so many black people, particularly black men, are still actively choosing to marry the lighter members of their own race, since this has been proven to be a means of assuring one's family heightened social status and economic success.

BEAUTY AND SOCIAL ATTITUDES

Society responds differently to persons who, by some culturally sanctioned standard, are considered more attractive, or better looking than others. This social response has certain effects on an individual's self-esteem and socialization, since humans are shaped by how others in this society respond or do not respond to them.

Research documents the influence that physical attractiveness has or is thought to have on behavior: children perceived as physically attractive are expected to achieve more than unattractive children and are also thought to be less likely to commit certain transgressions (Clifford & Walster, 1973); attractive adults are thought to have happier marriages than persons who are unattractive (Dion et al., 1972); opinions of attractive adults are more likely to be agreed with (Horai et al., 1974); and in disagreement, attractive adults are more likely to prevail over unattractive adults (Dion & Stein, 1978). In short, what is considered physically attractive is, by definition, good.

Thus, when examined in this context, it is not surprising that many women often behave as though beauty is something to be acquired by any means imaginable and at any cost necessary. The means include those sold over-the-counter, such as substances for coloring, permanenting, and straightening hair; dietary aids for losing and gaining weight; and pads for giving the appearance of fullness. Surgical methods for improvement are also considered fair play. Billions of dollars are being spent annually on products and services. Relentlessly pursued by "invisible insecurities," women spend countless hours precariously struggling to sustain their self-esteem (Brownmiller, 1984).

Although the majority of the research on physical attractiveness has been concerned with white subjects in the population, researchers have found that blacks were as likely as whites to attach certain values and favorable qualities to individuals based upon their outward appearance. Recently, Cash and Duncan (1984) conducted research on perceptions of physical attractiveness with black undergraduates. The findings indicated that the physically attractive were attributed more desirable personality traits than those considered unattractive. Attractive subjects were seen as more positive, more likeable, and more likely to have greater financial success. Moreover, attractive persons were often associated with higher levels of vanity and egotism, and they were considered less sympathetic to the oppressed, and more bourgeois in their attitudes.

Social scientists have bemoaned the preponderance of self-hatred believed to exist in the black community. The Clark doll-preference technique (Clark & Clark, 1952) has been frequently used to assess this purported phenomenon. The method consists of presenting a pair of dolls, one brown and one white, to preschoolers while asking questions about racial terms and attitudes. The Clarks concluded that black preschoolers suffered from negative racial identity since they seemed to be aware of and could use racial labels, yet preferred the white dolls as prettier and more desireable. Several decades of research supported the Clark Hypothesis; however, recently more careful studies by Porter (1971) and others, have questioned whether preference for a white doll necessarily meant rejection of the brown doll.

Psychiatrists have diagnosed and interpreted the black woman's problem with beauty and self-image. In their book, *Black Rage,* Grier and Cobbs (1968) expended great energy creating a context for and a full description of the black females' self-hatred. Various illustrations of her hair-straightening and skin-lightening efforts, which, despite the pain, achieve little degree of true success, exemplify the black female's never-ending struggle to approximate the white ideal of beauty. Grier and Cobbs contend that black women are the antithesis of American beauty. Femininity is out of reach for the black female, and, since her reference point is the enviously revered white woman, the despised and debased darker sister is relegated to the social role of ugly duckling. The psychiatrists concluded that, "there can be no doubt that she will develop a damaged self-concept and an impairment of her feminine narcissism which will have profound consequences for her character development" (p. 41).

Sociologist Calvin Herndon (1965) stated that intra-racial color discrimination among black women leads to sexual jealousy, with darker women resenting those lighter than they. The light-skinned Black women, he claimed, secretly take pride their skin color since it increases their chances for marriage and thus secures entrance into the middle classes. In fact, Herndon went so far as to posit that lighter skinned black women secretly abhor the idea of open integration and interracial marriage since either could force her to cease "playing white to prove herself as a desirable female" (p. 149).

Despite these conjectures, aside from the Clark doll studies, few studies exist assessing the relationship between the black woman's conception of beauty and her psychological development. Clearly, as members of this culture, blacks are affected by the dominant culture's values and meanings assigned to the illusive labels of beauty. Black women, as other women, have regularly used cosmetics mainly to improve their appearance.

Madame C. J. Walker, the first black female millionaire, amassed her fortune by inventing and marketing hair, scalp, and skin aids. While many have construed her efforts as having fed into the black woman's desire to approximate white standards of beauty, Walker herself denied such accusations, claiming instead that her goal was to enhance the overall physical appearance and health of black women (Giddings, 1984). Yet unsettling questions concerning the motivations behind the use of certain beauty aids continue to nag the black female community even seventy years since Madame Walker's success. Are these products utilized by women who possess a desire to approximate whiteness or who hold instead a more general female desire to "look one's best"? For example, a persistent practice that is yet to be clearly understood is the use of skin bleaching creme. Is it that black women use these cremes to "whiten" their skin or is it to smooth out the uneven skintone in normal black skin pigmentation? Or similarly, why do black women continue, despite the expense, inconvenience and discomfort, to straighten or perm their hair? Is it to stay stylish, or to look white?

RACISM AND SEXISM

While on the surface some of the suggestions of black female self-contempt may appear plausible, we contend that such conclusions are dangerously incomplete. In the pages below, we give attention to the effects of the *intersection of race and gender* to provide a more illuminating and comprehensive view of the psychological development of the black woman.

Earlier we stated that attractiveness affords certain tangible benefits to both men and women. Within the general category of "attractiveness" there exists a finer distinction, something called "beauty," that is generally based on a particular combination of hair, skin color, facial features, body size and shape. While appearance is important to all, personal beauty is frequently considered the most important virtue that a woman can possess (Lakoff & Scherr, 1984). It is, along with occupation and education, a status characteristic, affecting both behavior and cognition. In this culture, the advantages afforded to "the beautiful ones" have a qualitative component and involve varying types of subordination and superordination. Furthermore, personal beauty holds for women the same amount of importance as do the virtues of intelligence, political influence, or physical strength for men. However, unlike the male virtues that almost assure the holder real power in society, the power often associated with beauty is illusionary. Explain Lakoff and Scherr, " . . . women do not have power through beauty: beauty is power" (p. 279).

Undoubtedly, in this society, a woman's attractiveness "buys her more" than it does a man, since a woman's attractiveness is perceived to be associated with her ability to secure male companionship. However, it must be remembered that in a patriarchal society it is the man who chooses the woman, and not vice versa. In light of this inequity in social power, it is no wonder that a woman will do all she can to enhance her beauty, since her beauty is seen as one of the few ways in which she can gain social success.

The efforts undertaken to alter the asymmetric power relationship between men and women were due, in large part, to a new consciousness that emerged from the social struggles of the 1960s. Throughout the decades of the civil rights movements, a belief in the possibility of affecting substantive changes in power structures afforded many subordinated people the opportunity to change their ways of seeing themselves and their world.

Many assume the 1960s to have been a period in which black people transcended the pathology of colorism and stood back and analyzed its effect upon them. Clothing changed, and many black people wore Afro styles in an effort to actively define their newly politicized racial identity. Despite the inclusionary rhetoric of "black is beautiful," too often underneath this rhetoric, remained the old favoritism towards lighter-skinned women. Sexism, along with colorism, ran rampant and, as before; it was the lighter black woman who was, in a familiar way, favored. During the macho-revolutionary fervor of the sixties, to many black men, lighter sisters were still seen as the most desirable, most worthy, and most feminine, and thus, the most in need of (male) protection.

By the mid-1970s, the economy declined and inflation increased followed by a shift in attitude and an abandonment of the rhetoric of self-determination. The rising threat of unemployment within black communities led many to turn their attention towards securing for themselves and their families a piece of the dwindling economic pie. Daishikis and Afros were gradually replaced by tailored suits and hair permanents, as the idealistic goals of social change were substituted for more personal and individualistic concerns such as achieving economic and social success as defined by the dominant culture.

In addition to the pressures of economic survival, there were other reasons why the evolving process of self-determination was not carried into the 1980s. Some blacks simply could not deal with thinking about the upheaval that would result from the types of fundamental political and social changes proposed because the implications seemed so overwhelming. It had become too painful to analyze ourselves and the motivations behind our interactions critically. Those of us who were brave enough to do so came to understand how color consciousness has divided us, and how we, by perpetuating it, had contributed to our own oppression. If we had been able to sustain our critical position long enough to see what we had done to one another, then maybe we could have meaningfully altered our relationships. After all, is it not true that when we, as black women within a racist and color-conscious society, despise and degrade our darker sisters, we are doing little more than identifying with racist whites, the true oppressors? And when we as black women turn against our lighter black sisters, it is any more than acting out the frustration and envy we subconsciously hold towards a racist and sexist society that assigns status and power to one's race and gender? By hating our skin colors, we are buying into the notion that beauty and femininity are a black woman's most important virtue, and we are therefore relinquishing the power to define ourselves.

Black women of the 1980s are distinct in their variety of colors and choices of hairstyles. Sisters wear straightened hair, curly perms, and/or natural Afro styles. While the politically charged Afro has declined in popularity over the years, can this be said to reflect a regressive shift, a shift back to the era of imitating white standards of haircare and beauty? This question has no easy answer for the selections women make in their cosmetic options are obviously individualized. In general, we believe there are at least three major reasons why a black woman would choose certain hairstyles or cosmetics today. First, to enhance her beauty; second, to help her approximate the image that she believes might increase her chances for entrance and advancements in the institutions of the dominant society; or, third, to abdicate her racial identity and to look, as perhaps she may desire to be, white.

We believe the last reason to be far less frequent than is often asserted although analyses in the past have tended to focus on this third aspect of cosmetic usage — the wish to be white — when discussing black women and their attitudes regarding their hair and skin color. The psychological and sociological self-contempt hypotheses fail to acknowledge the larger sociopolitical sphere in which the black woman must do battle. Where else do the powerful influences of racism and sexism converge as they do in the lives of black women? Given both her color and her sex, she is presumed to have been twice victimized. For a black woman, the double jeopardy of race and gender complicates the problems of identity and choice because she must respond to the desires and expectations of black men and to white cultural values and norms. The messages given about what is attractive, acceptable, and necessary are often contradictory.

The double jeopardy of race and gender demands that black women negotiate these forces. Just as our black foremothers skillfully manipulated the social and political systems to their advantage, Black women today are finding it necessary and appropriate to do the same. Many have abandoned the Afro which is still often associated with Black militancy; and those employed in white businesses and institutions are straightening their hair to adopt a look acceptable to those who have power over them, and often over their family's economic survival. The politically astute Black woman recognizes the effect her presence has upon her white co-workers, and she makes the appropriate adjustments to fit the political climate. She does not necessarily buy fully into a white value system.

Undoubtedly, the legacy of being twice victimized by race and gender leaves in its wake a sense of self-hatred and racial resentment in some black women. However, we contend that the marginal position of black women in this society offers them the opportunity to repudiate the negative stereotypes, demands, and expectations imposed upon them by both white people and black men. Rising above externally sanctioned characterizations of womanhood, some black women are fashioning their identities based upon an analysis and understanding of their own struggles and successes. Further, Black women have united to support one another's efforts in the creation of newly defined roles and identities. Within this dynamic of self-determination, the black woman is proactive rather than reactive, aggressive rather than passive, and assertive rather than receptive.

The oppression of Black Americans originated with enslavement and was followed by centuries of their being denied access to advancement within the American socio-economic system. Having light skin and straight hair—looking closest to white—increased one's chances for economic and social success. Thus, the glorification of white standards of beauty grew out of a basic awareness of the few available means by which black people were able to improve their lot in life. As this nation grew, relationships between the races became increasingly strained: white supremacist ideology permeated nearly all social institutions to justify and to sanction the unequal social order that was being created.

The newly developing fields of behavioral science were shaped by racist ideologies as well. Inappropriate paradigms, such as the various deficiency models, were used to explain the behaviors and motivations of black people. Even today, many existing psychological and social theories have yet to rise above the self-contempt hypotheses which describe black women. These inaccurate conceptions of black female life need to be replaced by new and appropriate theories that can capture the unique dynamics of being both black and female. Literature, to some degree, has done justice in its depiction of these dynamics, illuminating critical themes and allowing readers to see the power of colorism in its fullness. Fortunately, many contemporary black female writers have succeeded in helping to tease out this complex issue, and, through their work, black women can share experiences.

Simplistic arguments and conclusions concerning the meaning of skin color and hair in the lives of black women fail to ascertain the reasons, motives, and intent behind most of the cosmetic practices women engage in. Furthermore, such conclusions serve more often to establish right or wrong judgments rather than to clarify the complexities of skin color and hair. Since the impulses behind these choices are complex, thus not easily identifiable, it is our contention that today's black women must gain an awareness of the roles racism and sexism have played in shaping their attitudes about skin color and hair.

Since black women have little political or economic power, survival needs often force us to make tradeoffs — to straighten our hair for that promotion which we believe will increase our family's income. Yet, at the same time, we must not allow our identities to be compromised.

In the post-60s decades, we have come to realize that nothing short of structural change will permanently alter our social relations in this society. As long as the traditional power-holders continue to define us and also to determine the definitions we take on, we cannot bring about real changes. We must first create powerful and positive identities for ourselves. We must gain a genuine sense of appreciation and love of our diversity, in all of our colors. Since colorism is a by-product of the effects of racism and sexism which underlie our social foundation, we as black women must continue to engage in activities aimed at social reconstruction. We as black women must become agents for social change.

REFERENCES

Brooks, G. (1975). If you're light and have long hair. M. H. Washington (Ed.), *Black Eyed Susans*. New York: Anchor Books.

Brown, W. W. (1970). *Clotel*. New York: Collier Books.

Brownmiller, S. (1984). *Femininity*. New York: Simon & Schuster.

Cash, T. S. & Duncan, N. C. (1984). Physical attractiveness stereotyping among black American college students. *Journal of Social Psychology, 1*, 71-77.

Clark, K. D. & Clark, M. P. (1952). Racial identification and preferences in Negro children, In G. E. Swanson, T. M. Newcomb, and E. L. Hartley (Eds.), *Readings in Social Psychology: The Revised Edition*. New York: Holt, Rinehard & Winston.

Clifford, M. & Walster, E. (1973). The effects of physical attractiveness on teacher expectations. *Sociology of Education, 14*, 97-108.

Dion, K., Berschid, E. & Walster, E. (1972). What is beautiful is good. *Journal of Personality and Social Psychology, 24*, 285-290.

Dion, K. & Stein, S. (1978). Physical attractiveness and interpersonal influent. *Journal of Experimental Social Psychology, 14*, 97-108.

Fauset, J. R. (1969). *The Chinaberry Tree*. New York: AMS Press Reprint.

Frazier, E. F. (1957). *Black Bourgeoisis*. New York: Collier Macmillan.

Giddings, P. (1984). *When and Where I Enter: The Impact of Black Women on Race and Sex in America*. New York: William Morrow.

Grier, W. & Cobbs, P. (1968). *Black Rage*. New York: Basic Books.

Guthrie, R. V. (1976). *Even the Rat was White: A Historical View of Psychology*. New York: Harper and Row.

Harper, F. (1971). *Iola Leroy*. New York: AMS Press.

Herndon, C. (1965). *Sex and Racism in America*. New York: Grove Press.

Horai, J., Naccari, N. & Fatoullan, E. (1974). The effects of expertise and physical attractiveness upon opinion agreement and liking. *Sociometry, 37*, 601-606.

Hurston, Z. N. (1984). My people, my people. *Dust Tracks on the Road*. Champagne, IL: University of Illinois, 215-237.

Lakoff, R. T. & Scherr, R. L. (1984). *Face Value: Politics of Beauty*. Boston: Routledge, Kegan, & Paul.

Morrison, T. (1970). *The Bluest Eye*. New York: Washington Square.

Mullins, E. & Sites, P. (1984). Feminist black Americans: A three generational analysis of social origins. *American Sociological Review, 49*(5), 672, October.

Porter, J. (1971). *Black Child, White Child: The Development of Racial Attitudes*. Cambridge: Harvard.

Thurman, W. (1970). *The Blacker the Berry*. New York: Collier Books.

Cognitive/Behavior Therapy for Agoraphobic Women: Toward Utilizing Psychodynamic Understanding to Address Family Belief Systems and Enhance Behavior Change

Iris Goldstein Fodor

During the past ten years with the advent of behavior therapy and the documented success of exposure treatment for alleviating the major symptoms of agoraphobics, there has been an increase in the research, theoretical, and clinical literature on agoraphobia (Beck & Emery, 1985; Chambless & Goldstein, 1982; Thorpe & Burns, 1983). While agoraphobia has been characterized as a high prevalence disorder for women and linked to a stereotypic female socialization experience (Brehony, 1983; Fodor, 1974), the treatment of choice has been some variant of behavior therapy and/or cognitive behavior therapy, which generally does not put women's issues in the foreground (Thorpe & Burns, 1983). In fact, anxiety disorders clinics and behaviorally oriented self help programs for agoraphobics, mostly female, have proliferated in recent years.

In spite of the popular claims of success, such programs may not be as helpful as promised. Recently, Emmelkamp and van der Hout (1983), among others, have called attention to failure rates following behavioral treatment, citing reports of high dropout rates, resistance to, and dissatisfaction with behavioral treatment.

In this paper, the author will take a close look at relevant aspects of the agoraphobic syndrome and cognitive/behavioral treatment

---

The author is a psychologist at New York University and in private practice.

program. She will also address familial and psychodynamic etiology, that are often ignored in the behavioral approach. The author will argue for an expanded cognitive/behavioral treatment for agoraphobics that takes into account psychodynamic variables, and presents a view of treatment as remediation of familial patterns. Given the importance of the therapist in teaching the female agoraphobic client new ways of behaving, additional attention needs to be directed to feminist issues and therapist/client process as an additional ingredient in fostering change.

THE AGORAPHOBIC SYNDROME

Woman age 41. . . . The patient was chronically anxious and feared death or sudden illness if she went out in the street, on trains, in cars, or to the theatre or church. She had reached the point at which she could not perform any of her duties and was helpless. Her husband had to remain home with her, and even then she continued to be frightened. (Terhune, 1949)

Terhune's characterization is still typical for today's agoraphobic. Most agoraphobics are female (75-85%) and the problem often begins soon after marriage or motherhood. Agoraphobics represent half of the phobic population and about 5% of a clinic population (more recent survey work would suggest that agoraphobia may affect many more women in the community) (Chambless & Goldstein, 1982; Thorpe & Burns, 1983).

The main features of agoraphobia according to the DSM III of the American Psychiatric Association (1980) are:

A marked fear of being in public places from which escape might be difficult or help not available in case of sudden incapacitation. Normal activities are increasingly restricted as the fears or avoidance behaviors dominate the individual's life . . . . (Examples of feared situations include busy streets, tunnels, crowded stores, elevators, or public transportation . . . Often these individuals insist that a family member or friend accompany them when they leave home. May or may not be accompanied by an anxiety attack. (p. 226)

Goldstein and Chambless (1978) have outlined the main features of the agoraphobic syndrome.

1. "Fear of fear" is central. Agoraphobics are afraid of becoming anxious or panicking. They are fearful when they are anxious about the physical symptoms emerging in a manner which is out of control.
2. Agoraphobics engage in avoidance behaviors. What they fear most are not the feared objects themselves (closed spaces, tunnels, etc.); they fear the feeling of being trapped in these situations. They fear most becoming hysterical and manifesting the physical symptoms (dizziness, hyperventilation, nausea) with no help or escape available. Avoidance helps them to maintain control.
3. Agoraphobics also suffer a lack in the development of self sufficiency. They usually rely on a significant other to be with them most of the time. They exhibit what Bowlby (1973) calls "anxious attachment," or anxiety about not being adequately taken care of or the possibility of being totally left alone, completely helpless.

   Another aspect of the lack of self sufficiency is the lack of skills to control themselves when they panic or try to negotiate the world as adults (Fodor, 1974; Goldstein & Chambless, 1978; Marks, 1978). Additionally, Foa and Chambless (1978) talk about their inability to solve problems when stressed.
4. Goldstein and Chambless (1978) describe the misattribution of emotions in agoraphobia. Agoraphobics exhibit a hysterical style of perception. They show a tendency to overgeneralize and to label most arousal as anxiety or panic. Research by Foa and Chambless (1978) suggests a real fear of arousal. The message is that anxiety is dangerous. Furthermore, agoraphobics show poor discrimination of other feelings (particularly anger). They are also reported to have widespread lack of assertiveness. They cannot express angry feelings or take risks in interpersonal confrontation because such expression elicits anxiety, and anxiety must be avoided at all costs.
5. Control is a central issue for agoraphobics. They fear loss of control during anxiety attacks and try to maintain control over themselves by controlling their significant other to be with them. Self esteem is linked to control. It is high when they feel in control and low when they feel out of control.

COGNITIVE/BEHAVIORAL TREATMENT
OF AGORAPHOBIA

Cognitive/Behavioral Treatment is built on the theoretical framework of social learning theory which stresses the interactions of behavioral, cognitive, and environmental factors. According to Bandura (1977):

> It is partially through their own actions that people produce the environmental conditions that can affect their behavior in a reciprocal fashion. The experiences generated by behavior also partly determine what individuals think, expect, and can do, which in turn affect their subsequent behavior. (p. 345)

Wilson (1984) in a recent review summarizes the cognitive/ behavioral approach as follows:

1. Most so-called problematic behaviors are learned in the same manner as all other behaviors; hence, therapy can be construed as the same kind of re-learning process involved in unlearning other kinds of behaviors.
2. There is an emphasis on the use of behavioral assessment to study the patterns of current problematic behaviors.
3. Treatments are individually designed. Each subproblem often calls for a specific treatment.
4. The therapist is viewed as a consultant/teacher/trainer who is there to help clients learn as much about themselves as possible in order to alter their maladaptive behavior patterns.
5. The behavior therapy component emphasizes corrective learning experiences in which clients acquire new coping skills and competencies in order to learn how to break maladaptive habits.
6. The cognitive component views emotional problems and maladaptive behaviors as a result of unproductive irrational thought patterns or dysfunctional thinking. Cognitive restructuring enables the patient to think differently about her problematic situations by identifying and analyzing these dysfunctional thought patterns and then attacking them by a form of socratic dialogue (Beck & Emery, 1985; Ellis & Harper, 1975).

7. Finally, there is an emphasis on pre-treatment assessment and posttreatment followup.

Much of the initial appeal of Cognitive/Behavioral Therapy in addressing women's issues in the mid-70s was based on the assumption that while learning took place within a social context, it was possible for women to transcend the constraints of their prior socialization experience and to become the agents of their own change. Hence, women could learn how to work on taking charge of themselves and thus be better able to realize their personal growth (Wolfe & Fodor, 1975). Agoraphobics were characterized as being reared as "stereotypically female" and behavior therapy was conceived as a model therapy for remediation of the avoidant, dependent behaviors, by teaching more independent coping strategies (Brehony, 1983; Fodor, 1974; Fodor & Rothblum, 1985; Padawer & Goldfried, 1984).

Chambless and Goldstein (1980), two major behavioral researchers and clinicians, have outlined a comprehensive cognitive/behavior treatment package for agoraphobia that fits the coping skills model for training and is also congruent with feminist treatment goals as outlined above. Most cognitive/behavioral programs for agoraphobia contain features of the Chambless and Goldstein treatment package, although they may emphasize one aspect of the program over another (e.g., flooding over a more cognitive component) (Beck & Emery, 1985; Chambless & Goldstein, 1980; Emmelkamp & van der Hout, 1983; Goldstein & Chambless, 1978; Thorpe & Burns, 1983).

The following are the components in a cognitive/behavioral treatment package for agoraphobia:

1. *Self assessment*. The client is taught a variety of assessment techniques, so she can begin to understand the pattern of her fears and avoidant behaviors.
2. *Treatment for fear of fear, anxiety, or panic attacks*. The client is taught anxiety management, that is, specific techniques for relaxation and breathing. The emphasis is on showing the client that she can learn about her patterns of anxiety attacks and how to handle herself when anxious. Sometimes anti-anxiety drugs are used as an adjunct to therapy to lower levels of anxiety.

3. *Treatment of avoidance behaviors.* Most of the training involves exposure to feared situations. The client is taught to confront rather than avoid. She works out a program of assignments to go out in the world. She is taught how to rely on herself as well as shown problem solving skills. This work could be carried out in a group.
4. *Assertiveness training.* The client is instructed in assertiveness techniques, and with graduated practice she is encouraged to be more assertive, particularly with significant others.
5. *Cognitive restructuring.* The client is taught to get in touch with her irrational or unproductive thinking about her anxiety and phobias (e.g., "I can't handle myself when anxious, I will never be able to get on a bus," etc.) and taught to either combat or substitute more productive thinking (e.g., "I can learn how to cope with anxiety," "with enough training I can learn to get on a bus," etc.) (Beck & Emery, 1985; Ellis & Harper, 1975).

TREATMENT OUTCOME

For the most part, behavior therapists have been very successful in designing short term treatments that feature exposure to the feared stimuli. Sixty to seventy percent of the cases are reported to be improved in most studies (Chambless & Goldstein, 1982; Emmelkamp & van der Hout, 1983; Marks, 1978).

However, as behavior therapists tackle more complex cases, problems arise. Agoraphobics have been reported to be very difficult to treat by therapists of different theoretical orientations (Emmelkamp & van der Hout, 1983). While psychoanalysts have a long history of difficulty in successfully treating agoraphobics, behavior therapists are beginning to report numerous treatment problems with agoraphobics (Fodor, 1974). For example, Barlow and Wolfe (1981) report a median dropout rate in their research program of 22% (range 10 to 40%). While behavioral treatment outcomes are reported to be successful in 50 to 70% of the cases, on close followup few clients are totally symptom free. Marks (1978) reports that only 40 to 60% are totally symptom free. Furthermore, agoraphobics are reported to have a high relapse rate.

RESISTANCE TO BEHAVIOR THERAPY

Recent developments in cognitive behavior therapy theory suggest that we need to look more closely at our failures and the complexity of people's issues. Recent work suggests a need to address patterns and underlying cognitive structures that operate out of awareness and are resistant to the piecemeal approach of current behavioral practice (Arnkoff & Glass, 1982; Fodor, in press). Foa and Kozak (1986), in an in-depth look at emotional processing of fear, propose that

> regardless of the type of therapeutic intervention two conditions are required for their reduction of fear. First, the fear relevant information must be made available in a manner that will activate the fear memory. Indeed, if the fear structure remains in storage but unaccessed, it will not be available for modification. Next, information made available must include elements that are incompatible with some of those that exist in the fear structure, so that a new memory can be formed. This new information which is at once cognitive and affective, has to be integrated into the evoked information structure for an emotional change to occur.

It seems likely that clients who drop out of or resist behavioral treatment may view their therapy or therapist in a negative manner and hence may not be open to learn new behaviors.

Emmelkamp and van der Hout (1983) interviewed patients who experienced difficulty following behavior therapy and cite the following comments by clients:

> When you feel terrible at the end of the exposure sessions, it is nonsense that the therapists are enthusiastic about your achievements.

> Treatment was a torment, anxiety did not reduce when I had to walk the street . . . having to walk on the streets was terrible . . . that was the most awful experience . . . it lasted much too long.

> People who suffer phobias always feel lonely . . . no one understands their feelings.

In studying the relationship between perceived therapist characteristics and outcomes of exposure therapies, Emmelkamp and van der Hout (1983) report that an empathic relationship was central.

In trying to understand the resistance of so many agoraphobic clients, mostly female, to the new learning in behavior therapy which emphasizes independence, going out in the world and mastery, we may need to take a closer look at what happens in therapy and how it may run counter to the familial learning experience. It may well be that the familial learning patterns are too well entrenched or are not adequately dealt with by the Cognitive Behavioral Therapy treatments. Further, following Emmelkamp and van der Hout's (1983) observation that behavior therapy is often very difficult for the clients, a much closer examination of the psychotherapy process seems warranted. What is really happening when a cognitive/behavioral therapist attempts to teach a phobic avoidant woman new modes of behavior that run counter to familial learning? What mechanisms does the client use to avoid the new learning?

Furthermore, we cannot assume that the past learning is still not current. We may need to assess how many of the same family patterns that may have contributed to the original avoidant patterns are still operating in the present. Chambless and Goldstein (1980) talk about continuing symbiotic issues in adult agoraphobics and report current interpersonal stress as contributing to the onset of symptomatology, while Barlow and Wolfe (1982), Hafner (1982), and Thorpe and Burns (1983) among others are suggesting an interpersonal focus in their behavioral treatment programs for agoraphobics.

AGORAPHOBIA AND FAMILY ISSUES

Given the resistance of many agoraphobics to accepting and responding to the new learning of cognitive/behavioral therapy, we need to more fully explore how the learning that occurred in the family of origin and the family ideology may still interfere with readiness to think differently and embrace a different way of being in the world. In this section, we will review agoraphobia and family issues.

While the symptoms of agoraphobia typically begin in young adulthood, it is likely that agoraphobics carry a dependent-avoidant pattern learned in childhood into adult life and that family interactions are central for encouraging and maintaining the symptomatology as adults. It is likely that agoraphobia also runs in families. Often agoraphobics are reported to have an agoraphobic mother, and there are reports of phobias and anxiety disorders in other family members. Furthermore, such families appear to create a family milieu that promotes dependency, inhibition of desire to move too far away from the nest as well as mistrust of the outside world.

School phobia which shares many features in common with agoraphobia could be considered a childhood version of agoraphobia (Bowlby, 1973). It is of interest that boys and girls develop school phobia with equal frequency. The male to female ratio is 49:51 (Gordon & Young, 1976). There are also reports of a high incidence of school phobia and/or fears of going to school in retrospective clinical studies of agoraphobics. Thorpe and Burns (1983) report that 30% of agoraphobics in their sample report childhood school phobia. In followup studies of school phobics, it is reported that 20-30% of them develop agoraphobia or neurotic disorders. Since agoraphobics are primarily female, it may be the female school phobics who are at risk for developing agoraphobia while male school phobics develop other symptoms later in life.

Generally agoraphobia runs in families. Agoraphobics are typically found to have mothers who are classified as agoraphobic or who have anxiety disorders. Beck, Solyom and Huger (1971) report that 34% of their sample had a phobic mother, whereas only 6% of their sample had a phobic father. Finberg-Orter and Fodor (1981) surveyed published case histories and report that a phobic mother is mentioned for 39% of females and 11% of males. Goldstein (1982) reports a number of cases with multigenerational agoraphobia in mothers, daughters, and even grandmothers.

There is little research or actual observational data on agoraphobic families. Almost all we know comes from clinical descriptions, single interviews with relatives, or retrospective questionnaires. Bowlby (1973) has studied agoraphobic families and reports that "it passes from one generation to another . . . it is vital that the neurotic difficulties of the parents of the patients should be looked at sympathetically in the context of their own experiences as children" (p. 304).

From the earliest clinical cases, it would appear that mothers of agoraphobics placed special demands on their children which may reflect their own agoraphobic tendencies.

Deutsch (1929) in the first psychoanalytic case description of an agoraphobic describes a mother who was making insistent demands upon her daughter to act as companion and caretaker to her.

Andrews (1966) provided an extensive review of the literature on phobia, including child and adult agoraphobic case descriptions from the psychoanalytic and behavioral literature, and presented strong evidence for the co-existence of phobic symptoms with personality patterns of dependency and avoidance. In a childhood case, where parental behavior was observed, parental overprotection was the rule. Andrews believed that phobics experience early interpersonal familial learning situations in which an avoidant-dependent pattern is an adaptive role for the child.

Wolpe (1958), whose pioneering work in behavior therapy for agoraphobics describes one client's symptoms:

> Miss K . . . 23 year old university graduate . . . apprehensive of walking outside unaccompanied lest she should fall . . . (her) range of activity gradually became more and more circumscribed. At one stage she would walk in the street only if her mother held her arm; later she entirely refused to leave the house and by the time I saw her, she was practically bedridden, apart from very tense wall-hugging journeys between her bed and a couch in the drawing room.

He then goes on to describe the overprotection as follows:

> An only child . . . she had been incredibly overprotected by her mother who insisted on standing perpetually in attendance on her. She was permitted to do almost nothing for herself, forbidden to pass up games lest she get hurt and even her final year at high school was daily escorted over the few hundred yards to and from the gates of the school by her mother who carried her school books for her. (p. 174)

Goldstein (1982) reports on a number of adult agoraphobic cases with a symbiotic mother-daughter relationship in his clinic sample.

The most frequent dyad is mother-daughter, and by far the most consistently difficult cases encountered are those in which the daughter, who is still living with the mother, is the identified client. Repeatedly we have seen the mother, who is usually also agoraphobic, deteriorate as the daughter improves. The daughter, being overwhelmed with guilt, relapses, and then the mother improves. . . . They are both highly resistant to any attempts to separate them from one another, although both give lip service to the necessity of more individuation. This relatively small subgroup alone accounts for the majority of our failures and early dropouts. (p. 200)

PARENTAL OVERPROTECTION: THE INCULCATION OF AGORAPHOBIC IDEOLOGY

These extreme cases, which are so resistant to change, highlight similar less extreme patterns that occur in high risk agoraphobic families. While a good deal of the clinical literature stresses maternal overprotection as central, there is little work on fathers and agoraphobia. What seems most likely, however, is that both parents create a climate for the inculcation and continued fostering of agoraphobic ideology.

Guidano and Liotti (1983), drawing on their own cognitive/behavioral treatment, and Bowlby's writing highlight patterns of interaction characteristic of agoraphobic parent/child interactions. They report that

agoraphobic patients report having experienced direct obstacles to autonomous exploration of the environment . . . . These include . . . being discouraged by the parents (usually their mother) from leaving home alone even for a short outing, . . . being kept at home for longer periods of convalescences than necessary after minor illnesses, . . . and not being allowed to go out and play with friends. (p. 219)

Guidano and Liotti (1983) emphasize that such parents set up agoraphobic belief systems indirectly. "The core of the agoraphobic cognitive organization is the tacit knowledge of an experienced limitation of their personal freedom to explore the world added to an emotional schemata in which the self-image has a hypothetical state of weakness. The need for freedom (autonomy) and the need for protection (dependency), or alternatively the fear of constraint and the fear of loneliness are the conflicting aspects of this ideational core" (p. 221).

Guidano and Liotti (1983) report that "the parents were not honest with the child about the reasons for the restrictions. . . . Clearly the mother (possibly herself agoraphobic) preferred to have the child nearby for her own companionship, but the reasons given to the child for prohibiting autonomy concerned the assumed weakness of the child. The child was given the following messages. 'You are fragile, you aren't healthy, you are not aware of the danger of the street. You don't know how to control yourself in front of strangers and the dangers of the outside world. There are bad boys out there, you mustn't play with them, it's dangerous, if you go out in the street, they could attack you, you might get hit by a car, get lost; no one will help you'." (p. 219)

Guidano and Liotti's (1983) work, from a cognitive/behavioral perspective, is reminiscent of recent psychoanalytic work in object-relations theory. While object relations theorists (with the exception of Bowlby) have not addressed agoraphobia as such, the work of Chodorow may enhance our understanding of some of the dependency issues so central to agoraphobics' socialization.

Chodorow (1978) views the sense of self as relational and that growth of the self and the lessening of dependency occur by differentiation from the mother.

> Children wish to remain one with mother and expect that she will never have different interests from them; yet, they define development in terms of growing away from her. In the face of their dependence, lack of certainty of her emotional permanence, fear of merging and overwhelming love and attachment, a mother looms large and powerful. . . . Analysts say that mothers come to symbolize dependence, regression, passivity and the lack of adaption to reality. Turning away from mother (and father) represents independence, activity, participation in the real world. (p. 82)

She then goes on to talk about how separation is particularly difficult for daughters and mothers because mothers identify more with their daughters. "At every stage of changeover of this separate-closeness dimension . . . the mother must be sensitive to what the child can take and needs. She needs to know both when her child is ready to distance herself and to initiate demands for care, and when it is unable to be distant or separate. . . . Because they are the same gender and their daughter and have been girls, mothers of daughters tend not to experience these infant daughters as separate from them in the same way as they do infant sons" (p. 84).

Following Chodorow's thinking, we can theorize that agoraphobic females may be suffering from an exaggerated case of the prototypical female separation experience. Furthermore, since some of the mothers of agoraphobics may themselves be agoraphobics, daughters of such women may have even more difficulty separating in that they identify with their mothers and therefore model agoraphobic behavior patterns.

TREATMENT ISSUES

Most phobic symptoms typically begin as agoraphobics are preparing to leave home, in the early years of a relationship, marriage, or when they have small children at home.

Chambless and Goldstein (1980) report that the onset of agoraphobia was related to high interpersonal conflict. They proposed that the phobic symptoms are the result of psychological avoidance behavior in conflict situations, "usually because of his/her unassertiveness the agoraphobic has found him/herself in an unhappy seemingly irresolvable relationship under the domination of a spouse or parent. The urge to leave and the fears of being on his/her own balance out, and the agoraphobic trapped in the conflict, is unable to move and lacks the skill to change the situation" (p. 324).

Since agoraphobics appear to carry over into adulthood the childhood patterns of relating and demonstrate ongoing problematic relationships with their parents and/or spouse which may contribute to the development of agoraphobic symptomatology, it is time for behavior therapists to address interpersonal issues in their treatment programs for agoraphobics. Cognitive behavioral programs need to be designed to address ways of remediating the childhood socialization experience. Given the powerful dependency needs of agoraphobics, cognitive behavior therapists need to be sensitive to how these issues are reflected in the psychotherapeutic interactions. Two different types of re-learning need to occur to undo the childhood patterns. One type of learning involves accessing the fear structure and enabling the client to be willing to tolerate high levels of anxiety to learn to face feared situations (Foa & Kozak, 1986). For this task, the therapist must be perceived as a strong person who can help the client master her fears and support her during the panic attacks. The second type of re-learning involves cognitive restructuring. The therapist challenges the world view of the family that views arousal, independence, and mastery as not safe or viable for this client. Since the clients are in a conflict over change and the therapist so often represents a very different perspective from the family's value system, it is important for the therapist to be aware of the differing value systems, the extent of the client's openness, readiness to change, and the ongoing pull of the family for no change.

THE THERAPIST'S DILEMMAS

"The agoraphobic's conflict seems to revolve around issues of dependency, autonomy and control. On the one hand, since she believes she cannot deal with the dangers in the outside world by herself, she is impelled to obtain help from a 'caretaker.' On the other hand, seeking succor may lead to surrender of sovereignty to another person. Because she 'needs' the other person, she has less claim to freedom or to exercising individuality" (Beck & Emery, 1985, p. 140). Thus, the therapist must expect that her strength and support, which may enable the client to venture out in the world, may also become problematic for the client. The therapist's attention to the way therapy is presented and perceived appears essential to enable the client to learn to resolve these issues of dependency, autonomy, and control.

Cognitive behavior therapy, particularly with a feminist therapist, represents a diametrically opposite set of values from those learned in the family. The therapist is giving the client messages that run counter to familial values. Examples of such messages include the following: "It's good to go out in the world, to be independent, to master, to be assertive, to be separate from the family. You are not helpless, you can handle yourself when you panic," etc. The therapist is also telling the client that she can learn new behaviors.

Another issue that must be addressed is that the therapist is most likely to be a person very different from the mother. In order to function effectively as a therapist, one is typically self reliant, independent, assertive, and skilled in tackling life's problems in spite of adversity. A therapist is also more likely to be career oriented and may not value being a full-time homemaker. Hence, the therapist's personality (even if achieved through struggling with issues similar to the client's) and philosophy is often at variance with the familial world view.

Hence, the learning climate of therapy could be characterized as a conflict between two sets of beliefs or ways of being in the world. The client often comes into therapy in conflict, experiencing the pull of both positions. The parental and therapist values can be characterized as follows:

Parental Beliefs

1. My daughter is a helpless child. She cannot take care of herself.
2. She cannot venture too far outside, because the world is dangerous and untrustworthy.
3. She is too weak, too much of a child to take care of herself out there in the outside world.
4. Security is to be achieved by staying close to mother/home.
5. I will not tolerate assertive behavior.
6. The worst thing that can happen is for my daughter to be independent, for I would lose the closeness to my daughter.

Therapist's Beliefs

1. The client can be taught how to handle her anxiety.
2. She can learn how to face her fears and handle being out in the world.
3. With my help, the client can learn how to rely on herself.
4. The client can only feel secure when she learns how to rely on herself.
5. The client can learn to be assertive and still remain close to significant others.
6. The client can learn how to be more independent and remain close to significant others.

The agoraphobic's conflicts could be characterized as reflecting both these belief systems.

Daughter's/Client's Conflicts

1. I am a helpless child, but I want to be able to handle my anxiety.
2. I cannot take care of myself too far from home, but I want to learn to be able to go out in the world and function more independently.
3. I can't be alone; I need my mother or mother substitute near. I would like to learn to be self sufficient.
4. Security is to be achieved by staying close to home. Security is to be achieved by learning competencies, so I can rely on myself.
5. I don't dare express my displeasure to significant others. I would like to learn to be more assertive.
6. The worst thing that can happen is to be separate from significant others, alone in the world. I would like the freedom to become more independent.

While I believe the etiology and underlying dynamics of agoraphobia can best be understood from an object relations/developmental perspective, research evidence would still suggest that the treatment of choice is some variant of cognitive/behavior therapy. However, such cognitive/behavioral treatments need to be sensitive to the underlying psychodynamic issues and therapist/client process. Through behavior therapy, the client is introduced to experiences that enable her to access and change her fear structures and through cognitive restructuring to question some of the childhood belief systems which are no longer viable for adult functioning and replace them with new beliefs about herself and the world as she learns new ways of behaving. The therapist needs to create a therapeutic climate where the client learns to try out these new behaviors and resolve cognitive conflicts.

STAGES IN THERAPEUTIC WORK WITH AGORAPHOBICS: THERAPIST/CLIENT PROCESS

As we work with agoraphobics using the cognitive behavioral procedures, we need to be ever mindful of therapist/client process. We need to keep in mind that we, as therapists, represent an alternative way of being in the world and that we are dealing with a client in conflict who is still very much in touch with her childhood patterns of interacting with significant others. The following is an outline for beginning work in attending to process. One becomes aware of how the agoraphobic patterning is revealed in the therapist/client interactions as one proceeds through the various stages of the behavioral treatment program (Fodor, in press).

1. The Therapist Is All Knowing and the Client Is the Ideal Student

During the first stage of behavior therapy, the agoraphobic wants the therapist to be strong, all knowing and wants to be dependent on the therapist. "With your tools, with your strength you will make me well, stronger." She has often chosen a behavioral approach because she wants the structure and is looking for guidance. She is only too willing to learn the various behavioral techniques.

2. Idealization of Therapist

As the various behavioral procedures are presented to the client, she begins to model the behavior of the therapist and talks about herself in a self disparaging way ("I'm such a baby, I'm so weak, afraid," etc.). She wants to be like the therapist (e.g., strong, brave, self supporting, independent, assertive etc.).

3. The Work Gets Hard—It's Not Going To Be Easy. Disappointment Sets In

After the client has learned some of the procedures and is being encouraged to go out more and face her fears, or after she has experienced anxiety as she is out there alone, the client begins to realize that therapy is hard work and that the therapist will not take away her discomfort or do the hard work for her. At this point she becomes angry at the therapist because "it's so hard." She also questions whether behavior therapy can really help her or if the therapist really understands how hard it is for her to use these techniques when she is so frightened. She also begins to question whether she can change, becomes somewhat hopeless and may also become more depressed. At this point resistance sets in.

As the client gets somewhat better, begins to do some things alone and masters anxiety a little, she becomes oppositional. She complains that nothing has changed and that the therapist has not helped. She asks for more techniques, but begins to belittle the techniques or oppose any suggestion. "Oh, I tried that already, it doesn't work. Is this another one of your Mickey Mouse techniques?" Typically, most behavior therapists work harder at this point. It is important to realize that the client is beginning to resent the therapist's power and needs to be more in charge.

4. Suggestions for Handling Opposition

a. To counter these traps, it is suggested that one puts the burden of change on the client's shoulders. (Since so many of my clients have a varied collection of tapes and self help books, when they ask you to come up with another intervention for them, insist that they do some research and come up with some ideas themselves.) The next session is used to help them make a choice.

b. Resist knowing all the answers. If they ask you for the best way to handle an anxiety attack, suggest several methods and let them explore these methods on their own and report back to you. Teach them how to be their own scientists, to assess and design treatments for themselves. Try to stay in a consultant mode.

c. "You don't understand how hard it is?!" One of the biggest complaints you have to deal with is the above. Often clients need your patience as they describe for the hundredth time their last anxiety attack. Agoraphobics feel it is very important for you to understand. Mother appeared to understand through merger. Listen and ask questions and acknowledge how hard it is, but you still believe they can change. Often self disclosure and modeling do not work with agoraphobics (e.g., if you tell them it was hard for you to get over your driving phobia, they see you as so different that they don't feel that your struggles have any application to their situation). Acknowledge that their struggle is hard, listening patiently to the details, and give lots of praise for change.

d. Be open to psychotropic drugs. For some clients, using drugs may be the only way they will expose themselves to new situations.

5. Family Resistance to Change

Often the behavior therapist is involved in a tug of war with significant others. Prepare the client early in therapy for signs of resistance, sabotaging of gains by significant others, or the development of symptoms in significant others (Hafner, 1982). An example is, the husband calls the therapist to complain that his wife is gone too much during the day and he wants accountability. One must remember that he married a woman who couldn't leave the house and he may need to be seen as the client improves. In another scenario, the agoraphobic daughter reports that her mother gets sick when she planned to take her first trip away. This is the point in therapy where it is important to spell out value polarities, and to help the client begin to choose what type of relationships she wishes to have with significant others. If she wishes to become more independent, this is the time to work on assertiveness issues and the ways one can remain in close relationships, yet be autonomous.

6. Helping the Client Make Choices, Set Goals, Learn To Spend Time Alone and Nurture Herself

As the client's symptoms become less of a problem, the therapeutic task approaches a more typical feminist psychotherapy, and there are many different ways to address the remaining problems. The author still utilizes the therapeutic relationship as the arena for new learning (for example, learning to be alone or with oneself). Since agoraphobics fear being alone and relying on themselves, a central feature of therapy is learning how to be alone, to be good company for oneself. Mini-experiments are devised and the client and therapist, using gestalt techniques, explore these issues.

Similar work is carried out for self nurturance. Many agoraphobics believe they need to be with someone else to be nurtured, or they are being selfish if they give as high a priority to meeting their own needs as taking care of their families. For many agoraphobics, who are out of touch with their own feelings, who view any arousal as anxiety provoking, gestalt awareness training is utilized. They are taught to listen to themselves, to be aware of what they may need at a particular moment in time and are encouraged to explore ways of satisfying their needs and supporting themselves while being emotionally open to a range of feelings and experiences. A fuller discussion of the integration of gestalt awareness work with focused behavior therapy has been described elsewhere (Fodor, in press).

For goal setting, visual imagery is utilized. The agoraphobic client is encouraged to construct her own fantasy about a life without phobias. She is encouraged to explore all future possibilities and to learn enough about herself to be able to choose a reasonable path.

This paper is the beginning of work in designing behavioral interventions that are sensitive to underlying psychodynamics and interpersonal issues for agoraphobics. In spite of the problems, current research suggests that behavioral techniques are still among the most effective tools for changing of anxiety based symptoms and given the proliferation of anxiety disorder clinics and behavioral self help programs in the community, there is no doubt that the behavioral approach still has wide appeal. More and more agoraphobics, mostly women, will be offered behavioral interventions, often in short-term treatment packages as the treatment of choice. Therefore, much more work needs to be done to understand how and why these interventions work or do not work, to design research that addresses some of the underlying psychodynamic and familial issues taking into account that agoraphobia is mainly a female syndrome, and to incorporate these variables into treatment programs. In addition, much more attention needs to be given to what actually occurs between the therapist and client during cognitive/behavior therapy. By studying therapist/client process, one should be able to make effective use of the therapeutic alliance to foster change.

REFERENCES

American Psychiatric Association (1980). *Diagnostic and Statistical Manual of Mental Disorder* (3rd ed.). Washington, DC: Author.

Andrews, J. D. (1966). Psychotherapy of phobias. *Psychological Bulletin, 66,* 455-480.

Arnkoff, D. B. & Glass, C. R. (1982). Clinical cognitive constructs: Examination, evaluation, elaboration. In P. C. Kendall, *Advances in Cognitive Behavioral Research and Therapy,* Vol. 1, New York: Academic Press.

Bandura, A. (1977). Self-effacy: Toward a unifying theory of behavioral change. *Psychological Review, 84,* 191-215.

Barlow, D. H., & Wolfe, B. E. (1981). Behavioral approaches to anxiety disorders: A report on the NIMH-SUNY, Albany, Research Conference. *Journal of Consulting and Clinical Psychology, 49,* 448-454.

Beck, A. K. & Emery, G. (1985). *Anxiety Disorders and Phobias: A Cognitive Perspective.* New York: Basic Books.

Bowlby, J. (1973). *Separation Anxiety and Anger.* New York: Basic Books.

Brehony, K. A. (1983). Women and agoraphobia: A case for the etiological significance of the feminine sex role stereotype. In V. Franks & E. Rothblum (Eds.), *The Stereotyping of Women: Its Effects on Mental Health.* New York: Springer.

Chambless, D. & Goldstein, A. J. (1982). *Agoraphobia: Multiple Perspectives on Theory and Treatment.* New York: Wiley.

Chambless, D. L. & Goldstein, A. J. (1980). Agoraphobia. In A. J. Goldstein & E. B. Foa (Eds.), *Handbook of Behavioral Interventions.* New York: Wiley.

Chodorow, N. (1978). *The Reproduction of Mothering.* Berkeley: University of California Press.

Deutsch, H. (1929). The genesis of agoraphobia. *International Journal of Psychoanalysis, 10,* 51-59.

Ellis, A. & Harper, R. A. (1975). *A New Guide to Rational Living*. Englewood Cliffs, NJ: Prentice-Hall.

Emmelkamp, P. M. G. & van de Hout. (1983). A failure in treating agoraphobia. In E. B. Foa and Paul M. G. Emmelkamp, *Failures in Behavior Therapy*. New York: Wiley.

Finberg-Orter, B. & Fodor, I. G. (1981). A survey of published case histories of male and female agoraphobics, unpublished manuscript.

Foa, E. B. & Chambless, D. L. (1978). Habituation of subjective anxiety during flooding in imagery. *Behavior Research and Therapy, 16,* 391-399.

Foa, E. B. & Kozak, M. J. (1986). Emotional processing of fear: Exposure to corrective information. *Psychology Bulletin, 99*(1).

Fodor, I. (1974). Sex role conflict and symptom formation in women: Can behavior therapy help. *Psychotherapy: Theory, Research and Practice, 2*(1).

Fodor, I. G. (1974). The phobic syndrome in women. In V. Franks & V. Burtle (Eds.), *Women in Therapy*. New York: Brunner-Mazel.

Fodor, I. G. (in press). Moving beyond CBT: Integrating gestalt therapy to facilitate personal and interpersonal awareness. In Jacobson, N. (Ed.), *Behavior and Cognitive Therapists in Clinical Practice*. New York: Guilford Press.

Fodor, I. G. & Rothblum, E. D. (1985). Strategies for dealing with sex role stereotypes. In C. Brody (Ed.), *Women Therapists Treating Women*. New York: Springer.

Goldstein, A. J. (1982). Agoraphobia: Treatment successes, treatment failures, and theoretical implications. In D. L. Chambless and A. J. Goldstein, *Agoraphobia: Multiples Perspectives on Theory and Treatment*. New York: Wiley.

Goldstein, A. J. & Chambless, D. L. (1978). A reanalysis of agoraphobia. *Behavior Therapy, 9,* 47-59.

Gordon, D. A. & Young, R. D. (1976). School phobia: A discussion of etiology, treatment and evaluation. *Psychological Reports, 39* (3, Pt. 1), 783-804.

Guidano, V. F. & Liotti, G. (1983). *Cognitive Processes and Emotional Disorders*. New York: Guilford Press.

Hafner, R. J. (1982). The marital context of the agoraphobic syndrome. In D. L. Chambless and A. J. Goldstein, *Agoraphobia: Multiples Perspectives on Theory and Treatment*. New York: Wiley.

Marks, I. (1978). Exposure treatments: Clinical studies in phobic, obsessive compulsive and allied disorders in W. S. Agras (Ed.), *Behavior Therapy in Clinical Psychiatry* (2nd ed.). Boston, MA: Little Brown.

Padawer, W. & Goldfried, M. (1984). Anxiety-related disorders, fears and phobias. In E. Blechman, *Behavior Modification with Women*. New York: Guilford.

Solyom, I., Beck, P., Solyom, C. & Hugel, R. (1974). Some etiological factors in public neurosis. *Canadian Psychiatric Association Journal, 19*(1), 69-79.

Terhune, W. (1949). The Phobic Syndrome: The Study of Eighty Six Patients with Phobic Reactions. *Archives Neurological Psychiatry, 62,* 162-172.

Thorpe, G. & Burns, L. (1983). *The Agoraphobic Syndrome*. New York: J. Wiley.

Wilson, G. T. (1984). Behavior therapy. In R. J. Corsini (Ed.), *Current Psychotherapies*. Itasca, IL: F. E. Peacock Publ., Inc.

Wolfe, J. L. & Fodor, I. G. (1975). A cognitive/behavioral approach to modifying assertive behavior in women. *The Counseling Psychologist, 5*(4).

Wolpe, J. (1958). *Psychotherapy by Reciprocal Inhibition*. Stanford, CA: Stanford University Press.

Beyond Homophobia: Learning to Work with Lesbian Clients

Rachel Josefowitz Siegel

A special kind of learning can take place between lesbian and nonlesbian[1] women within the therapy relationship. All therapists, lesbian and nonlesbian, have absorbed the pervasively heterosexual assumptions of our society, the fear of homosexuality, the ignorance and denial of lesbian existence. Male-centered cultural messages insist on an uneven division between homosexual and heterosexual, female and male, consistently oppressing and devaluing the homosexual and the female. The resulting polarization permeates our experience, keeping women separated from each other in mutually exclusive categories and denying our rich and caring connections with each other. Inner conflicts and denials mirror the external divisions and keep us from enjoying the full range of human sexuality and creativity.

Working together in therapy relationships, we have an opportunity to integrate the polarized parts of our personalities and to name and eliminate some of the ways in which we project them. This paper, written by a nonlesbian feminist therapist, focuses on

The author is a feminist therapist in private practice in Ithaca, New York. She is co-editor of *Women Changing Therapy*, Haworth Press, 1983

The author wishes to thank Sandra F. Siegel for her help in clarifying language and ideas; also to Marilyn Frye, Candace Widmer, Beverly Burch, and Lauree Moss for critical and responsive readings of early drafts.

An earlier version of this paper was published in Walker, L. and Rosewater, L. B., eds. (1985), *Handbook of Feminist Therapy: Women's Issues in Psychotherapy*. New York: Springer. Reprinted by permission.

1. The terms "lesbian" and "nonlesbian," ambiguous as they are, are used quite simply according to the client's or therapist's self-definitions.

growth and development she has experienced in the first 10 years of her work with lesbian clients. Her goal, beyond the best interests of her clients, has been to overcome her own ignorance and fear of lesbian reality, to lift the veil of invisibility imposed by the male heterosexual power structure, and to break the taboo of silence that helps to perpetuate the myths and distortions surrounding our love of women and our fear of that love. This writer's lesbian clients have had a chance to form a deep, nonsexual relationship with a caring, nonlesbian therapist, based on the kind of trust and respect that society, and often their own families, have denied them.

The therapist's learning, alternately frightening, painful, or exhilarating, took place in four modes: in her own therapy, through literature, with lesbian colleagues, and from lesbian clients. This last and most important mode will be explored most fully.

LEARNING THROUGH THERAPY

In her own therapy the therapist can best uncover the complexity of her sexual feelings and the particularity of her attractions and aversions to women. She can sort out the feelings and issues triggered in her by lesbian clients. However, if her own therapist is not a lesbian, the therapy will be reduced to the limits of lesbian consciousness in both therapists. In my therapy, the uncovering and exploration of sexual feelings toward women produced a deeper level of comfort with myself and eased my initial communications with lesbians in and out of therapy. The courage to explore the topic further grew out of my therapy; a fuller understanding of the lesbian experience came from other sources.

LEARNING FROM THE LITERATURE

I found the older literature about lesbians of limited use; it is based on heterosexist assumptions and on inferences drawn from studies of male homosexuals (Escamillo-Mondanaro, 1977; Ries, 1974). Although lesbianism is no longer officially considered a pathological entity, the bulk of current psychiatric literature does not reflect any significant change in attitude (Goodman, 1977; Sang, 1977). Some recent studies aim to dispel the myths of lesbian pathology. Ries (1974), surveying psychological studies of lesbians, finds no research evidence of increased pathology among lesbian women or their families of origin than among heterosexual samples of women in similar circumstances. Kirkpatrick, Smith, and Roy (1981) find that lesbian mothers treat their children very much like other mothers; gender development problems and types or frequency of pathology are similar for children of lesbian mothers and nonlesbian mothers. Hoeffer (1981) finds no significant differences among such children in acquiring sex-role behavior. Goodman (1977) observes that lesbian mothers "have helped their children to be more sensitive and accepting of differences between people and to have respect for these differences" (p. 20). Lyons (1983) finds the fears surrounding custody issues to be the only significant differentiating factor.

Research that consistently finds more similarities than differences between samples of lesbian women and heterosexual women in similar circumstances is obviously important in counteracting the still prevailing attitudes and traditional training of mainstream psychiatry. Yet the need to disprove "lesbian pathology" and to prove the lesbian mother's harmlessness to her children indicates how far we are from seeing each other as equally human and complex, in a world that divides us into "normal" and "other," "deviant," "queer," and "unacceptable."

Recent feminist publications identify some of the blatant offenses perpetrated against lesbians in the name of therapy, such as denial of the client's reality, coercive cures through aversive therapy (Litwok, Weber, Rux, DeForest & Davies, 1979), and therapists collaborating with parents in the involuntary treatment of lesbian adolescents (Escamillo-Mondanaro, 1977). Lesbian accounts of homophobic persecution are often trivialized or misdiagnosed as paranoia. Psychiatric hospitalization can be especially harmful to lesbians, as the heterosexist milieu is bound to increase her sense of alienation from the world at a time when she is most in need of affirmation for her own feelings and lifestyle (Frye, personal communication, November 1982).

More subtle are the errors of therapists who attribute all of a woman's problems to her lesbianism or who refuse to focus on her lesbianism because they consider it a symptom that will disappear when other underlying problems are resolved (Sang, 1977).

Lesbian therapists offer new insights and helpful suggestions. Litwok, Weber, Rux, DeForest, and Davies (1979) state, "The lesbian faces problems and stresses not encountered by any other group of individuals in our society. . . . Lesbians may *act* just like everyone else, but the stressors which they face are unique to their situation." Other writers (Cummerton, 1982; Escamillo-Mondanaro, 1977; Goodman, 1977; Litwok et al., 1979) advocate changes in clinical training programs and in mental health agencies that would educate therapists to the needs of lesbian clients and would make the atmosphere in these institutions hospitable to lesbian colleagues as well as clients. They urge nonlesbian therapists to confront their own biases, to become comfortable with all aspects of their own sexuality, and to learn as much as possible about the complexity of lesbian existence and the available lesbian community resources.

Gradually, my own reading moved beyond the professional literature and into the richness of lesbian culture. I began to appreciate the immense contributions to feminism made by lesbian thinkers. Adrienne Rich (1979, 1980) and Marilyn Frye (1981) had profound effects on me. I began to read lesbian novels, short stories, and biographies. I absorbed a deeper, more direct sense of the lives of lesbian women by reading such varied fare as *Rubyfruit Jungle* (Brown, 1978), *Sappho Was a Right-On Woman* (Abbott & Love, 1973). *The Coming Out Stories* (Stanley & Wolfe, 1980), *Nice Jewish Girls* (Beck, 1982), and *The Color Purple* (Walker, 1982). A Meg Christian concert introduced me to the sense of humor and joyousness of a lesbian celebration.

LEARNING FROM LESBIAN COLLEAGUES

Learning among colleagues, in consultation, supervision, or at professional meetings entails an engagement and dialogue between lesbian and nonlesbian therapists that is essential to our work with lesbian clients but often has been avoided. Difficulties emerge. The risk of self-exposure and rejection are deeply felt. It is easier to interact within the safe territory of our commonalities or to avoid each other than it is to identify and explore our differences. It appears easier to deny expression to important aspects of ourselves and to maintain the distance between each other through "lies, secrets, and silence" (Rich, 1979). This kind of avoidance is a familiar survival tactic for women in a male world and for lesbians in a heterosexual world. The growth and healing that occurred when I learned to interact more openly with lesbian therapists has deepened and facilitated my therapeutic work with lesbian clients more effectively than any amount of reading or personal therapy.

LEARNING FROM LESBIAN CLIENTS

I learned most directly from lesbian clients, listening carefully during the therapy hour, asking for clarification when the client's needs called for it or when I felt confused or uninformed. Gradually, as I learned to identify the homophobic and heterosexist content of the psychological theories and assumptions that had been part of my professional training, I grew more open to factual input from lesbian clients.

Together, within the safety of the therapy room, we began the slow process of exposing the layers of cliches, myths, fears, and fantasies that surround the taboo of homosexuality.

My lesbian clients unfolded the day-to-day patterns of their lives. The innumerable denials, exclusions and insults that engulf them individually and as couples and diminish their sense of worth and well-being in the world. I became aware of my own heterosexual privileges. I recognized the immunity conferred upon me by my married state, the public support and acceptance of being coupled that increases my sense of worth by association and opens the door to daily advantages. I learned to appreciate the complexities, fears, and rewards of the long coming-out process as well as the consequences of not coming out, and to respect each client's individual pattern and timing in making these decisions. I also learned to sort out the many aspects of a woman's concerns that were related to heterosexist oppression from those that were not.

There were changes in my attitude toward lesbians as my feminist consciousness became more sophisticated and my identification with women more profound. Early on, I accepted and validated the sexual preference of women for women as an alternate lifestyle and offered my lesbian clients a benign therapeutic antidote to the "heterosexual imperatives" (Rich, 1980) of our culture, along with large doses of consciousness raising about the politics and economics of institutionalized homophobia. I then went through a phase of envy and admiration, idealizing lesbian women who had the courage to separate themselves from the aggressively sexist relationships that prevail in the heterosexual mainstream of society. It was a long time before I sensed that the bestowing of idealizations can be a way of holding onto the power of defining the other person. No matter how well intentioned, it can still interfere with the client's process of self-discovery and self-definition.

THE LESBIAN COUPLES GROUP

Recently, I came to the emotional and intellectual realization that our mutual learning and acceptance was limited to the degree that my interpretations of lesbian reality came out of my own reality. Like male definitions of women, my heterosexual observations of lesbians are necessarily self-limited. They may fall short of the individual lesbian's reality and run the risk of being experienced as external and judgmental, even when not intended to judge or to define. I began to search for more sensitive and equalitarian ways of interacting that would allow us to work through the varied aspects of the lesbian/nonlesbian, woman-loving/fear-of-woman-loving split.

I am indebted to the six women who trusted me to facilitate a lesbian couples group, for confronting me and challenging me to move beyond my familiar and unintentionally condescending leadership style.

Group interaction was intense. We played out an inverted version of the ancient female drama of not living up to each other's idealized expectations. There was much pain and anger. One member said, "I am not the lesbian you want me to be," and I felt, "I am not the perfect therapist/mother/friend you want me to be." My urge was to try harder, to provide a "strong woman" model capable of contradicting the "not-good-enough" messages. I wondered if the drama we were reliving was that of the "inadequate mother" being blamed for her daughter's "deviant" sexuality, by a society that misunderstood and devalued both. Another lesbian client in individual therapy was able to express similar feelings when she blamed her mother for not teaching her to be more feminine, more "normal." The roles were reversed in the group: The therapist/mother/heterosexual was excluded — she was the deviant, the other — but the interaction was the same. We worked through the "not good enough" feelings that every woman experiences in being "other than" the male norms of our society, and which every woman internalizes and projects onto mother, daughter, lover, sister, colleague, friend. We challenged each other, became real to each other in our individual complexities, and began to deal with our differences in a more honest and accepting way.

I began to sense how deeply and how often we treat ourselves and each other as society has treated us. We reject, criticize, or fail to acknowledge or to value in each other those aspects of our lives and of our personalities which society devalues in women, including our friendships with and our love of women. In matters of sexuality and sexual choice especially, we mirror society's values by imposing silence and invisibility on the reality of our sexual feelings and activities. When lesbians interact with non-lesbians, this can take the form of imposing social or political judgments on each other's sexual choices.

It also seemed more difficult to be specific about sexual activity with lesbian clients than with most other clients, even when sexual functioning had been identified as a reason for seeking therapy. When I opened the subject, asking the usual questions, I was at times perceived as seductive or as a voyeur; when I did not mention sex, my silence was interpreted as disapproval. Aware of the sexual tension between women in the therapy room and the enormous silence that surrounds it in a heterosexual environment, I learned to respect the special sensitivity of lesbian women to being seen as sexual oddities, depicted in ways that are intended to arouse and titillate or in ways that deny their sexuality and reject it as odious. Language was also a problem, since the words we use in describing sexual functioning are based on a male-centered and heterosexual perspective, and the language for describing sexuality is inadequate.

REFLECTIONS

When the doors that seal off the lesbian experience are opened, women find new ways of relating to each other, of making significant connections.

The dialogue between lesbian and nonlesbian women in individual or group therapy, in consultation and supervision, at conferences and among friends can build a bridge of trust and understanding, overcoming some of the barriers between us. The opportunity to recognize and accept the differences and commonalities between us in a supportive atmosphere can facilitate the process of differentiating ourselves from the stereotypes imposed by a patriarchal hetero-sexual culture and lead to a deeper level of self-awareness and self-acceptance.

UPDATE 1986

When I presented this material at the ORTHO Women's Institute in 1984, it was in an atmosphere of predominantly heterosexual assumptions. Only a handful of the 80 women present had previously considered the possibility that homosexuality could be as "normal" or as positively valued as heterosexuality. The workshop format elicited open discussion of therapist's attitudes. Questions were raised about the biological or cultural causes of homosexuality and even about the moral consequences of accepting lesbians in the community. Rejections and idealizations got stuck in a rhetoric of deviance or otherness. The lesbians among us felt the pain of becoming visible among the distorting mirrors of non-lesbian colleagues' responses. The non-lesbians struggled with the visibility of our own biases. We all felt the guilt and anger that keeps us apart and the need for much more understanding and genuine communication.

Since this article was first published there have been more workshops and more publications on this topic by lesbian and non-lesbian feminists. We continue to struggle against the prevailing and overwhelmingly elitist forces that would keep us divided against each other, and prevent us from mutual empowerment. We have begun to explore the connections between homophobia, heterosexism, and all other "isms," and learned to appreciate and respect the differences among us.

REFERENCES

Abbott, S. & Love, B. (1973). *Sappho was a right-on woman: A liberated view of Lesbianism*. Briarcliff Manor, NY: Stein & Day.

Beck, E. T. (Ed.) (1982). *Nice Jewish girls: A lesbian anthology*. Watertown, MA: Persephone Press.

Brown, R. M. (1978). *Rubyfruit jungle*. New York: Bantam Books.

Cummerton, J. M. (1982). Homophobia and social work practice with lesbians. In A. Weick & S. T. Vandiver (Eds.), *Women, power, and change*. Washington, DC: National Association of Social Workers.

Escamillo-Mondanaro, J. (1977). Lesbians and therapy. In E. I. Rawlings & D. K. Carter (Eds.), *Psychotherapy for women*. Springfield, IL: Charles C Thomas.

Frye, M. (1981). To be and be seen: Metaphysical misogyny. *Sinister Wisdom, 17*, 57-69.

Frye, M. Personal communication, November 1982.

Goodman, B. (1977). *The lesbian: A celebration of difference*. Brooklyn, NY: Out & Out Books.

Hoeffer, B. (1981). Children's acquisition of sex-role behavior in lesbian-mother families. *American Journal of Orthopsychiatry, 51*(3), 536-544.

Kirkpatrick, M., Smith, C. & Roy, R. (1981). Lesbian mothers and their children: A comparative study. *American Journal of Orthopsychiatry, 51*(3), 545-551.

Litwok. E., Weber, R., Rux, J., DeForest, J. & Davies, R. (1979). *Considerations in therapy with lesbian clients*. Philadelphia: Women's Resources.

Lyons, T. (1983). Lesbian mothers' custody fears: Facts and symbols. In Robbins, J. H. & Siegel, R. J. (Eds.), *Women changing therapy: New assessments, values & strategies in feminist therapy*. New York: Haworth Press.

Rich, A. (1979). *On lies, secrets and silence*. New York: W. W. Norton.

Rich, A. (1980). Compulsory heterosexuality and lesbian experience. *Signs: Journal of Women in Culture and Society, 5*(4). 631-660.

Ries, B. F. (1974). New viewpoints on the female homosexual. In V. Franks & V. Burtle (Eds.), *Women and therapy*. New York: Bruner/Mazel.

Sang, B. E. (1977). Psychotherapy with lesbians: Some observations and tentative generalizations. In E. I. Rawlings & D. K. Carter (Eds.), *Psychotherapy for women*. Springfield, IL: Charles C Thomas.

Stanley, J. P. & Wolfe, S. J. (Eds.) (1980). *The Coming Out Stories*. Watertown, MA: Persephone Press.

Walker, A. (1982). *The color purple*. New York: Harcourt Brace Jovanovich.

SECTION II

Arenas of Power

Every aspect of our lives is an arena of power with a history and a set of social usages that we strive to become aware of and, when necessary, to change. This section explores our workplaces, professional organizations, and bodies as such arenas of power.

Autobiography is one of the tools the women's movement uses for "consciousness raising" or increased self awareness. In my article I use an autobiographical statement to describe how the political and the professional have become the personal for me.

Each arena of power has its social and historical context. For example, when Deanna Pearlmutter writes about the relationships of women staff in a teaching hospital, she writes from her experience as a director of nursing at Massachusetts General Hospital, the teaching arm of Harvard University Medical School.

This institution has a long record of sexist practices which are detailed by Mary Roth Walsh (1977). From 1850 on, Harvard University turned down many applications to medical school from qualified, and sometimes distinguished, applicants. In 1915 they admitted a few women with the proviso that their degrees be given from Radcliffe College. It was not until 1945 that women were permitted to enter Harvard medical school as equals with men.

A male privileged professional and social organization has been so completely the context of our lives that often we do not fully

135

perceive how it limits us. Hamilton, Alagna, King, and Lloyd's analysis of sexism in the workplace makes a major contribution to our knowledge and awareness of the full extent of the harm done to us by sexual discrimination and abuse in our workplaces.

The American Psychiatric Association is a major battleground for women's issues. What is biological, what is interpersonal, what is considered part of a personality disorder, what is caused by trauma, and what is gender-related are subjects of major impact on concepts applied to women and treatment of women. These battles, described by Paula Caplan and myself are described against the background of an organization which has about a fifteen percent woman membership. In its early years it permitted no women members.

One of the significant contributions of the women's movement in the last twenty years has been to make the physical abuse of women a major area of study. Jan Leland-Young and Joan Nelson add to this knowledge by offering a prevention model for physical assault of women. Erica Rothman and Kit Munson, under the guidance of Elaine Hilberman Carmen and others at Chapel Hill, North Carolina, describe the realities of battered women and are pioneers in developing programs to help them. In this paper the authors document how the authority of the court is used to involve the violent husband in a treatment program.

Martha Zuehlke writes of the powerful psychological and social consequences of enabling young women to take leadership and power over their reproductive lives. She is also describing a step in a long struggle which has proceeded since the turn of the century when contraceptive information was illegal. Nurse Margaret Sanger (1971) went to jail for opening a birth control clinic in 1916. She devoted her life to one of the major transformations of our society by establishing an organization for research in family planning and the establishment of clinics throughout the United States. It has made family planning available to many and thus enabled those women to take an essential kind of power over their lives. This paper describes an extension of the power to young and poor women.

Susan Johnson and Susan Guenther write about the necessity for lesbians to be honest with their physicians about their sexual orientation in order to receive appropriate care. Basically, they are concerned about relationships: about the need for openness, trust and connection between physician and patient.

There are two papers about childbearing and rearing. The creation of a new person is the most profoundly personal and relational of experiences. In our society it occurs in the hospital, which is a highly technologized environment oriented to disease and the treatment of emergencies. The flow of birth as a natural, spiritual and personal event is largely destroyed. Martha Livingston analyzes this clash and the creative practices that work to preserve the personal. She gives us an in-depth picture of the realistic forces which mold the experience of childbirth in our society today and describes some of the realities which any one of us needs to know when we must deal with these forces.

Mechaneck, Klein, and Kuppersmith demonstrate in their paper on single mothers that women who decide to have and raise children of their own and have the freedom and the resources to do so, can cope quite successfully. In fact they may be better off than women whose relationships with their children's fathers do not work out and who seek divorce (Chester, 1986).

REFERENCES

Chesler, P. (1986). *Mothers on trial*. New York: McGraw-Hill.
Sanger, M. (1971). *Margaret Sanger: An autobiography*. New York: Dover Publications, Inc.
Walsh, M. (1977). *Doctors wanted: No women need apply*. New Haven, CN: Yale University Press.

A Woman's Experience

Marjorie Braude

I cannot separate my development as a psychiatrist from my development as a political and social individual. If there has been one major change agent it has been the conceptualizations and development of the women's movement during my adult life.

I had a very wonderful basic and medical education at the University of Chicago, but one flawed with some major anachronisms. While I became imbued with the ideals of basic scientific thinking and general truth, I could see many anachronisms between the principles taught and the way humans, both medical personnel and patients, were treated, and somehow felt these anachronisms must bear on the health of the patients.

I also discovered a number of the ways in which women could be discriminated against and harmed. I learned that men who failed a clinical quarter in my medical school could repeat it, but women could not. I learned that few hospitals would take my application for internship seriously because I was married and the hospital that accepted me did so only after I swore in front of a committee to not become pregnant. I learned from the treatment of women patients, particularly on obstetrical and gynecological services. On the one hand they were expected to accept the word of the gynecologist as absolute, with little explanation of courses of action that had major consequences for their lives and health, and on the other hand information they brought about themselves and their bodies was usually considered not reliable. Treatment was dogmatic and I witnessed treatment that was unnecessarily harmful. Many of my fellow students were able to close their eyes to the bad parts but I was never

The author is a psychiatrist in private practice in Los Angeles, California and senior attending staff at Westwood Hospital. She is Vice-President, Association of Women Psychiatrists, and past Treasurer, American Medical Women's Association. She was Co-Chair in 1983 and Chair in 1984 of The Women's Institute, American Orthopsychiatric Association.
Reprinted with permission from *Psychiatric Annals,* February 1983.

able to do so. However, I was a reasonably happy member of the system until an event made the political become the personal for me. Three seconal pills changed my perspective and alienated me from my chosen profession.

The occasion of the three seconal pills was the birth of my first child. Having delivered sixty-five babies I had an accurate idea of obstetrical procedures and hazards. The obstetrician whom I had counted on was away when my child was born at Cedars of Lebanon Hospital in Los Angeles in 1953. The obstetrician who took over insisted on giving me drugs which I did not need and was angered by my protest. I had observed the blue color and slow responses of children who were born drugged and did not want this for my beloved child. Not only were the standard doses of demeral and scopolomine given me but I was forced to take three seconal pills at the same time. The combination would have been prohibited at either of the hospitals at which I had trained, but my regular contractions every four minutes made it impossible for me to get up and leave or protest with effectiveness. I hoped that my child would not be born until the drugs had worn off but she was born two hours later at the height of the action of the drugs. I have no memory of her birth.

I have never been able to fully deal with the damage and insult of this experience. The knowledge, powers, and ethics that I had acquired as a physician were abused (Seiden, 1978). I was in psychoanalysis at the time which deepened my perceptions of myself but my analyst was a German male physician who upheld the perceptions of other male physicians. I did not receive a realistic kind of empathy or support and eventually became alienated from him. I became somewhat of an isolationist in my field of psychiatry and experimented with the uses of power in another field. I helped my husband carry out a movement to form a large park in the Santa Monica Mountains. He then decided to run for elective office, and I dropped most of my practice for five months to help him. He won the election and has been a professional politician for sixteen years.

I have learned many things during the sixteen years. I have learned that if one conceptualizes a project well, articulates it clearly, works had and utilizes the access to decision making which is possible in our democracy, one can do a great deal. In 1962, we published a plan for a 25,000 acre park in mountains which few people knew about. Twenty years later it is a national recreational area with 32,000 acres in public ownership and more planned. It has involved the energies of thousands of people who don't even know about its beginnings. I have learned a great deal about political processes, the kinds of people who become politicians, the kinds of pressures under which they operate, and the kinds of approaches which are likely to be effective with them.

I have used my knowledge in various community causes with considerable success. I served on a Narcotics and Dangerous Drug Commission for Los Angeles County and used my office to help establish drug abuse treatment facilities. I was the prime mover in founding and developing a drug abuse treatment agency in my community.

The women's movement gave voice to events which I had experienced as an individual but did not know how to conceptualize or articulate. Once again, the political became the personal when I walked into a feminist women's workshop at a psychological meeting. I felt good. I was at home. I was understood. I spent a weekend meeting with the women psychologists who had given the workshops and I was on my way, reading women's literature and joining women's committees. I co-chaired the women's committee for the Southern California Psychiatric Society, and discovered that it was hard for the woman's committee in an 87% male organization to develop any consistent sense of purpose. We kept falling into some of the same patterns of adapting to male leadership which have impeded our creativity in the past, often with men who wished to be of assistance to us. A big step forward came for me in the APA meeting in San Francisco when a group of women organized a powerful campaign to ask the APA to observe the ERA boycott and cancel its meetings in New Orleans. The campaign was beautifully and powerfully organized. It was a major consciousness raising experience for those of us who participated. In our many organizing meetings we made some important personal discoveries. Many of us had been very lonely and isolated at national meetings. In our sexist tradition men either related to us as sexual objects or avoided us because somebody might think they were relating to us as sexual objects and did not treat us socially as friends and colleagues. We discovered the joys of being with each other and vowed to have women's events and social meetings at future APA meetings.

The re-emergence of women's studies has been momentous for me. Why in a college where John Stuart Mill was revered, did we study "On Liberty" and did not even know that "The Subjection of Women" existed. And why did we not know the wonderful story attached, that he had a long romance with feminist Harriet Taylor,

who he eventually married in a pioneering non-sexist marriage and
whose writings are side by side with his (Mill & Mill, 1970). I
mention this as an example of the discoveries that scholars of
women make. There is now a significant and important literature of
women's studies which has not been incorporated in most of education. Since my own discovery of the woman's movement the dimension of the courage, creativity and scholarship of women have
opened up to me book by book.

My daughter who is a historian wrote a paper on nineteenth century American women and the rise of the gynecology profession and
opened up to me the whole field of the history of women in medicine, both as practitioners and patients. As I studied I understood
the historical and social derivation of the dogmatic attitudes and
practices of the men who had taught gynecology, purporting to
teach scientific truth, and my experiences began to make rational
sense (Ehrenreich & English, 1978; Walsh, 1977).

This has had the impact upon me of a realization that the division
of women's experience into medical specialties creates some artificial kinds of separation into mind, body and social context. I no
longer, for instance, think that I understand the early psychological
experience of an infant without knowing about the actual birth experience for mother and child. I am studying the lives of two women
who have become famous as both creators of social change and as
patients. One is Bertha Pappenheim who created a Jewish feminist
movement in Germany (Kaplan, 1979) and who is also known as
Anna O. in Joseph Breuer's classical case of hysteria (1957). The
other is Charlotte Perkins Gilman, a powerful American feminist
and writer, who was a patient of S. Weir Mitchell and who wrote her
own case history as a small novel called *The Yellow Wallpaper*
(1973). The fact that these women were psychiatric patients in their
young adult lives at a time when their personal aspirations were
denied, and that they emerged from illness into positions of leadership, self expression, and power make them persons of great interest.

This has had two kinds of impact on my practice. It has made me
take up women's battles and has made working with patients much
more enjoyable and productive. Many of the women who come to
me have a depressed and demeaned view of themselves. I can often
perceive clearly how they have simply not appreciated the strength
of their struggles or the reality of their potential. Some come from
prior therapists who persisted in devaluing them. It is a pleasure to

watch them grow and enjoy themselves as they awaken to their own worth and potential.

Right now I am particularly enjoying getting to know a woman in her fifties who had her first mental breakdown as a teenager and has been under almost continuous psychiatric care ever since for depression. She had been seriously beaten by her father as a child. Her prior psychiatrists did much to reinforce her depreciated view of herself. One even had sex with her for several years while he did it, and she did not object. To see this woman gradually awaken to the fact that the same energy she had put into surviving in a depressed and angry way is an asset that she can put into creative activity, and to watch her begin to do this gives me much satisfaction.

The second kind of impact is that I have been asked to take up women's battles in a number of court cases. Some of them have involved the long term consequences of rape or molestation, some have involved sex between psychiatrist and patient, and some have involved custody issues in which the mother was a single professional woman, whose adequacy as a parent was contested when the father remarried and could provide a nuclear family. In most of these situations I have been the therapist first and then called upon by the court to present testimony. To use the rape situation as an example, working with the patient uncovered severe long term consequences to her psyche and ability to function. The few studies available in this area tend to support that this occurs, but the studies are sparse and not fully adequate. Since rape is a common event in our society, why are there not more studies? Each of these cases brings me back to the same concern. Why are not more resources devoted to important problems of women?

My current chapter is a fascination with women physicians. I became active in our local group. We put out a directory of women physicians and began to have meetings. As we discover each other's identities and abilities, we enjoy and strengthen each other. Considering that we are a small minority in our profession with many unique struggles, the strengths and energy of many of the women is amazing. I have been the treasurer of the American Medical Women's Association. I am part of a group that is reorganizing the organization to become a strong voice for women's needs and participation in medicine. I find the women who are active are a remarkable group who have led creative lives in spite of strong difficulties. I enjoy this group in a way that I never enjoyed working in predominantly male medical organizations. I know that we can become much stronger within the medical profession, and that we can be in a key position to use our insights to improve women's health care.

In my adult life my perceptions and energies became somewhat fragmented as I tried to adapt to a world that did not clearly perceive me and my kind. Through women's studies I have been able to reorganize those perceptions in a clear and coherent way. Most of the women's studies of importance are occurring in fields and journals outside of psychiatry and medicine where women have achieved greater access to research tools and positions. I would like to see these studies more fully incorporated into medical and psychiatric teaching and more resources allocated to them within psychiatry and medicine.

It would be logical for me to combine my knowledge of women's studies with my experience in the political arena. I have done so in one area of controversy, which is to write and testify before legislative committees on the medical and psychological consequences of government policies on abortion.

Medicine, including psychiatry, is a powerful political arena. It plays a major role, which is only partially delineated and recognized, in the social control or liberation of women. It can determine or influence government politics. We women need to assert ourselves more fully in this arena. We need to delineate our issues, raise them at every opportunity, and take leadership of them in all of our professional organizations.

Bertha Pappenheim (Anna O.) wrote a prayer with the line, ". . . thanks . . . for the hours when I found words to express the things which touched me, so that I could influence others. To feel power is to live — to live is to desire to serve."

REFERENCES

Breuer, J. & Freud, S. (1957). *Studies on Hysteria*. New York: Basic Books Inc.

Ehrenreich, B. & English, D. (1978). *For Her Own Good*. New York: Anchor Press.

Gilman, C. P. (1973). *The Yellow Wallpaper*. Westbury, NY: Feminist Press.

Kaplan, M. A. (1979). *The Jewish Feminist Movement in Germany*. Westport, CN: Greenwood Press Inc., 30-57.

Mill, J. S. & Mill, H. T. (1970). In A. Ross (Ed.), *Essays on Sex Equality*. Chicago: University of Chicago Press.

Pappenheim, B. *Prayers*. New York: Forcheimer E. Collection of Leo Baeck Institute.

Seiden, A. M. (1978). The sense of mastery in the childbirth experience. In M. T. Notman, C. Nadelson, (Eds.), *The Woman Patient Medical and Psychological Interfaces*. New York: Plenum Publishing Corp.

Walsh, M. R. (1977). *Doctors Wanted. No Women Need Apply*. New Haven, CN: Yale University Press.

Gender and Roles
in a Hospital Setting:
Affiliations or Alienations
Among Women Health
Care Providers

Deanna R. Pearlmutter

INTRODUCTION

Hospitals have traditionally been viewed as the true power base, the castle or home of the physician. Women in hospitals were there to serve the master, or physician, in caring for the sick. Initially this work was done predominately by nurses. Other health professions, and thus professionals, have joined nurses in the hospital setting. These include social workers, psychologists, teachers, dietitians, occupational therapists, recreational therapists, speech therapists, and physical therapists to name but a few. A major proportion of these professionals are also women.

Hospitals will be used as the focus for this paper. However, much of what occurs in a hospital setting is duplicated in other organizational systems and settings because what is really being considered are the dynamics operant in women regardless of the setting. Such dynamics are primarily due to the socialization of women. The resultant attitudes and behaviors, primarily in their interactions with each other, exist in all settings. One theme is power. Three basic concepts regarding power will be employed in exploring the affiliations or alienations among women health professionals. These are: (1) Women do not need to discount other women in order to obtain

The author is Chair of the Psychiatric Nursing Service, Massachusetts General Hospital.

power. (2) The first step in getting power is to resist domination. (3) Women can bring more power to power by not using it inappropriately. Ways women do deal with each other in light of these concepts are important to consider.

In talking about health care, one usually refers to the health care team. In this context a team is a group of people each of whom possesses particular expertise and each of whom is responsible for making individual decisions. Together they hold a common purpose. The health care team meets together to communicate, collaborate, and consolidate knowledge from which plans are made, actions determined, and future decisions influenced. This definition of a team infers an equal relationship among team members. Speaking of her work with families, Virginia Satir once commented that whenever there was some dysfunction, the relationship always followed some form of hierarchy. Never did she see equality. However, introducing equality healed the relationship.

Perhaps that simple intervention should be the message of this paper. Women health professionals must first view each other with respect for one another's knowledge and position. One aspect of feminism is equal rights and opportunities at work. Women together are strong. But, women in the health care professions haven't been together. And, they haven't been strong. Certainly there is the power issue and problems of status and authority. These are evident in professional isolation/identification; competition in peer relationships; and difficulties in establishing authority relationships.

In the health care field there are many shared areas of responsibility and accountability. But the structure also designates specific responsibilities and areas of accountability. These boundaries expedite team functioning and prevent role diffusion and confusion. For example, in a psychiatric setting one might find nurses, social workers, psychologists, activity therapists, and psychiatrists who all have responsibility for "psychotherapy." However, when looking at specific responsibilities, the nurses focus on the milieu and nursing care; the social worker focuses on family care work; the psychologist does psychological testing; and the psychiatrist has responsibility for medical care. All comprise the health care team.

Nursing is a "female" profession yet the administrative positions within nursing are often held by men. It is true that many men and even women are reluctant to be subordinate to a female. Social and cultural mores condition women so that they have a difficult time seeing themselves as hierarchical superiors to both men and women. Women have been kept in relatively powerless roles. They have been valued for their "nurturing" which is viewed as female. Thus when in a position of authority they face a major discrepancy between learned social requirements and the requirements of their position. This contradiction is also confusing to subordinates. Respect for position and credentials conflicts with socially conditioned expectations for female behavior and status. Thus such women are often labelled as "cold and hard" while a man in a similar position is most apt to be viewed as "ambitious and industrious." Nurses are often criticized for their deference but there are reasons for such behaviors. First of all, most physicians are male and most nurses are female. The socialization process is difficult to reverse. Secondly, I place blame on nursing educators for their selection and socialization of students. Too often the very ones most needed to effect change are culled out before they graduate because they are too questioning or rebellious. Third is level of education and social class. It is fairly recent for nursing education to occur in the academic setting. It was formerly thought of as a field with social mobility for women from lower socioeconomic groups, who sometimes brought with them low self-esteem and poor academic backgrounds, which their nursing training had not improved.

Certainly the women's movement has had an impact. Beliefs regarding the role of women have changed. Peer relationships have been established with other health disciplines as practice roles expand and autonomy increases.

Certainly the problem of the non-physician/physician relationship has exacerbated as the status of women in society has changed. Predominately female staffs in hospitals are asking for more rights and responsibilities from predominately male physicians and administrators. But, predictably, attempts to change the role of the nurse have met with resistance from both outside and within the nursing profession.

There are personal qualities vital to interdisciplinary team functioning. These are:

1. Being able to accept and tolerate differences and different perspectives of others — including members of your own discipline.
2. Being able to function interdependently.
3. Being able to trust the knowledge and abilities of others.
4. Being able to negotiate roles with other team members.

5. Being able to be problem- or patient-oriented, rather than status- and profession-oriented.
6. Being able to form new values, attitudes, and perceptions.
7. Being able to tolerate constant review and challenge of ideas.
8. Being able to be a risk taker.
9. Being able to accept a team philosophy of care.
10. Possessing personal identity and integrity.

Before women can conquer the corporate world of hospitals, they need to have a greater understanding of themselves. Acceptance of women in positions of organizational authority has been slow and occurs at different rates according to hierarchical levels. Acceptance has been greater at the lower levels of authority and least at the higher levels of authority. It is still very common for Directors of Nursing, especially if female, to be without voice and vote on hospital boards.

Power is an issue for women by virtue of the fact that women have very little of it. For centuries women have been taught to consider themselves powerless relative to men and societal forces. Most women have yet to discover their ability to handle power. They are reluctant to take control. Power implies control. Traditionally this has meant male domination and control of women. Power can also mean the ability to control oneself. Women need to take the initiative for this rather than waiting to be asked to share the power with physicians and hospital administrators. Women who are successful in using power expect to be treated as equals. Women are finally coming into their own: rising in power as well as developing new modes of power strategy. There are power strategies that women must know. Included would be power coalitions, power caucuses, power shifts, power cliques, and power games. A firm foundation is needed. This can be gained by:

1. Developing interpersonal and persuasive techniques.
2. Building group alliances and coalitions.
3. Choosing proper leadership styles.
4. Taking risks and learning confrontation/negotiation techniques.
5. Phasing out ineffective leaders.

Nurses have traditionally felt powerless versus physicians who have felt themselves all powerful. Lewis Thomas (1983), in his book *The Youngest Science: Notes of a Medicine Watcher,* speaks of nurses' professional "feud" with doctors, their wish to have their professional status enhanced, and doctors being infuriated by their claims to be equal professionals. Dr. Thomas ends by stating that he is on the nurses' side. Challenging interaction with other professionals is frequently as necessary to creative work as is the opportunity for solitude and thought. The one minority group behavior which is rarely seen among women is the strengthening of in-group ties. This is needed.

A survey of female resident physicians yielded some interesting data. The residents reports as "helpful" interactions with "outstanding" women from other professions. Such interactions occurred most often at national meetings. but, interactions with females from other professions in their own institutions were not of note.

It would be helpful for women to stop taking "assistant" titles. This is important in order to effect a cultural image change from subordinate servant. Thus women must learn to: (1) Deal with bureaucratic mechanisms. (2) Deal with the diverse needs of the allied health professions. (3) Compete within a new setting. (4) Define their role in the organization. (5) Determine how to gain and use power and authority.

Why hasn't this happened? There are psychological characteristics common in oppressed minorities. And, women are an oppressed minority. The work socialization of women does not encourage achievement and competition. Women are competitive with each other because their power is often considered to be dependent on their personal or physical attributes rather than their skill or competence. Power is not viewed as a universally available resource which all can tap and share. Rather, power is viewed as a sum-zero commodity. If one person has power, another must lose it.

Women enter the power system of the hospital with in-grained gender-role socialization handicaps. They relate to power differently than men. Because of their female mental set regarding power, female nurses often sabotage nursing as a whole in order to feel adequate as individuals. One sees the class "pecking order" emerge. When the exercise of power is thwarted or blocked, and one is rendered powerless in the larger arena, a power hierarchy is established where one does have some control, i.e., over subordinates. It is interesting that nurses leave for medicine, social work, or psychology to name most common career shifts. But, rarely do people in these fields leave them for nursing.

Both powerless women and powerful women react against their own colleagues. Women in power often feel precarious and insecure because they have risen through a system wherein power may have been acquired through covert and often subversive styles. Women frequently adopt the style of male leaders as one means of securing their positions. Women learn the lessons of any minority. They admire and emulate the power group while mistrusting themselves. Approval of the higher status group is most important to the second-class group. Thus they tend to tear down one another rather than the dominant group. This is common among professional women, particularly those who have achieved high status. Denying membership in their own female group, such women take on the attitudes of men which include negative attitudes about women.

It has been said there is a narcissistic fit between medicine and nursing. Identifying features of a narcissistic relationship or system involves three major ingredients: (1) an overvaluing of one part of the system; (2) simultaneous devaluing of another; (3) intolerance for any difference or separateness among the parts. Traditionally medicine has been overvalued and nursing has been undervalued. Nursing sought refuge in merging with medicine and thus becoming the handmaiden or narcissistic extension of physicians. Nurses must gain strength from within by learning to cultivate an affirmative sense of their own value.

The obstacles of sexual discrimination in the work world are multiplied by women's socialization and attitudes toward themselves. Three major destructive self-perceptions of women's socialization are:

1. Inability to make a full commitment to a career. The professional role of the female-dominated professions is most compatible with the female gender role. Teaching, nursing, and social work are viewed as semi-professions by many. They are preparation for marriage or "something to fall back on." Nursing often refers to "appliance" nurses. These are women who go to work for money to buy a refrigerator, stove, and/or dishwasher! Thus it is assumed that women are more committed to feminine role responsibilities than to a career. This certainly helps prevent disruption of the currently male-dominated occupational and familial systems.

2. Women are in competition with one another. Two factors contribute to such competition. These are territoriality and the fact that

women are comfortable competing with other women. They are socialized to be in competition with other women for the attention of men. Thus they learn *not* to help one another. This has probably been why women had a tendency not to act as colleagues with or mentors for other women.

Gilligan (1982), in her book *In a Different Voice,* describes how men learn to argue issues while remaining effective teammates in order to accomplish a goal. Women, on the other hand, interpret differences of opinion as a form of personal rejection and divide over issues into separate camps. Thus they withdraw and form new cliques rather than dealing with conflicts and resolving them. Because women are often insecure and discontented with themselves, they have little esteem for others like themselves. Such insecurity emerges in women fighting defensively rather than supporting each other. Women may fail to seek support, affirmation, and/or guidance from other women because they fear making themselves vulnerable to colleagues whom they distrust and underrate. Thus competition and distrust among women prevent their meeting their personal needs for mutual support and their professional needs for unity. Social workers tend to have a strong group identification. Although this is supportive, it can also lead to greater aggressiveness and territoriality in relation to other disciplines.

3. Women are less valued than men. The socialization of women is key in their development and later beliefs. Female children are often less desirable. From birth, girls and boys are treated differently. Girls learn to be passive and dependent. They have problems with self-esteem. Thus girls desire things *male*—not just a penis. Girls need to identify with other females, especially mother. But, it's hard to identify with what is not valued. Ambivalence, low self-esteem and a disparaging attitude to one's own kind develops. Gender-typing reflects gender-ranking. Men's work, whatever it is, tends to be more highly regarded. Women's work has lower prestige and lower financial compensation. Achievement counts for less when it occurs in a primarily female, gender-typed occupation.

Women in health professions face the same opposition and discrimination that all women in society face. But, these women are in double-jeopardy. They are women in a male-dominated society *and* female professionals in a male-dominated health care delivery system. Nurses are viewed by the health care bureaucracy as powerless, predominately white, middle-class females thought to be submissive, docile, and pleased to be governed by men.

One might expect that the stress of professional training would generate a camaraderie of support and sharing amongst women. But strangely, the reverse is true. Consider, the prejudice frequently developed by women physicians toward another woman's professional performance. In trying to forge a professional identity in a masculine field, women may find themselves absorbing the prejudices that exist against their own gender and thus they devalue the competence of other women. Many women enter medical school with negative self-images, and feeling less adequate than men. These feelings are projected onto their female peers. Thus they then believe no woman can be as competent as a man. Studies of the female "fear of success" and books such as *The Cinderella Complex* (Dowling, 1985) support this theory. This unfortunate phenomenon occurs at a time when women could benefit from supporting each other and sharing their common experiences.

Although the Women's Movement has resulted in the development of support systems and feelings of camaraderie among many women who previously felt isolated and insulated from one another, much work has yet to be done. Most nursing leaders already network to make professional contacts and gain more resources. But, these networking skills are seldom used to form supportive, sharing relationships. There is still more competition than cooperation at the top of nursing's ladder.

Support systems for women which encourage collaboration are one means of keeping women from turning against one another. Men are good team players. They stick together. Women are stereotyped as not sticking together. Peer alliances, that work through the exchange of favors, are often neglected in the striving of women for power. Men are good at collecting such "chits."

Facilitating the good performance of others and affording them opportunities for recognition provides a climate of good will which, in turn, increases power. Such behavior requires that one view power as an entitlement all may share and enjoy. It is not a sum-zero commodity. If all members of the health care system experience a sense of power, the effectiveness of the group as a whole is enhanced. Colleague behaviors must be fostered. These include showing competence, giving feedback, recognizing skills and competencies of one another, showing respect for one another, and consulting with one another.

Women health care professionals need to form networks with one another. We need to form ties and become colleagues and resources to women in fields other than our own. We cannot afford to be isolated. We must share information, problems, solutions, and hopes. We need to help one another manage the stresses and frustrations engendered by the patriarchal systems in which we find ourselves. Such behaviors serve to strengthen in-group ties.

Sisterhood *is* powerful.

REFERENCES

Dowling, C. (1985). *The Cinderella Complex*. New York: Pocketbooks.
Gilligan, C. (1982). *In a Different Voice*. Cambridge: Harvard University Press.
Thomas, L. (1983). *The Youngest Science: Notes of a Medicine Watcher*. New York: Bantam Books.

The Emotional Consequences of Gender-Based Abuse in the Workplace: New Counseling Programs for Sex Discrimination

Jean A. Hamilton
Sheryle W. Alagna
Linda S. King
Camille Lloyd

Health programs for women will be improved when specific gender-related health risks and treatment needs are better identified (Hamilton, 1985). One type of life crisis that disproportionately affects women is gender-based abuse (Carmen, Russo & Miller, 1981). The spectrum of gender-based abuse encompasses physical and sexual violence against women (Russell, 1984), as well as the psychological abuse of unequal and devalued social roles and employment discrimination. Women are the primary victims of all forms of gender-based abuse. There is speculation that gender-based abuse is related to the excess of depression in women as compared to men (cf. Carmen et al., 1981; Russo, 1985; Weissman & Klerman, 1977).

In recent years, health care providers have more closely examined the emotional correlates and consequences of certain specific

Jean A. Hamilton is a psychiatrist in private practice, and Scientific Director, Institute for Research on Women's Health (IRWH). Sheryle W. Alagna is a psychologist and Associate Professor, Medical Psychology, Uniformed Services University of the Health Sciences, Bethesda, Maryland. Linda S. King is a clinical social worker in private practice and IRWH, Washington, DC. Camille Lloyd is a psychologist and Director of Student Counseling Services, University of Texas Health Science Center, Houston.

forms of abuse, including rape, battering and incest. However, one area of abuse that has received much less attention, in terms of the identification of health risk and treatment needs, is sexual harassment and the other forms of sex discrimination that occur frequently in the workplace. The purpose of this paper is to clarify what we know — and what we do not know — about the psychological correlates and consequences of gender-based discrimination in the workplace. The implications for future research, and for developing new treatment programs for women will be discussed.

BACKGROUND

Employment discrimination on the basis of sex was originally added to the 1964 Civil Rights Act in order to sabotage the Act by making it appear ridiculous to Congress (Pendergrass, Kimmel, Joesling, Petersen & Bush, 1976). The courts now recognize, however, that discrimination in the workplace is expressed in differential hiring, work or training assignments, promotions, salary (Dolkart, 1983), and by other forms of disparate treatment such as the conditions of work or work-related training (Shapiro, 1983; Wolman & Frank, 1975; Women in Computer Science at MIT, 1983).

In 1980, the Equal Employment Opportunity Commission (EEOC) issued final guidelines regarding sexual harassment as one specific type of employment discrimination. Harassment on the basis of sex consists of unwelcome sexual advances, requests for sexual favors and other verbal or physical conduct of a sexual nature, as these occur under specified conditions affecting employment (cf. Simon & Crocker, 1983). As shown in Table I, specific forms of sexual harassment, listed roughly in order of increasing severity, include: pressure for dates, sexually suggestive words or gestures, and sexual remarks, deliberate touching, pressure for sexual favors, letters and calls, and actual or attempted rape or assault (U.S. Merit Systems Protection Board, 1981; discussions of sexual harassment in educational settings are beyond the scope of this paper but are available elsewhere).

Perhaps because it is more easily identified and measured than other types of discrimination, the mental health literature has focused almost exclusively on sexual harassment. (The exception has to do with discussions of sex-discrimination in *academia*.) Conse-

Table I

Forms of Sexual Harassment*

A. Less severe

1. pressure for dates (55%)
2. sexually suggestive looks or gestures (73%)
3. sexual teasing, jokes, remarks, questions (77%)

B. Severe

4. letters, phone calls, or materials of a sexual
   nature (42%)
5. pressure for sexual favors (52%)
6. deliberate touching, leaning over, cornering,
   pinching (62%)

C. Most Severe

7. actual or attempted rape or assault (20%)

D. Others (e.g.; "Quid Pro Quo" in the workplace, where a
   women who sleeps with the boss obtains advantages, while
   similarly situated women are less advantaged).

Other Forms of Employment Discrimination

(e.g., disparate treatment, or discrimination in the
conditions of work include but are not limited to:
exclusion from social or peer networks in which
business occurs, information is shared, or decisions
are made; inappropriate or differential work assignments; differential assignment of resources or
assistance).

* Severity and percents for females, from U.S. Merit
Systems Protection Board, 1981.

quently, much of the data cited here will pertain to sexual harassment, although we are also interested in the many other forms of
employment discrimination that have received less research attention. In fact, our clinical experience leads us to believe that sexual
harassment is merely more obvious, overall—whereas other types
of employment discrimination may occur together or independently,
but may be of greater harm.

Despite legal efforts over the past fifteen years to improve the
status of women in the workplace, women's jobs continue to have

low status, little autonomy or opportunity for growth, and generally low pay (cf. Fuchs, 1986; Kanter, 1981; Women's Bureau, 1984). Although some believe that sex discrimination is a thing of the past, others believe that discrimination has merely been "modernized": i.e., it is less blatant, and more subtle and covert (Benokraitis, 1986). The persistence of discrimination is perhaps best summarized in a single statistic: women usually make around 60 cents on the dollar, compared to men (Fuchs, 1986).

METHODS

We have reviewed much of the legal, sociological, educational, and mental health literature pertinent to gender-based abuse in the workplace. Additionally, we refer to our informal and clinical experiences (J.H., L.S.K., C.L.) with more than 34 women. This group included: (1) ten female patients who believed themselves to be the victims of some type of employment discrimination on the basis of sex, but who did *not* file a formal complaint; (2) eight female patients who filed some type of formal complaint based on sex discrimination; (3) group discussions in 1982 with nine women members of the "NIH Committee for Women in Research," as well as discussions with other participants at the Workshop on Clinical Research Careers for Women, sponsored by the National Institute for Child Health and Human Development in 1984 (J.H.), and with other colleagues; and (4) seven women who identified themselves as victims of employment discrimination on the basis of sex and who filed complaints. The 34 women, aged about 22-55 years, were employed in a wide variety of occupations, ranging from "white" to "pink" (secretarial/clerical) collar types of employment.

We believe that our participation as facilitators (J.H. and L.K.) for the latter group, which identifies itself as the "Complainant's Support Group," provides a unique addition to the literature in this area. Although this was not a treatment group, per se, we will briefly discuss our understanding of this group from a clinical perspective.

And finally, we have begun to collect reports of symptomatology in self-identified victims of employment discrimination as confirmed by various assessments (e.g., attorney evaluations), using standardized, clinical research measures. These measures include a symptom checklist, the SCL-90 (Derogatis & Cleary, 1977); a screening measure for depression, the CES-D (Weissman & Myers, 1978); and a measure of Post Traumatic Stress Disorder, the "Reaction Index, (A) Adult Form" (Frederick, 1985). Only very preliminary data is available from this ongoing study.

PREVALENCE

The only systematic data on prevalence is for sexual harassment. Despite methodological flaws that include non-random subject selection and differences in severity and definition of cases (e.g., lifetime vs. point prevalence over differing time periods), we have reason to believe that verbal and physical sexual harassment is widespread (Safran, 1976), with risk estimates for women ranging from about 40-90%. Perhaps the best data on prevalence comes from a carefully designed, random-sample survey of Federal government employees in 1981, where 42% of the approximate 10,648 women responding (representing 694,000 federally employed women, with an 85% overall return rate) reported that they had been sexually harassed on the job in the two years immediately prior to the survey (U.S. Merit Systems Protection Board, 1981). In the U.S. Merit Systems Study (1981), 62% of women had experienced *severe* sexual harassment (e.g., deliberate touching), and 20% reported actual or attempted rape or assault. Unfortunately, we know virtually nothing about the prevalence of other types of employment discrimination.

SERIOUSNESS

As MacKinnon (1979) observed, even if sexual harassment — as one example of gender-based abuse in the workplace — was not prevalent, it might still be a serious problem. Given the actual prevalence, however, we are particularly concerned by the neglect of this topic in the psychiatric literature. This neglect appears to stem partly from the erroneous belief that gender-based abuse in the workplace is an insignificant life event. For example, the psychiatrist Chief of a National Institute of Mental Health (NIMH) administrative unit, remarked that women might be "demoralized" by employment discrimination, but not "depressed" (Personal Communication to J.H., 1984).

The trivialization of sex discrimination by mental health professionals is documented anecdotally by a series of recent, informal discussions with four other NIMH clinical researchers. These individuals failed to see, or else specifically denied the connections between: (1) routinely calling women stereotyped, derogatory names in a professional work setting; (2) discriminatory attitudes or behaviors; and (3) a hostile work environment. It is alarming that these clinicians do not understand that attitudes are reflected in gender-stereotyped words, and that descriptions of personality in women often reflect gender-related stereotypes.

That these attitudes intrude in therapy is documented by the report of an NIH female physician who was severely physically and verbally harassed on the basis of sex. Her career was threatened by her male physician supervisor. When she sought advice from an NIMH staff psychiatrist, she was told: to pull up her hair, to wear glasses, and to appear less attractive — as if she were provoking the man's illegal behavior. This type of victim-blaming advice is similar to that once given to rape victims, but it has long been known to be inappropriate, ineffective, and harmful.

Despite these unfortunate blind-spots and biases among the "experts," who are entrusted to perform research on women's mental health and who offer women psychiatric treatment, what women actually report is that discrimination has severe and far-reaching consequences. In one study, using a non-randomly selected sample, 42% of the victims of sexual harassment reported leaving jobs where they were harassed, either because they were unable to stop the harassment, or because they were retaliated against for complaining. Another 24% of that sample had been fired as a result. This means that 66% (2/3) of that group of women were driven out of at least one job by sexual harassment (Working Women's Institute, 1978). Even with a random-sample, 9% of women (projected to total 24,660 persons) reported changing jobs under adverse circumstances in association with sexual harassment, and another 16% reported suffering in terms of side-effects, such as adverse working conditions, or diminished opportunities for advancement (U.S. Merit Systems Protection Board, 1981). Some degree of *emotional distress* is reported by up to 96% of sexual harassment victims (Working Women's Institute, 1975), and a variety of sexual harassment related stress effects have been documented (Crull, 1982; Gutek, 1985).

For the individual women who leave jobs under duress, the costs include: loss of income, loss of seniority, a disrupted work history, problems with references for future jobs; and, there is often a failure to qualify for unemployment benefits, at the same time that a loss of confidence interferes with seeking another job.

Research confirms that the life changes commonly associated with sexual harassment, as one type of employment discrimination, can have harmful sequelae. As shown in Table II, the 43-item "Social Readjustment Scale" (Holmes 1978; Masuda & Holmes, 1967), includes eight items (nearly 20%) that pertain to employment. Based on rankings of "life changes" associated with these

Table II

Employment-related Items from The
Social Readjustment Rating Scale

Number	Life Event	Mean Value (Life Change Unit)	Comparable Event in terms of LCU
31.	Major change in working hours or conditions	20	like a change in residence (20)
30.	Troubles with the boss	23	
32.	Major change in responsibilities at work (e.g., promotion, demotion, lateral transfer)	29	like foreclosure on a mortgage or loan (30)
18.	Changing to a different line of work	36	
16.	Major change in financial state (e.g., a lot worse off, a lot better off than usual)	38	like one death of a close friend (37)
15.	Major business readjustment (e.g., merger, reorganization, bankruptcy, etc.)	39	
10.	Retirement from work	45	
8.	Being fired at work	47	

events by large numbers of people, it has been shown that greater life change units (LCU) are moderately linked to the subsequent occurrence of illness (cf. Raskin & Struening, 1976, however for methodological concerns; and, newer instruments may better evaluate stressors in women's lives). Based on the life changes reported above, a total of about 161 LCU would be commonly associated with sexual harassment (e.g., #31, 32 and 22 or 18, and 16 or 15, and 10 or 8). This level of change is defined as a *mild life crisis*, and one study suggests that this level of change may be associated with adverse health affects in 37% of subjects (see also Tabor, 1982; and Crull, 1982, 1984, on the stress of sexual harassment as one form of employment discrimination). Especially for women who are deeply committed to their careers, severe employment discrimination is likely to be as stressful as a divorce, a major illness (Pendergrass et al., 1976), or other (with LCUs of 73 and 53, respectively).

Alternatively, the severity of psychosocial stressors are routinely indicated on Axis IV of the DSM-III. These ratings are based on the clinician's assessments of the stress experienced by the "average" person in similar circumstances. Based on the guides for making these ratings, on a scale from 1-7 (1 = none, and 7 = catastrophic), we believe that workplace abuse would commonly warrant ratings of severe to extreme (5-6); moreover, both occupational and legal, as well as abuse-related stressors, are recognized in DSM-III ratings (American Psychiatric Association, 1980).

SPECIFIC SYMPTOMATOLOGY

In order to bring the negative consequences of gender-based abuse in the workplace into the mainstream mental health literature, we must clarify the type, severity, and duration of sexual harassment and other employment discrimination-related symptoms in relation to the symptoms of medically recognized disorders. Unfortunately, discrimination-related symptomatology has not yet been adequately assessed. Where systematic data is available, it is again restricted to sexual harassment. For example, in the U.S. Merit Systems Protection Board (1981) random-sample study, 21-82% of women reported that their "emotional or physical condition" worsened, depending on the severity of sexual harassment. However, the survey did not assess specific symptoms in a more detailed way.

As evidence of the likely seriousness of sexual harassment-related symptoms, we have summarized the findings from a variety of less controlled and non-clinical surveys. Although ratings of *severity* are not available, the *types* of symptoms, such as feeling frightened, angry, helpless, guilty, along with somatic symptoms, and difficulty concentrating—are of serious concern to mental health professionals (Safran, 1976; Working Women's Institute, 1975, 1979). These and additional sources (e.g., Silverman, 1976/1977; Wehrli, 1976; Crull, 1984) document, at least anecdotally, that the emotional consequences or correlates of sexual harassment include almost all of the types of symptoms required to diagnose a "Major Depressive Episode" (American Psychiatric Association, DSM-III, 1980, see Table III).

For these reasons, we believe that some women suffer clinically significant emotional symptoms as a result of gender-based abuse in

Table III

On the Likelihood that Employment-related
Symptoms are Clinically Significant

Abridged
Diagnostic Criteria:

Major Depressive Episode	Symptoms Reported by Victims of Sexual Harassment
A. Dysphoric Mood <u>or</u> Loss of Interest . . . in usually activities or pastimes. (e.g., depressed, sad, blue, hopeless, low, down in the dumps, irritable).	+
B. At least four of the following (present nearly every day for at least two weeks).	
1. poor appetite or weight loss	.+
2. increased or decreased sleep	.+
3. psychomotoractivity, increased or decreased	.?
4. loss of interest or pleasure or decreased sexual drive.	.+
5. loss of energy; fatigue.	.+
6. feeling of worthlessness, guilt.	.+
7. decreased concentration.	.+
8. thoughts of death.	.?
C.-E. Rule-out other disorders.	.?

the workplace. The occurrence of clinical depression has been documented in relation to another type of gender-based abuse, rape (Frank & Stewart, 1983). The psychological impact of social and situational factors in women's lives is further discussed by Russo and others (1985).

The hypothesis of post-discrimination depression needs further evaluation, however, since at present there is too little symptom-specific empirical data from which to draw firm conclusions. While only preliminary data from our ongoing study are currently available, the CES-D measure of depression and the SCL-90 symptom checklist support our impression that the type and severity of reported symptoms are of clinical significance.

HOW WOMEN ARE HARMED BY EMPLOYMENT DISCRIMINATION

Some experts have assumed that women cannot be seriously harmed by verbal harassment and by other forms of discrimination in the workplace as long as these experiences fall short of physical violence. Besides ignoring the bulk of psychiatric theory about emotional harm, this perspective ignores the subordinate social role status and the continued devaluation of women in our society. That is, sexual harassment and other forms of gender-based employment discrimination are manifestations of, and reminders to women of their ascribed social roles (cf. Evans, 1985). In addition to reinforcing women's social roles, gender-based abuse in the workplace serves as a threat as to the consequences of deviation from those roles.

We have found a victimization model to be useful in understanding the effects of workplace abuse on women's mental health. There is a growing body of knowledge about common responses to sudden trauma, whether by crime or by natural disaster. Many victims exhibit a post-trauma syndrome characterized by shock, emotional numbing, constriction of affect, reliving by waking or sleeping images, and by other manifestations of anxiety or depression.

The symptoms of post-traumatic stress disorder (American Psychiatric Association, 1980) are present in some victims of severe sex discrimination (Titchener, 1986). Especially for the 20% of women who experience actual or attempted rape or assault on the job (U.S. Merit Systems Protection Board, 1981), flashbacks are not uncommon. As examples, one of the victims of Employment

Discrimination in the "Complainant's Support Group" was sexually assaulted at work, leading to a seriously injured arm and it was not unexpected for her to have flashbacks; and a patient's white-collar employer screamed at her abusively and threatened to hit her in the workplace, a financial institution, when she refused a date with him — subsequently, she experienced recurrent nightmares of this event.

Certain aspects of the victimization of women may be relatively specific or unique to the trauma of gender-based abuse. The key to understanding the more specific aspects of harm comes from recognizing the internalization of social stereotypes and prejudices that devalue women, along with the subsequent activation of these attitudes by victimization. As a normative aspect of women's psychological development in this society the learned, self-devaluation tends to engender low self-esteem, self-doubt and a reliance on the opinions of others.

The internalized psychological oppression is reinforced by threats of physical or sexual violence, which are so prevalent as to be normative life experiences. For example, in a randomized sample of 930 women, Russell (1984) found that 44% were the victims of rape or attempted rape, and that 38% were the victims of at least one incestuous or extrafamilial experience of child sexual abuse before the age of 18 years. Psychologically, these experiences come to represent the societal prediction of what we can expect, and of who we are, and what we *deserve*, as women: i.e., to be used, devalued, and humiliated. A sense of unworthiness may thus become part of the organizing nucleus of women's self-esteem, and may contribute to the unconscious background of our experiences in the workplace. Moreover, because sexuality is such a private experience, all forms of sexualized-abuse are likely to be deeply humiliating, which creates a conflict between getting help and keeping the secret.

THE REALIZATION OF HARM
BY DISCRIMINATION

Because sexual harassment and other forms of employment discrimination are so prevalent, these experiences are likely to fade into the background of our lives as women at work. Since we as women have also been taught to devalue our talents (Roos, Gaumont & Colwell, 1977), and to lower our expectations, the realization that we have experienced even *profound* discrimination is often slow in coming. Instead of conceptualizing our experiences as "discrimination," most women initially report confusion and bewilderment (cf. Bumiller, 1984; Crosby, 1982; Crull, 1984; Nielson, 1982). Many women react with disbelief and resist accepting what appears to be extremely irrational. Isolation and a lack of validation and reality-based feedback also undermine trust in one's own perceptions. The victim's minimization or denial interferes with taking action, and, inadvertently colludes with the aggressor/discriminator. For example, the discriminator will likely explain what has happened as a "joke," an "oversight," or the result of a "budget cut," and so on. The woman will have a vested interest in affirming the discriminator's point of view, because it is so dangerous to realize that those you depend on are not benevolent or trustworthy.

A specific incident such as an unexpected termination or nonrenewal, or a lack of promotion may finally spark a woman's anger. As Pendergrass and her colleagues (1976) have observed, a woman often decides to fight when she realizes that there is nothing else to lose. Unfortunately, women are left fighting from a position of weakness, not strength. This situation reaffirms the fact that women generally respond from a socially disadvantaged position.

Once the realization of *profound* discrimination sinks in, there is generally the gradual recognition of a large number of inequities that occurred previously but were deflected. In addition to experiencing isolation and confusion, the woman may begin to understand the price she's paid for working in a discriminatory environment: the cumulative erosion of her self-confidence by inappropriate negative or stereotypic feedback about herself as a woman and the absence of the ordinary positive feedback received by her co-workers who are not being subjected to discrimination. The acute effects of activating the accumulated pain and rage may give rise to emotional flooding and disorganized behavior. The heightened awareness of harm is a mixed blessing because it is often accompanied by a profound sense of disillusionment, guilt, and despair.

In order to survive once the realization of harm occurs, the woman must rely on protective mechanisms that include renewed efforts at denial and the suppression of affect. One reaction to her own increased sensitivity to the chronic abuses she formerly overlooked, will be to try viewing these incidents in isolation, as if each act of discrimination really did occur separately — out of the context of the overall pattern of the abuse, and apart from women's devalued social role.

At this point—because of the despair and efforts at denial—the woman's controls are likely to be erratic. It is common for a woman to express extreme ambivalence. She may both curse the unfair way she's treated, and alternately discredit her own abilities (cf. Pendergrass et al., 1976). There are few, if any, role models for successfully responding to severe discrimination (cf. Miller, 1976, for a discussion of subordinate role status; Sparks & Bar On, 1985). The woman is in a difficult situation: being a victim she can't afford to act like one. To appear victimized (even hypersensitive or irritable) is risky because it may be taken by crucial decisionmakers or potential supporters as evidence that the woman is not suffering from discrimination, but that she is really incompetent, and deserves whatever she gets.

REACTIONS TO DISCRIMINATION MAY APPEAR TO JUSTIFY THE ABUSE

The "Catch-22" in gender-based employment discrimination is that reactions to the discrimination may appear to justify the abuse. The *internalized* devaluation of ourselves as women is furthered by victimization, and runs along several lines. After all, haven't we all been "warned" to stay at home; or that we as women "couldn't" succeed" in certain fields? Since we don't deserve much and we get what we deserve, we come to feel responsible for our own pain and "unrealistic expectations." Further, we are trained to feel responsible, as nurturers, for the behavior of men, and to wonder why we couldn't "handle" whatever happened. The resultant self-doubt and blame give rise to guilt and humiliation, which are draining and demoralizing.

A central issue becomes the woman's sense of control. If we believe that we are being harmed irrationally, then we may feel even more helpless and out of control. One alternative is to believe that the abuse is justified—then at least it appears "rational"; and perhaps we could learn to change it. One way to achieve a sense of control is through identification with the aggressor.

The stress of being devalued internally *and* externally, by powerful authorities, can push intelligent, rational, and otherwise well-functioning women to an extreme crisis of self-doubt. Consider the following hypothetical example:

One woman in academics was told that she was denied a promotion because she had not produced a single publication. In fact, she knew rationally that she had more than ten relevant publications, which was greater than average for similarly situated males. Yet she tearfully spent night after sleepless night sorting through the *reprints* of her actual publications, rechecking the dates and authorship, trying to hold on to the very reality of her perceptions that she indeed had publications.

In this example, the woman's work was devalued to the point of *invisibility* in the eyes of powerful authorities.

The hypothetical example described above may appear extreme, and the reader may find it *hard to believe* that this kind of reaction occurs in an otherwise well-functioning woman. But we believe that the example is both fair and representative of: (1) the extraordinary *irrationality* that fuels and maintains gender-based discrimination, and (2) of women's difficulty in coping with the profound self-doubt that it engenders (cf. Nielsen, 1982; Raymond, 1982). The first step forward is for each of us to overcome our disbelief.

Ironically, the hypothetical example would probably be easier to handle than many situations of actual discrimination because the "lie" in our example was so clear and concrete. An even more insidious assault, would have been for the discriminator(s) to admit to a few of the woman's publications, but to label them as mediocre — which would be much more difficult to refute.

Taken together, all of these processes begin to undermine the victim's actual performance. The woman's ambivalence, intermittent denial, and self-doubt heighten her struggle to suppress the rage and to protect herself by continuing to perform her job. It requires tremendous self-respect to function at work — rather than to cry out in pain and indignation. This is true especially at a time when one's self-esteem is under attack.

The woman feels powerless or helpless because the feedback is not contingent on her actual performance (Peterson & Seligman, 1983). Her job satisfaction and ambition are eroded and she may begin to question her career choice as well as her abilities. To some extent, the self-doubt that is set in motion by the discrimination functions as a self-fulfilling prophecy. Even if a woman maintains adequate performance at work, it is accomplished only with a great deal of effort, at an enormous personal cost, as expressed in stress-related symptoms.

THE IMPOSSIBLE DECISION:
CHOOSING BETWEEN THE FRYING PAN AND THE FIRE?

To the extent that women have a decision about discrimination, it is fundamentally a choice between miserable alternatives: to speak out, and become a pariah, or to suffer in silence. To choose between alternatives such as the "frying pan" versus the "fire" has been called a non-choice, choice. In the words of a woman who settled a sexual harassment case out of court:

> I felt like I was standing on the 15th floor of a burning building . . . I had a choice of standing there and being eaten by the flames or jumping out of the window and maybe ending up dead or very injured or walking away alive. I had to jump. I just had to. I could not stay there and be eaten by the flames. (Rosenberg, 1985)

In addition to the more tangible losses, there is also the loss of one's actual *job performance* as a result of being literally handicapped in the workplace. Especially for professionals or other women who are highly invested in their work, this may mount to lost ideas, programs, discoveries, and publications.

And then there are the non-tangible losses; the loss of confidence in one's abilities; the loss of enthusiasm in seeking another job, as one has now become sensitized to discrimination and dreads encountering it again. And ultimately, there is lost time, living through a crisis that often consumes years of one's life. These losses must be *mourned*, regardless of whatever action one decides to take or not take.

From our experience with the Complainant's Support Group, we have observed that the victims who speak up feel that it is their only choice, as though a level of injustice has been reached that can't be ignored. A sense of *integrity* is what seems to drive the complaint process. The problem with speaking up is that about half of the complaints provoke negative responses, such as retaliation, and half fall on deaf ears (cf. Crull, 1984, Evans, 1985). The emotional costs of pursuing a complaint are high (Boring, 1982), perhaps even higher than those ensuing from the original abuse. In the words of a woman who won an out of court settlement "this has been a living hell, and its changed me forever" (Rosenberg, 1985).

On the other hand, sexual harassment, as one form of discrimination, tends to get worse if ignored (Crull, 1984). Doing nothing tends to reinforce feeling victimized. If one stays silent, the "choice" is to remain in a constant state of vigilance; to experience chronic intermittent stress and a sense of helplessness, to suppress one's anger toward the harasser so as to avoid providing him with further ammunition to use against you; and to deny your realistic fear that the attacks may escalate (cf. Crull, 1984). Needless to say, this amounts to a prescription for depression, or for behaving like an emotionally—if not physically—battered woman. Hence the costs of pursuing a complaint must be weighed against the costs of endurance, which are far from negligible (Farley, 1975; MacKinnon, 1979).

Similarly, the costs of "simply leaving" — as some therapists routinely advise—are profound in terms of the loss of seniority and job continuity, as well as the loss of self-respect. As one woman said, the bottom line is that when you have children and no support payments "you can't keep quitting" (cf. Evans, 1985).

One of the barriers to speaking up is the woman's socialization to put the needs of others above her own (Miller, 1984). To speak up threatens the woman's relatedness, and threatens to make others highly uncomfortable, as well as accusatory. Because of the woman's socialization, the woman's sense of herself as a "caring" person is at stake. But what is also at stake are male and female social roles (e.g., I can't hurt my boss after all he's done for me; his wife and family would be so embarrassed; I don't want to hurt the organization after all the good it's done). Other women, as well as men, are likely to punish the woman who speaks up, for her deviation from the ascribed female role (e.g., its called "unprofessional" and "unladylike" to file a complaint; or the attacks may be of a sexualized nature, which are meant to punish, blame, or discredit the woman, e.g., to question her seductiveness, or her sexual preference).

EMOTIONAL CONSEQUENCES
OF THE COMPLAINT PROCESS

If a woman decides to file a complaint, there are several predictable consequences. The decision to speak up changes her status from
simply that of a victim, to a victim-turned "whistleblower." In addition to punishment for blowing-the-whistle (Glazer, 1983), the institutional responses are typically defensive, along these lines:

1. It didn't happen (e.g., there was no discrimination, simply a
   neutral event such as a budget cut);
2. If it did happen, it wasn't intentional (e.g., it was a joke, or an
   oversight); and the corollary,
3. Even if it did happen, the woman brought it on herself due to
   her peculiar personality (e.g., she's seductive, hypersensitive,
   or prone to misinterpretation — although the "data" to support
   this is often gathered in the time period after she filed the
   complaint); and
4. Even if it did happen, the good work done by the discriminator
   or the institution outweighs the bad (as if the law therefore
   does not apply).

Second, if the work environment has been bad before, it is likely
to get worse. In order to defend its self-image or lessen its feared
liability, the institution generally retaliates by increased criticism,
character assassination (often of a sexualized nature), unfair work
assignments and standards, or outright sabotage. Because retaliation is so stressful, we recommend that women explore other job
possibilities, and when possible change jobs, before filing a complaint.

Depending on one's field, the organizational response can be extraordinarily hurtful and disappointing. For example, women in science may discover the extent to which scientists are prejudiced, and
when confronted, both lie and falsify the data, shaking the founda-
tions of the woman's belief and trust in scientific objectivity
(Gornick, 1983); and women in the church may discover that ministers are not the role models of altruism they appeared to be, thereby
shaking the woman's religious faith (Complainant's *United Method-*

ist Church, Sexual Harassment Church Trial, Washington, DC, 1985). Experiences such as these pose a severe threat to one's assumptions about living in a just, orderly, meaningful world (Silver, Boon & Stones, 1983).

This sense of betrayal is the tip of the iceberg. Only by speaking up does the woman encounter a whole set of continuing institutional abuses; lying, distortion of the truth, omission of information and deliberately misleading statements.

If the victim seeks validation or support, much less truth-telling, from co-workers, she risks further punishment as the messenger of bad tidings. The refusal of co-workers to come forward with corroborating information is often experienced as collusion and betrayal. When co-workers confide the truth privately but cower publicly, the victim feels insult added to injury. The realization that others will benefit from her actions is bittersweet, especially because the colluding female co-workers frequently have the most to gain. (In some cases, the victim must watch as her work, which was devalued, is taken over and exploited by those who remain, and who are credited with its true value.)

In addition to the "second injury" at work, the victim may perceive rejection by—and lack of support from—family and friends, as well as from legal and mental health professionals (Symonds, 1980). The resultant anger may reach debilitating proportions, and may be directed at anyone who does not immediately understand and sympathize with her plight (cf. APA Task Force Report, 1984). As is common in the families of rape victims, one example of a genuinely hurtful response is to "blame" the victim (e.g., "this kind of thing happens all the time; why couldn't she handle it?"; "it's *unbelievable* that anyone would sabotage her work the way she says, it would be so irrational for her boss to do that—she must have brought it on herself").

EFFECTS ON THE FAMILY

The more the woman manages to restrain the anger at work, the more it may spill-out at home. Family members who are male are likely to identify to some extent with the male-managers at work. The victim may also confuse males in her family with the aggressor, thereby displacing fear and anger onto other males. Female children may over-identify with the mother, and internalize her crisis as a warning about their own future as women in the workplace.

Reciprocally, victims often have difficulty in discussing workplace abuse with their own mothers, partly because of the humiliation surrounding the sexualized nature of both the abuse and the retaliation (e.g., one of the Complainants feared her mother's response to learning that she'd been called everything from promiscuous, to Lesbian). Effects on the mother-daughter relationship can be profound.

For example, one of us treated the mother of a victim of severe sexual harassment:

> The mother developed a full-blown major affective disorder in response to learning of her daughter's lengthy experience of sexual harassment. In this case, the mother experienced considerable guilt, wondering if she had failed to adequately prepare her daughter for the world's injustices. Her daughter's revelation of victimization further disrupted the mother's previous defenses against the pain of her own sexual harassment/discrimination in the workplace. She could thereafter no longer deny her own anger and sense of self-devaluation. She felt guilty for her failure to protest her own workplace-related abuse, wondering if her own collusion and silence had in some indirect way made her own daughter's victimization more possible. It was as if she grieved because she felt that her own behavior must have encouraged her daughter's prolonged silence and endurance of the abuse.

The strain on the family cannot be exaggerated, often leading to sexual and other relationship difficulties, and impatience with children (Crull, 1984; Pendergrass et al., 1976).

At home as well as at work the victim is likely to be punished for inadequate nurturing and to feel guilty, even though she is exhausted. Unlike women with physical injuries, most victims of workplace abuse carry "invisible wounds," which fail to elicit the appropriate sympathy and support.

The strain at work and at home is compounded by the fact that work on a complaint case amounts to at least another part-time job. For example, the already burdened victim must collect and prepare data for her attorney. The financial costs of even a modest complaint are also burdensome.

GUIDELINES FOR DISCRIMINATION
COUNSELING PROGRAMS

Particularly on the first interview, the client may appear extremely unstable, histrionic, paranoid, or depressed. This has been termed "legal psychosis" (Berger, 1980). Clinicians must assess the cause of the symptoms: is the intense affect or extreme behavior the *cause* of the abuse, or are these symptoms a *response* to the abuse. Naive counselors may do more harm than good, inadvertently revictimizing the victim by confounding distress, with the causes of stress.

We believe that the available data supports the counseling strategies recommended by Pendergrass and her colleagues (1976). Specifically, the counselor is advised to adopt the following assumptions: (1) the woman actually has experienced discrimination (most women have); (2) she probably has an adequate or better work history; (3) she has probably *reacted* in some way to the discrimination, which has probably been rubbed in by the time she realizes it; (4) if she has complained in any way, there has likely been retaliation; (5) extreme affect and behavior should be interpreted in terms of victimization, until proven otherwise (though even "difficult" persons may be discriminated against).

The most important therapeutic tasks are: empathy, validation, and helping the woman to resist the internalized tendency to devalue herself. The woman needs to be believed, encouraged and trusted (Pendergrass et al., 1976; 1979). Informationally, the therapist must be aware of the data that ignoring sexual harassment does not make it go away (Crull, 1984; cf. Simon & Crocker, 1983). Specific recommendations for employment discrimination can be summarized as follows: *assertive responses are the most effective* (U.S. Merit Systems Protection Board, 1981; Lindsey, 1977; Simon & Crocker, 1983).

While it is non-traditional, the therapist must take an active role. The therapist must be alert to the risk of victimization triggering self-devaluation. The victim will struggle against identifying with the aggressor's devaluation of herself and her work. The therapist must repeatedly clarify the victim's tendency to "shoot-herself-in-the-foot."

The woman must be encouraged to contain her anger and hurt in the workplace out of *self-respect*. The damage to supportive relationships must be continually assessed, and the possible use of maladaptive strategies for managing stress by the victim and her family must be monitored (e.g., the partner's alcohol usage may increase, as well as the victim's). The therapist should be sensitive to predictable crises in the complaint process. The stress of administrative or legal proceedings is one example. Complainants have reported lying awake all night imagining "being interrogated" before depositions. The stress of "just waiting" during long delays in the administrative or legal process is another example. These delays reinforce the patient's sense of powerlessness. And concurrent life crises must be assessed (e.g., one of the Complainants had to avoid looking tearful in a hostile work environment, despite the fact that her sister was dying).

PARALLELS TO INCEST

Several parallels to incest may be useful. As with incest, the victim of employment discrimination is economically, if not emotionally, dependent on the aggressor. In both cases, the gender-based attack is an abuse of power, and a betrayal of trust, which confuses the victim (Silver, Boon & Stones, 1983). As with physical and sexual violence against women within the family, sexualized abuse against women in the workplace is often *humiliating*, which encourages women to keep it a secret.

Unfortunately, in the case of discrimination, the administration or legal complaint process may replicate the harm that occurs in the incestuous family or the community—where other adults are indifferent to or actually perpetuate the harm (cf. Swanson & Biaggio, 1985). For example, members of the Complainant's Support Group have felt that administrative procedures which are *internal* to a company or a government agency have the appearance of being "under the thumb of management," and that these investigations too often feel like a sham.

An incest-like version of *second injury*—which feels like the "investigator, judge and jury" collaborate with and protect the "criminal" (alleged discriminating official) and overlook the harm—has been a major topic of discussion in the Complainant's Support Group. Several Complainants have felt more wounded by the deciding officials' erroneous findings of "fact," than by the discrimination itself. To continue our previous hypothetical example: despite acknowledged evidence in the file, the availability of reprints, and sworn testimony by a co-author, suppose that the deciding official upheld the alleged discriminators, finding that the woman had *no* publications. Despite the acknowledgment of corroborating, sworn testimony by co-workers, who openly stated that women were *routinely* called stereotyped, derogatory names, suppose that the official found that there was *no evidence* of a hostile work environment.

Again, the hypothetical example may strain belief, but case histories that demonstrate a blatant disregard for the facts by higher level supervisors, or deciding officials have been detailed elsewhere (Evans, 1985). For example, in *Bundy* v. *Jackson*, 641 F.2d 934 (D.C. Cir, 1981), the female plaintiff was repeatedly harassed by male supervisors who requested that she engage in a sexual relationship. When she sought assistance from a higher level supervisor, he answered her with a sexual proposition and the comment "any man in his right mind would want to rape you." In this case, the truth is on a par with Kafka's fiction.

Both the discrimination itself and the "second injury" embodied in the complaint process, appear to reactivate previous experiences of gender-based abuse for victims of child sexual abuse, rape, and spousal abuse such as battering (cf. Crull, 1984). In our experience, for example, the abuse of power by a respected official felt like incest to a former incest victim. And a former rape victim reported feeling that the only experience emotionally comparable to her victimization by the complaint process was when she had been physically raped. Given the relatively high prevalence of child sexual abuse and rape reported by Russell (1984), the reactivation of prior experiences of abuse may be common.

POSSIBLE POSITIVE ASPECTS
OF THE COMPLAINT PROCESS

While we have focused mainly on the negative consequences of discrimination and the complaint process, the silver-lining consists in the woman's sense of integrity. The women in the Complainant's Support Group have demonstrated a remarkable desire to translate their pain into a better work environment for other women. Taking action on behalf of one's self or others, i.e., trying to make the institution a better place for women, can be part of the healing process (Boring, 1982; Nielsen, 1982). This may also be a reflection of women's psychological development, where anger is seen as justified when action is taken "in relation" to others (cf. Miller, 1984). By analogy to incest, the refusal to collude by means of secrecy (Herman, 1977) — that is, the active stance of "blowing-the-whistle," of not sacrificing one's own integrity for the comfort of others — is critical to using the crisis as an opportunity for growth.

While there is no systematic data specifically on the employment discrimination victim's satisfaction with having filed a complaint, we have examined the literature for other types of gender-based abuse. For 150 cases of patient-therapist sexual abuse, virtually all of the reports by the client or a significant other revealed that making the complaint was beneficial to the client's resolution of the experience (Schoener, Milgrom & Gonsiorek, 1983). And Glazer (1983) documents that virtually all of the whistleblowers he interviewed (admittedly a non-random sample of males and females) were able to rebuild their careers, and a belief in their own competence, and integrity. A member of the Complainant's Support Group said that she was "delighted that I didn't let them walk over me." For at least some women, an active stance in terms of the complaint appears to be an important part of the "re-building" process (cf. Tichener, 1986).

On the other hand, for rape victims, the extended legal process may exacerbate symptoms, and inflict additional demands on victims, although the long-term sequelae are unclear (Sales, Baum & Shore, 1984). One individual in the Complainant's Support Group, whose case has gone on for over eight years, "would not advise anyone to file a complaint." While the time-course of symptom resolution is unknown, Crull (1984) has suggested that the emotional consequences of employment discrimination may persist for several years (cf. Pendergrass, 1979).

ALTERNATIVES OR ADJUNCTS TO INDIVIDUAL COUNSELING: SUPPORT GROUPS AND SOCIAL ACTION STRATEGIES

To our knowledge, our experiences with an ongoing support group for complainants who are victims of gender-based employment discrimination is unique. The group setting is clearly advantageous in validating women's shared experiences. For some women, peer counseling will be adequate to buttress over-burdened support systems. However, others will clearly require individual psychotherapy.

Several of the women in our group experienced difficulties in setting limits on counseling their peers. It was not uncommon for group members to spend hours on the phone attempting to assist others who were in crisis. An experienced facilitator from the local Rape Crisis Center was a valuable resource-person who assisted group-members in clarifying the role of the group. The needs of several individuals who were in crisis eventually exceeded the resources of the group, and resulted in drop-outs.

A focus of the remaining group is to find ways of helping other women who are victims of gender-based employment discrimination. As suggested by Sparks and Bar On (1985), the group believes that new programs are needed that provide "girls and women training and practice in handling all forms of violation" — street harassment, job harassment, and social harassment.

ON THE NEED FOR COUNSELING PROGRAMS

Employment discrimination is a prevalent and serious stressor in the lives of women. As women increasingly enter the workforce, they are at risk for the emotional consequences of discrimination and the complaint process. While relatively few women go through the complaint process, those who do may require long-term supportive psychotherapy and/or some type of support group. The defensive tactic of long delays by the discriminating institution often wears the victim down, delaying the *emotional* as well as the legal resolution of the case. The delays become a chronic stressor, overburdening even the best support system, and adding to a sense of helplessness. The emotional consequences of discrimination and the complaint process include: (1) victimization, and in some cases a post-traumatic stress reaction; (2) re-victimization, and chronic intermittent stress, and (3) a degree of stress, loss, and attacks on self-esteem that are consistent with depression.

The morbidity associated with severe workplace abuse almost certainly exceeds that from relatively rare psychiatric syndromes, such as obsessive compulsive disorder, where the estimated point prevalence is only 1.3-2% (Insel, 1984). Yet we undoubtedly fund more clinical research and treatment programs for obsessive compulsive disorder than we do for the psychological sequelae of gender-based employment discrimination. And there has been no support for a systematic examination of the complaint process.

The need for developing new counseling programs for sex discrimination is documented by: (1) our experiences with the Complainant's Support Group; (2) Women's Legal Defense Fund legal counselors, who have identified a need for support resources for many of the 50-60 victims of workplace abuse who call each month (Personal Communication, Donna Lenhoff, Esq., Associate Director, WLDF); and (3) by staff members of the local Rape Crisis Center (Personal Communication, Nkenge Toure, 1985), who have recently responded to requests for counseling from victims of severe sexual harassment in the workplace—suggesting that women are in need of somewhere to turn.

While peer counseling and other grassroots, community-based programs will be useful for many victims of workplace abuse, individual or group psychotherapy with trained mental health professionals will likely facilitate the victim-to-survivor process, as well as the victim's capacity to respond to the crisis as an opportunity for growth. Particularly for the small proportion of women who pursue some type of complaint process, we believe that there is a critical need for the type of validation provided by mutual-support groups.

NOTE: Additional recommendations for and concerning working with attorneys are available by writing directly to Jean Hamilton, MD, Institute for Research on Women's Health, 1616 18th Street, NW, #109B, Washington, DC 20009.

Parts of this paper, in previous versions, were presented at: 16th National Women and the Law Conference, New York City, 1985; Women and Health Round Table, Washington, DC, February 1986 and the Annual Meeting of the American Psychiatric Association, Washington, DC, May 1986.

This paper is based on: (1) our clinical experiences (J.H., L.S.K., C.L.) with women in psychotherapy; (2) discussions (J.H.) with Members of the "NIH Committee for Women in Research" (1982), as assisted by the NIH Clinical Director's Office, and discussions at the Workshop on "Clinical Research Careers for Women," sponsored by the National Institute for Child Health and Human Development (1984); and (3) our work (J.H. and L.S.K.) with victims of employment discrimination who formed a "Complainant's Support Group." The latter grew out of a series of Educational/Discussion meetings that were co-sponsored by: The Women's Legal Defense Fund (WLDF), The Institute for Research on Women's Health (IRWH), and the Committee on Women, of the Washington Psychiatric Society (WPS) in 1985-86.

In addition to those who have shared their experiences with us, we especially wish to thank: Attorneys Donna Lenhoff and Claudia Withers of WLDF; Psychiatrists Heloise DeRosis, Elizabeth Morrison and Molly Strauss of WPS; Dr. Henry Segal of Chevy Chase, MD; Sarah Burns, Attorney and Assistant Director, Georgetown University Law Center, Sex Discrimination Clinic; and Attorneys Larry Latto and John Rich, of the law firm of Shea and Gardner, Washington, DC; Attorney Suzanne Meeker, formerly of Shea and Gardner, and now with the National Women's Law Center, of Washington, DC; and, Attorney Jane L. Dolkart of the law firm of Dolkart, Langer and Zavos, of Washington, DC.

REFERENCES

APA Task Force on the Victims of Crime and Violence. (1984, November). Kahn A. S. (Ed.), Washington, DC.
American Psychiatric Association. (1980). *Diagnostic and Statistical Manual of Mental Disorders*.
Benokraitis, N. (1986). *Modern Sexism: Blatant, Subtle, Covert*. Englewood Cliffs, NJ: Prentice-Hall, in press.
Berger, M. (1980). Litigation on behalf of women: A review for the Ford Foundation. New York: The Ford Foundation.
Boring, P. Z. (1982). Filing a Faculty Grievance. In M. L. Spencer, M. Kehoe, and K. Speece (Eds.), *Handbook for Women Scholars*. San Francisco: American Behavioral Research Corporation, pp. 124-126.
Bumiller, K. (1984-6). Antidiscrimination Law and the Enslavement of the Victim: The Denial of Self-Respect by Victims Without a Cause. Working paper, 1984-6. Disputes Processing Research Program, Law School. University of Wisconsin-Madison, 53706.
Carmen, E. (H.), Russo, N. F., Miller, J. B. (1981). Inequality and Women's Mental Health: An Overview. *Am. J. Psychiat., 138*(1), 1319-1330.
Crosby, F. J. (1982). *Relative Deprivation and the Working Woman*. Oxford U. P.
Crull, P. (1984). Sexual Harassment and Women's Health. In Chavkin, W., *Double Exposure*. Monthly Review Press.
Crull, P. (1982). The Stress Effects of Sexual Harassment on the Job. *American Journal of Orthopsychiatry, 52*, 539.
Derogatis, L. & Cleary, P. (1977). Confirmation of the Dimensional Structure of the SCL-90: A study in construct validation. *J. Clin. Psychol., 33*, 981-989.
Dolkart, J. L. (1983). Discrimination on the Job. In B. A. Burnett (Ed.), *Every Woman's Legal Guide*. New York: Doubleday, 277-316.
Evans, L. J. (1985). Sexual Harassment: Women's Hidden Occupational Hazard. In J. R. Chapman and M. Gats (Eds.), *The Victimization of Women*. Beverly Hills: Sage Publications, pp. 203-223.

Farley, L. Testimony before the Commission on Human Rights of the City of New York, Hearings on Women in Blue-Collar, Service, and Clerical Occupations, "Special Disadvantages of Women in Male-Dominated Work Settings," April 21, 1975.

Frank, E. & Stewart, B. D. (1983). Treatment of Depressed Rape Victims: An Approach to Stress-Induced Symptomatology. In P. J. Clayton and J. E. Barrett (Eds.), *Treatment Approaches to Depression: Old Controversies and New Approaches*. New York: Raven Press, p. 309.

Frederick, C. J. (1985). Children Traumatized by Catastrophic Situations. In E. Spencer and R. S. Pynoos (Eds.), *Post Traumatic Stress Disorder in Children*. Washington, DC: American Psychiatric Press, pp. 71-99.

Fuchs, V. R. (1986). Sex Differences in Economic Well-Being. *Science, 232*, 459-464.

Glazer, M. (1983). Ten Whistleblowers and How They Fared. *The Hastings Center Report, 13*(6), 33-41.

Gornick, V. (1983). *Women in Science*. New York: Simon and Schuster.

Gutek, B. A. (1985). *Sex Role Stereotyping and Affirmative Action Policy*. Monograph and Research Serv., No. 32, Univ. Calif., Los Angeles, Industrial Relations.

Hamilton, J. A. (1985). Avoiding Methodological and Policy-making Biases in Gender-Related Research. In: Report of the Public Health Service Task Force on Women's Health. Vol. II (Commissioned Papers), Washington, DC, Supt. of Docs., U.S. Govt. Print. Off., pp. IV 54-56.

Herman, J. & Hirshman, L. (1977). Father-daughter incest. *Signs, 2*, 735-756.

Holmes, T. H. (1978). Life Situations, Emotions, and Disease. *Psychosomatics, 19*(12), 747-754.

Kanter, R. M. (1981). Women and the Structure of Organizations: Explanations in Theory and Behavior. In O. Grusky, G. A. Miller (Eds.), *The Sociology of Organizations*. New York: Macmillan.

Lindsey, K. (1977, November). Sexual Harassment on the Job. *MS*, pp. 47-48.

MacKinnon, C. A. (1979). *Sexual Harassment of Working Women*. New Haven: Yale University Press.

Masuda, M., Holmes, T. H. (1967). Magnitude Estimates of Social Readjustment, *J. Psychosom. Res., 11*, 219-225.

Miller, J. B. (1984). The Development of Women's Sense of Self. *Work in Progress*. Stone Center for Development Studies, Wellesley College, Wellesley, MA.

Miller, J. B. (1976). *Toward a New Psychology of Women*. Boston: Beacon Press.

Nielson, L. L. Alchemy in Academe: Survival Strategies for Female Scholars. In M. L. Spencer, M. Kehoe, K. Speece (Eds.), *Handbook for Women Scholars*. San Francisco: American Behavioral Research Corporation, pp. 113-120.

Pendergrass, V. E., Kimmel, E., Joesling, J., Petersen, J., & Bush, E. (1976). Sex discrimination counseling. *American Psychologist, 31*, 36-46.

Pendergrass, V. E. (Ed.). (1979). *Women Winning. A Handbook for Action Against Sex Discrimination*. Chicago, IL: Nelson-Hall.

Peterson, C., Seligman, M. E. P. (1983). Learned Helplessness and Victimization. *Journal of Social Issues, 2*, 103-116.

Raskin, J. G., Struening, E. L. (1976). Life Events, Stress, and Illness. *Science, 194*, 1013-1020.

Raymond, J. (1982). Mary Daly: A Decade of Academic Harassment and Feminist Survival. In M. L. Spencer, M. Kehoe, and K. Speece (Eds.). *Handbook for Women Scholars*. San Francisco: American Behavioral Research Corporation, pp. 81-88.

Rosenberg, H. (1985, Friday, June 28). CBS Settles Suit on Sex Harassment. *Los Angeles Times*, pp. 1, 19.

Russell, D. E. H. (1984). *Sexual Exploitation, Rape, Child Sexual Abuse and Workplace Harassment*. Beverly Hills: Sage Publications.

Russo, N. F. (Ed.). (1985). *Developing a National Agenda to Address Women's Mental Health Needs*. Women's Programs Office, American Psychological Association, 1200 17th Street, N.W., Washington, DC 20036.

Safran, C. (1976, November). "What Men Do to Women on the Job," *Redbook Magazine*, 148.

Sales, E., Baum, M. & Shore, B. (1984). Victim readjustment following assault. *Journal of Social Issues, 40*(1), 117-136.

Schoener, G., Milgrom, J. & Gonsiorek, J. (1983). Responding Therapeutically to Clients Who Have Been Sexually Involved with Their Psychotherapists. Minneapolis, MN: Walk-In Counseling Center.

Shapiro, E. (1982). A Survival Guide. In M. L. Spencer, M. Kehoe and K. Speece (Eds.), *Handbook for Women Scholars*. San Francisco: Americas Behavioral Research Corporation, pp. 121-122.

Silver, R. L., Boon, C., & Stones, M. H. (1983). Searching for Meaning in Misfortune Making Sense of Incest. *Journal of Social Issues, 2*, 95-96.

Silverman, D. (1976-77). Sexual Harassment: Working Women's Dilemma. *Quest: A Feminist Quarterly, III*(3), 15-24.

Simon, A. E. & Crocker, P. L. (1983). Sexual Harassment on the Job. In: B. A. Burnett (Ed.). *Everywoman's Legal Guide*. New York: Doubleday, pp. 317-330.

Sparks, C. H. (1985). Bar On, B-A, A Social Approach to the Prevention of Sexual Violence Toward Women. Work in Progress. Stone Center, Wellesley College, Wellesley, MA (No. 83-08).

Swanson, L. & Biaggio, M. K. (1985). Therapeutic Perspectives on Father-Daughter Incest. *The American Journal of Psychiatry, 142*(6), 667-674.

Symonds, M. (1980). The second Injury. In L. Kivens (Ed.), *Evaluation and Change: Services for Survivors* (pp. 36-38). Minneapolis, MN: Minneapolis Medical Research Foundation.

Titchener, J. L. (1986, May). Discrimination and Harassment as Psychic Trauma. Presented at the Annual Meeting, American Psychiatric Association, Washington, DC (Abstract).

Trubeck, D. M. et al. (1983). *Civil Litigation Research Project: Final Report*. Law School, University of Wisconsin-Madison.

Weissman, M. & Myers, J. (1978). Affective disorders in a U.S. urban community. *Archives of Gen. Psychiatr., 35*, 1304-1311.

Weissman, M. M. & Klerman, G. L. (1977). Sex Differences and the Epidemiology of Depression. *Archives of General Psychiatr., 34*, 98-111.

Werhli, L. (1976, December). Sexual Harassment in the Workplace: A Feminist Analysis and Strategy for Change. M.A. Thesis, Mass. Inst. Technol.

Wolman, C. & Frank, H. (1975). The Solo Woman in a Professional Peer Group, *American Journal of Orthopsychiatry, 45*(1). 164-171.

Women's Bureau, U.S. Report of Labor (1984). *20 Facts on Women Workers*, pp. 2-3.

Women in Computer Science at M.I.T. (1983, February). Barriers to Equality in Academia. 545 Technology Square, Cambridge, Mass. 02139.

Working Women's Institute (Hodgson, L.) (1975). Sexual Harassment on the Job: Results of Preliminary Survey. New York: Working Women's United Institute.

Working Women's Institute (Crull, P.) (1979). The Impact of Sexual Harassment on the Job: A profile of the experiences of 92 women. New York: Working Women's Institute Research Series, Report No. 2.

U.S. Merit Systems Protection Board (1981). *Sexual Harassment in the Federal Workplace: Is It a Problem?* Washington, DC: U.S. Government Printing Office.

Women Psychiatrists Change the American Psychiatric Association

Marjorie Braude

In 1979 women organized at the American Psychiatric Association's annual meeting. For several years the APA had supported the ERA. The Board of Trustees had backed the ERA economic boycott of unratified states but had been overturned by referenda of the membership three times on issues related to the ERA boycott. Last year the APA met in non-ratified Chicago and most of the women unhappily went along. Next year's meetings were scheduled for New Orleans and when this was approved by one of these referenda it was too much for some of the women members. Several determined women formed a group called "Psychiatrists for ERA" and they planned a campaign for this year's annual meeting in San Francisco. They asked each concerned member to contribute the amount that a psychiatrist charges for one psychiatric session to Dr. Jean Baker Miller, treasurer. With the six thousand dollars that were raised they acquired space in the exhibit center for a woman's information center, arranged for Gloria Steinem to address the APA and planned two demonstrations. They planned a petition campaign in which members were asked to sign that they would not go to New Orleans next year. A newspaper explaining the issues was distributed all over the convention. Members were encouraged to submit their papers for next year's meetings to the Orthopsychiatric Association or the Academy of Psychoanalysis rather than APA. The application forms for doing so were circulated. These organizations

The author is a psychiatrist in private practice in Los Angeles, California and senior attending staff at Westwood Hospital. She is Vice-President, Association of Women Psychiatrists and past Treasurer, American Medical Women's Association. She was Co-Chair in 1983 and Chair in 1984 of the Women's Institute, American Orthopsychiatric Association.

Reprinted with permission from the *Journal of the American Medical Women's Association*, January 1981.

183

plan to meet in ratified states. Many women were notified of these plans in advance through their district branch women's committees, and many came prepared to spend some time staffing the women's center, circulating petitions, and participating in the demonstrations.

Our planning meetings and caucuses brought us together and we met and spoke with others who felt strongly and similarly. We stopped submerging our opinions as we usually did in groups that are all or mostly male. We realized that we all had a deep sense of isolation and that it was very important to come together, to share our perceptions and to make them known. On the opening Monday, the APA had an "extraordinary" meeting at which three speakers, two from the Board of Trustees and one from Psychiatrists for the ERA, made eloquent and powerful statements about the urgency of ERA and the need to support the boycott. The opposition was invited, but declined to speak and merely circulated a typed statement. The meeting was preceded by women of the organization and our friends marching with signs expressing our views in front of and through the auditorium. For many of us it was the first time we had ever picketed about anything. The depth of our feelings and our sense of rightness grew as we marched and as we spoke our minds. Also, on Monday the elected representatives of the APA Assembly met and passed a group of resolutions pledging to commit organization resources to educating members on the issues for psychiatry involved in ERA.

Our information center did a continual business circulating petitions and information. Many a spouse could be seen escorting her husband to the information center and requesting that they not go to New Orleans next year. Spouses also helped circulate petitions. Three thousand signatures were collected in three days. On Wednesday Gloria Steinem spoke to an overflow audience in a large ballroom, after our second demonstration and news conference. Her analysis of women's and men's situations in our society was clear and thoughtful. She mentioned that women will of course wish to ask their psychiatrists what their views are on ERA, and of course will want to know if their psychiatrists will attend a meeting in unratified Louisiana.

Thursday morning the Board of Trustees met. Many of us were in the audience. Dr. Jean Shinoda Bolen, as leader of Psychiatrists for ERA, made a clear set of demands and included a request that the names of psychiatrists who attended the New Orleans meeting be listed so that women patients could know who did not support ERA and the boycott. The trustees voted to change their plans and not go to New Orleans.

In a historic statement they said that

the members of the Board of Trustees and the Assembly of the APA are convinced that ERA is a psychiatric issue. The fact that women do not have equal rights has been demonstrated to affect their mental health. The APA will courageously lead this effort to bring this message to the world by not meeting in a state which has not ratified ERA. Although this will be distressing to those members of APA who recently voted against economic boycott, both the Board and the Assembly felt that a vigorous effort is absolutely essential.

They also voted to appropriate $25,000 from association funds to be spent on educating legislators and the public on the importance of ERA from a mental health point of view. They asked for contributions to defray part of this and received checks for $3,400 during the meeting. We women formed the beginning of an ongoing organization to be called "Association of Women Psychiatrists." In doing this we recognized that while a Women's Committee appointed by the President of APA has an important role, it cannot fill the functions of an ongoing organization whose leadership and functions and concerns are defined by its members. We plan women's meetings and social occasions at next year's meeting. We have learned how valuable we are to each other. We have a tremendous feeling of having stepped out of our isolation, having used our abilities for our equity, and a new sense of identity and power with our organization and ourselves as women in psychiatry.

The actual triumph was brief. One month later the Board of Trustees of the American Psychiatric Association rescinded its action and the meeting was actually held in New Orleans. The ERA failed to be ratified. Does that mean the campaign was a failure? Several years later we can look back on it and find that the following events have occurred.

There has been an ongoing social and professional network of women psychiatrists who have met at the annual meeting in a women's caucus and formed "The Association of Women Psychiatrists."

There has been an increase in programs, books and articles by women on issues of concern to women. These have included programs on professional concerns of the woman psychiatrist, gender identity, on rape, battering and incest. A task force has done a survey on psychiatrist patient sex and an educational workshop on this subject has been worked out. The psycho-sexual development of women has been reevaluated. The American Psychiatric Association's own publication, an annual volume entitled "Psychiatric Update 1983," has included an article by Ethyl Person, entitled "The Influence of Values in Psychoanalysis: The Case of Female Psychology" which reexamines basic issues from a feminist point of view. There is now a newsletter for women psychiatrists. Women have obtained leadership positions in APA, culminating with Carol Nadelson becoming the first woman president of APA in 1985. She has made a priority of encouraging women to leadership. Above all, there is a dedicated group of women in APA who communicate, support each other on important issues, and have a clear consciousness of women's issues and a developing articulateness and assertiveness about stating them. Their presentations have become an important part of each year's scientific program. Women are still only fourteen percent of the American Psychiatric Association but a vocal and influential fourteen percent.

What does this history have to say to other women? Women, in any large national organization which has been predominantly and traditionally male, need to develop their own clear consciousness of their women's issues; women also need a caucus or gathering place of their own in which to recognize those issues and develop clear strategies to implement them. Women need to develop their own communication organ and network within the organization. Women need to work together on these issues. It takes a clear consciousness and an ongoing effort to influence a large, well-financed body. Now that women are entering the medical and other professions in much larger numbers, there is an opportunity to do this, but it will not be automatic. It will take the same process of conceptualization, organization, energy and work that any social change requires.

The Name Game:
Psychiatry, Misogyny, and Taxonomy

Paula J. Caplan

INTRODUCTION

The American Psychiatric Association's *Diagnostic and Statistical Manual of Mental Disorders* (Third Edition) (1980) is an extremely important book. Known as *DSM-III*, it has been translated into many languages and is sold all over the world. It is the bible of psychiatrists and many other mental health professionals, who during their training learn about the varieties of mental disorders largely by reading and studying the *DSM-III*. As noted in a December 2, 1985, *Time* magazine article, "the . . . *DSM-III* is of crucial importance to the profession. Its diagnoses are generally recognized by the courts, hospitals and insurance companies" (Leo, 1985, p. 76). Therefore, any attempt to add new diagnostic categories to it should be considered with profound gravity. For many people, the elimination of homosexuality per se from the *DSM-III* meant that it was no longer considered a mental disorder, and this helped to liberate and legitimize homosexuality for many delighted people. The words of the *DSM-III* have at least as much power to damn and ostracize as to liberate and legitimize. The struggle described in this chapter is important, because it is a struggle against what is, at best, the major North American psychiatric association's insensitivity to women's experience and, at worst, its profound and powerful misogyny. It is a struggle which provides sad evidence that we women

---

The author is a clinical psychologist who is Head of the Centre for Women's Studies in Education and Associate Professor of Applied Psychology, Ontario Institute for Studies in Education. She is an assistant professor of psychiatry and lecturer in women's studies, University of Toronto, Canada.

Printed with permission from the author; also in press as an added section paperback edition of Paula J. Caplan, *The Myth of Women's Masochism*, scheduled for Spring, 1987, publication by New American Library. The author wishes to thank Russell C. Maulitz, MD, for suggesting the title of this paper.

must still keep up our guard, that those on whom many would rely for protection of our psychological well-being can be precisely those who continue to be deeply enmeshed in victim-blaming and other practices that are harmful to women and who continue to be blinded to the realities of women's lives.

I had used parts of the *DSM-III* in my teaching and had found those parts to be helpful. Little did I dream that I would one day be part of a struggle to prevent the APA from adopting a diagnostic category for its manual (see Appendix 1), which was already unofficially used and had profoundly harmed women. In October, 1985, my book, *Myth of Women's Masochism,* was published, and shortly before this, feminist psychiatrist Jean Baker Miller had informed me that the American Psychiatric Association's (APA) Work Group to Revise *DSM-III* had proposed "masochistic personality disorder" for inclusion in *DSM-III-R* (the revised version), and APA's Committee on Women (chaired by Dr. Teresa Bernardez) was going to try to defeat the proposal before it went to the APA Board of Trustees for approval. I was glad to work with the Committee on Women, since the proposed category would go against everything I believe and would perpetuate the harm that I had seen therapists and others do to women in the name of their belief that women are masochists.

First, I shall briefly summarize some of the basic ideas from my book. Then, I shall discuss some of the enormous number of useless and dangerous aspects of the proposed diagnostic category of "masochistic personality disorder."

THE MYTH OF WOMEN'S MASOCHISM

In my article, "The Myth of Women's Masochism" (1984), and my 1985 book of the same title, I argued as follows: Because many mental health professionals and laypeople believe that women are masochists—taking pleasure in pain, seeking out suffering—when they see an unhappy woman they are quick to blame her for her own misery. Rather than seeking to identify, understand, and promote changes in the factors that make her unhappy or keep her in an upsetting situation, they bring out some form of the myth of women's masochism; they may say explicitly, "You're a masochist," or they may use a more subtle form, such as "Do you see how you are the architect of your own unhappiness?" "You must have a fear of success," or "Why do you do this to yourself?" The myth blinds people to the true causes of women's unhappiness. There have been two main tributaries to the myth: (1) the belief that women's anatomically-based pain (menstrual cramps, labor pains, the possibility of being raped, women's allegedly passive and suffering sexual experiences, etc.) reflects our *enjoyment* of pain; and (2) the mislabelling as masochistic of much of women's learned behavior, especially being nurturant and self-denying, putting others' needs ahead of one's own, etc. The mislabelling has placed women in a devastating Catch-22 situation: In order to *avoid* the pain of rejection and disapproval, girls and women behave in self-denying ways, but then that selfless behavior is used as "proof" that they are masochists. It would be possible to admire and appreciate unselfish, giving behavior or to relieve women of the need to be *endlessly* nurturant; however, the most common responses to women's selflessness are a simple failure to notice or appreciate it and a readiness to mislabel it "masochistic." To a woman and a man displaying the same behavior different motives will be attributed. Rather than being called "masochistic," a hardworking father is likely to be admired as a good provider, for example, and the husband of a difficult wife is likely to be called tolerant for putting up with her.

INADEQUACIES, RISKS AND DANGERS

The word "masochistic" was later changed to "self-defeating" for the proposed *DSM-III-R* category. In this section, I shall begin with an assessment of "self-defeating personality disorder" in light of the aims of the *DSM-III* and shall then describe the risks and dangers of the diagnosis.

The DSM-III's Aims

The diagnostic categories in *DSM-III* are supposed to be vast improvements over other systems of nomenclature because the former are to (1) have a solid research base, (2) minimize subjectivity in judging whether a label is appropriate, and (3) be atheoretical.
    A. *The research base.* Spitzer's "Introduction" to *DSM-III* includes the following statement: ". . . *DSM-III* reflects an increased commitment in our field to reliance on data as the basis for under-

standing mental disorders" (1980, p. 1). But before February, 1986, there was nothing at all in the literature on attempts to measure anything called "masochistic" or "self-defeating personality disorder," nor is there even now the one thing needed as a beginning for such measurement and documentation — an attempt to reach consensus on a definition and to ensure that the terms are not misnomers, that they do not mask or distort the problems of the people under study. Despite this, the December, 1985, Report of the Ad Hoc Committee includes the sentence: "Changes [for *DSM-III-R*] were proposed based on the best available scientific data" (p. 2).

An article published in February, 1986, (Kass, MacKinnon & Spitzer, 1986), is the closest thing to actual, systematic research on this topic that has been published. It is co-authored by Spitzer, the prime mover of the *DSM-III* and *DSM-III-R*, and by Frederic Kass, a member of the American Psychiatric Association's Advisory Committee on "Personality Disorders." Spitzer chairs the American Psychiatric Association's Work Group to Revise *DSM-III*, and Kass is a member of that Work Group. Nine of the major problems with this article are described below.

1. In this article, the only thing that the authors "prove" is that "masochistic personality" is applied consistently by a few Columbia University Psychiatry Department staff and residents (most or all of whom may have known that one of the authors was spearheading the revisions of *DSM-III* and perhaps that he was proposing "masochistic personality disorder" as a new category) to a cluster of traits which come from very old clinical — and no research — literature.
2. The authors begin by pointing out that "Axis II in *DSM-III* represents an advance in the diagnosis of personality disorders, as categories were chosen to reflect and enhance clinical work and were defined by clear criteria to achieve better standardization" (p. 216). They claim that "masochistic personality" "may have particular diagnostic importance because of a reported association with negative therapeutic reaction and poor treatment outcome. . . . " (p. 216). I suggest that a major reason for the negative therapeutic reaction and poor treatment outcome is not the nature of the disorder itself but rather the serious, destructive misdiagnosis as "masochistic" or "self-defeating" of depressed people and people with poor self-esteem, who lack the energy, the social support, and the

belief system to identify, avoid, and get out of unhappy situations.

3. Their theoretical background for considering these patients, as reflected in their literature review, is based heavily on old clinical literature from work ranging from 1916 through the early 1950s.

4. Kass, MacKinnon, and Spitzer used as judges of the patients they studied eight attending physicians and seven residents of unspecified gender in the Department of Psychiatry at Columbia University College of Physicians and Surgeons. They had each one select three to five of their own patients (from a total of how many, we are not told) for a total of 59, 38 (64%) of them female. They do not say whether they provided any guidelines for selecting those patients and, if so, what they were.

5. They report that "Using their own respective personal criteria, the therapists diagnosed eight patients, 14% of the sample, as having masochistic personality disorder" (p. 217). That 14% sounds like a substantial part of a psychiatric patient population, except that the authors do not say how they instructed the psychiatrists to choose their patients. Of the eight patients, six were female, a sex difference the authors say is not statistically significant. However, the lack of a statistically significant sex difference in a group of eight patients (and with such a tiny sample it hardly is worth doing a statistical comparison) cannot reassure us that the diagnosis is not — and will not be — applied in a sex-biased way.

6. The authors do not say whether the eight patients came from only two of the psychiatrists, whether about half of the psychiatrists each identified one "masochistic" patient, or whether the number was distributed in some other way. This is a crucial question, since the already small number of allegedly masochistic patients comes from a very small (one is not told exactly how small) number of therapists, and one would also want to know how many of the alleged masochists were labelled by attending physicians and how many by residents.

7. Kass et al. asked the unknown number of psychiatrists to decide whether ten items selected by the authors were descriptions of the "masochists" and concluded that "the clinicians' concept of masochism was reflected well by the content of the items" (p. 218). This is no doubt true — but it tells us no more

than that between two and eight psychiatrists and/or residents from the same department in the same institution tend to (mis) label in the same way, a finding which is not surprising, particularly within the same institution.

8. It is interesting, too, that the *DSM-III* Advisory Committee eliminated from their proposed category of "masochistic personality disorder" two of the ten criteria included in the Kass et al. study, one because it was "not thought to be central to the construct of masochistic personality" (p. 218) and the other "because many members of the committee felt that the item was more reflective of one of the paraphilias, sexual masochism." The first of those two items was "Often prides self on being ethically or morally superior to others," and the second was "Often sexually excited by fantasies, stories, or pictures of being humiliated, punished, hurt, or coerced." As the words of Kass et al. indicate, this is construction of diagnostic category by opinion (of an unspecified number of members of an Advisory Committee). It is a far cry from the empirically-based category or research-based category construction that the *DSM-III's* authors have claimed is one of their major aims.

9. Kass et al. conclude their article by recommending that "it would be feasible to study the relationships among masochistic personality, negative therapeutic reaction, and poor outcome" (p. 218). In any undergraduate methodology course, one learns that before examining relationships among phenomena, one must first determine whether each of the phenomena is a legitimate construct, is clearly and correctly defined, and has been shown to exist. None of these things has been done in regard to either "masochistic" or "self-defeating personality disorder."

Furthermore, as Frances M. Newman (1986) has observed, countertransference may play a large part in both negative and therapeutic reactions and poor treatment outcome with the so-called "masochistic personality." Many psychiatrists and psychoanalysts lead rather privileged lives and achieve financial success. Often, they have learned to "accept" their positions of privilege through analysis, in which they learn to "work through" their own "masochistic" needs to please others, to put themselves second, and to do without some of the material rewards of a consumer society. Indeed, many psychiatrists, psychoanalysts and other professionals pride themselves on being able to deal with money – to charge high fees and to charge for patients' missed appointments and holiday times.

Asks Newman, how does such a professional react when confronted with a patient who is selfless, self-sacrificing or just plain unwilling to do some of the things necessary to make it, to succeed, to acquire? No doubt some are uncomfortably reminded of their own struggles to overcome these very feelings in themselves. This puts the patient in the very sticky position of being made to feel bad about not being selfish. And there follows from that the negative therapeutic reaction, in which the patient feels worse and, in order to regain a sense of control and well-being, begins to battle the psychiatrist's attempts to make the patient over into his or her own image.

Here, notes Newman, we have a clash of values rather than the manifestation of psychopathology. This clash in an unequal relationship can have one of three outcomes: The patient can "agree" with the psychiatrist and work to take on the psychiatrist's values, leading to a "successful" treatment outcome. Or, the patient can appear to agree with the psychiatrist by suppressing the very material that occasioned the therapy and resulted in the clash. Or the patient will be unable to proceed in therapy.

In a related vein, Bob Metcalfe (1986) has made the following assessment of the Kass et al. article. He notes that the authors have made it clear that the category "masochistic personality disorder" is unofficially being widely used, and therapy with individuals so labelled is not working. Metcalfe points out that this failure may be due to:

1. Incompetent treatment by the psychiatrist;
2. Misdiagnosis, leading to misdirected – and, therefore, poor – treatment; and/or
3. Interference with the therapy by the therapist's enjoyment of the therapist/patient power differential, in which case the therapist gains a greater sense of power the longer s/he interprets and "works through" the patient's behavior, (mis)interpreting it as motivated by the need to be powerless or mistreated. Thus, the patient's presumed motive perfectly complements the therapist's power motive.

One further misguided attempt to create a research base for "self-defeating personality disorder" was initiated in January, 1986. At that time a letter co-signed by Spitzer, Kass, and Janet Williams, a member of the Work Group to Revise *DSM-III*, went out on APA letterhead, accompanying a questionnaire "to obtain data that will help determine how many of the eight diagnostic criteria are necessary to make the diagnosis" (Letter from Work Group, 1986). According to the letter, the questionnaire was sent to APA members who had indicated an interest in personality disorders in the APA biographical survey; however as feminist psychiatrist Marjorie Braude pointed out in her letter to the editor of the official APA journal, the questionnaire was constructed in a way that guaranteed dramatically skewed responses:

> The questionnaire . . . asks if I believe that the diagnosis of self-defeating personality disorder should be included in the revised *DSM-III*, and that none of the existing personality disorders are adequate for this purpose. If I answer yes I am asked to go on to describe characteristics of specific cases. If I answer no I simply return the questionnaire without my clinical data. By including only data from psychiatrists who think there is a need for this diagnosis one will obtain skewed rather than random results. . . . (Braude, 1986)

Thus, the people asked to select the definitive criteria for the diagnosis are only those who already believe (on an unknown variety of potentially conflicting grounds) that this is a valid diagnosis. Noting that she has "seldom seen a case in which abuse of one category or another did not emerge upon careful questioning," Braude predicts the following sequence of events: The skewed sample of respondents will powerfully push the diagnosis toward inclusion in the *DSM-III-R*; the exclusionary clause that means ruling out this diagnosis if the behavior is in response to abuse will be rendered useless, because the psychiatrists most likely to have helped develop and/or to assign the "self-defeating" label will be those *least* likely to ask about abuse in their history-taking; and "victims of abuse will be treated as masochistic which will only victimize them further."

Ironically, one large body of research that *does* exist indicates that females are far more likely than males to have poor self-esteem and low levels of aspiration, a pattern that virtually ensures that "self-defeating personality disorder" would be overapplied to females.

In view of the total absence of valid research on this diagnosis, it is curious that Spitzer said "Basically . . . [the feminists are] against what we are trying to do. . . . They are so enmeshed in spouse abuse that they can't focus on what we see as a problem — that there are people whose pain and suffering can't be explained by objective reality" (Leo, 1985, p. 76). Similarly, were it not so dangerous, it would be amusing that psychoanalyst Richard Simons, agreeing with Spitzer, said "It's not scientifically valid to throw out a category merely because it might be misused" (Leo, 1985, p. 76). Ironic, that science would be invoked in this context. Indeed, it would seem that it is Spitzer and his group who are unable not only to see "objective reality" but even to plan a methodologically sound way to research the reality that might bear on the proposed category. In view of this, as was noted in a report of the APA Committee on Women, "The diagnosis . . . does not represent a clear, concise entity which would help either to discriminate one treatment group from another or to alleviate the patient's suffering. Furthermore, it is useless in estimating prognosis" (Committee on Women, 1985). Thus, the proposed diagnosis is based on no good research and is at worst destructive and at best useless.

B. *Elimination or minimizing of subjectivity.* A second major aim of the *DSM-III* is to eliminate, or at least minimize, the role of subjectivity in assigning diagnostic labels. One reason for this aim is the lack of agreement among psychiatrists about how patients should be labeled. Another is that prevention and useful treatment are the ultimate goals of mental health workers, high-quality research is necessary to determine workable techniques of both prevention and treatment, and decent research cannot be grounded on the shifting sands of highly subjective labels. But, as Jean Baker Miller compellingly demonstrated in her May 13, 1986, presentation at the APA symposium, every one of the criteria for the proposed "self-defeating personality disorder" leaves unusually wide space for subjective interpretation and application (Miller, 1986). Miller explained how many of her patients who are the wives of successful men (including psychiatrists), as well as the men themselves, could easily be assigned this label. For example, in regard to Criterion 1, she noted that our society teaches women that becoming a doctor's wife is a pinnacle of achievement; thus, psychiatrists' wives might well have felt when they married that they had made the best possible choice. When many such women now find that their husbands are rarely home and are minimally involved with the family, asked Miller, are we now to consider them self-defeating? Further, Miller noted, those husbands—who in choosing to become hardworking psychiatrists were clearly selecting highly desirable, high-status alternatives—could be considered "self-defeating" because their involvement in work and uninvolvement in the richness of family life could well be regarded as undesirable alternatives. She made similar comments about the other criteria. Many of the criteria are very accurate descriptions of behavior that has been required of women and also interpreted as signifying mental disorder, so that, depending on one's subjective view, they could be interpreted as signs of mental disorder or signs of an understandable, safe adaptation to powerful social influences. Thus, for example, in regard to Criterion 1, Carmen (1985, p. 2) has noted that "When clinicians focus on internal motivation as the primary explanation for destructive or maladaptive behaviors and fail to take into account the social origins of these conflicts, they will see 'opportunities to alter the situation' where none exist." Criterion 7, in addition to being vague, is often simply a sign of naivete. Criterion 9 could be construed as pathological, but in fact often it is simply a sign of good reality testing in women, in view of society's general devaluation of women compared to men and its specific devaluation of the roles of housewife and mother. This lack of objectivity, this openness to gross distortion in interpreting people's motives, is a problem for all of the criteria.

C. *Maintenance of an atheoretical stance.* DSM-III categories are supposed to be atheoretical, so that professionals and researchers from various theoretical orientations can use them for clinical and research purposes. "Self-defeating personality disorder" is quite simply *not* atheoretical, since it does not include the criterion, "Patient acknowledges having a need to do self-defeating things" (in the way, for example, that patients are asked if they hear voices). If that is not included, how does one know if the person is self-defeating (especially if the patient denies wanting to be self-defeating)? To make such an interpretation, one has to assume that the self-defeating motivation is unconscious; one has to make inferences about the motives behind the patient's behavior, and the moment one makes an inference, one abandons an atheoretical stance.

D. *Risks and dangers.* Some of the risks and dangers involved in the proposed diagnoses have been mentioned earlier or are implicit in some of the points already made. The following is a no-doubt incomplete list of the dangers it poses.

  1. Although "self-defeating" or "masochistic personality disorder" is not currently a *DSM-III* category, the term as used both clinically and informally has already done a great deal of damage, making both women and their therapists needlessly and unjustifiably pessimistic about the ability and motivation of many unhappy women to change their situations. It causes one to focus on the patient's unhappy situation as if it were desired by the patient rather than on factors within the patient and within the environment that could be modified. At its best, psychotherapy opens new possibilities. At its worst, it closes them down. The proposed diagnostic category tends powerfully to stop inquiry, both on the part of the patient and on the part of the therapist, about the nature of the patient's problems. It is already clear that this is the case, even though the category is not official, because large numbers of us have heard reports from patients about their therapists telling them such things as "You are the architect of your own misery" or "Do you see how you bring all your problems on yourself?" Even feminist therapists have misguidedly said such things. Patients have found themselves both more depressed after "therapy" than before and also hopeless, now having not only the problem for which they sought help but also the added problem of having a therapist who persuades them that there is a sickness inside them that leads to their problems. I have received numerous letters and had countless interviews with women who have said that their therapists used this type of approach and left them feeling more powerless than before to change their behavior, since they feel, "If I bring it on myself, I might as well give up and stop trying." If they are told it is unconsciously motivated, it's even more frightening, because it means they can never be sure why they are doing anything, making any choice. Such interpretations as "self-defeating" or "masochistic" are presented—and received—as though they were explanations in and of themselves. By contrast, a therapist who diagnoses a problem as due to the patient's poor self-esteem thereby finds and offers a way for the patient to probe toward greater self-understanding and greater possibilities for making real changes. Furthermore, this category of

self-defeating personality disorder is *not* parallel or complementary to "sadistic personality disorder," in which the *goal* of the behavior is to inflict suffering on others. Nevertheless, "self-defeating personality disorder" is highly likely to be paired with "sadistic personality disorder" — as indeed the authors of the diagnoses have done — and "self-defeating" will be mistakenly assumed to be the aim of the behavior listed in criteria 1 through 9. Where there is scope for misinterpretation, there *will* be misinterpretation, as the original *DSM-III* authors warned.

2. Much of the behavior included in the criteria is a combination of adaptation to the misogyny in our society and an obedient execution of the traditional female role. Women trying to avoid or minimize rejection and risk in our culture learn to put other people's needs ahead of their own and to ignore their own needs. Indeed, from developmental psychology textbooks we learn that increasing emotional maturity involves being able to delay gratification, put other people's needs ahead of our own, behave in selfless ways, and so on. It seems bizarre and destructive now to call such behavior an indicator of serious psychopathology, to label as sick what women have been trained to do and punished for *not* doing. Most of the criteria are features of traditional feminine behavior which women have learned in order to win approval and acceptance, to get what they want. This is the *opposite* of self-defeating behavior, since they know that *rejection* awaits them if they do *not* behave in these ways. For many groups of people (most notably, women), criteria 1, 2, 3, 5, 7, and 8 are substantial parts of the roles that society *prescribes* for them, indeed often punishes them if they refuse to behave in these ways. To call people self-defeating for behaving in self-denying, self-effacing ways in order to *avoid* punishment and rejection — and in order to receive approval and love — is to insist that their behavior be regarded as pathological whether or not they follow the socially prescribed route. As Carmen (1985) observes, "In its confusion of cause and effect, the diagnosis of masochistic personality disorder provides a good description of the female *response* to inequality, powerlessness, and second class status at home and in work-settings. The criteria for masochism reflect the survival strategies of subordinate group members in their relationships with dominants (Miller, 1976, p. 3)." It is

relevant to note here that Spitzer wrote in the DSM-III intro-
duction that in *DSM-III* "there is an inference that there is a
behavioural, psychological, or biological dysfunction [in the
disorders in *DSM-III*], and that the disturbance is not only in
the relationship between the individual and society" (1980,
p. 6). Furthermore, as noted in a Committee on Women report: "The criteria and the diagnosis are an additional burden
on women and minority groups where racial and gender stereotypes involve socially reinforced behaviors such as self sacri-
fice, submission, deferring one's own needs and interests, patience and constancy which are positive traits in traditional
roles but are labelled pathology under these criteria" (Committee on Women, 1985).

3. The *DSM-III* Work Group's exclusion of abuse victims is an
indication that its members acknowledge the inappropriateness
and unfairness of "self-defeating personality disorder" for
such victims. However, a serious danger related to this point
remains: As Braude (1986) and Miller (1986) have noted, psychiatrists often fail even to inquire about a history of abuse,
and abuse victims are notoriously reluctant to reveal or acknowledge it even when asked. This makes the exclusionary
clause woefully inadequate. Furthermore, many of the criteria
are cardinal features of the traditional female role, and the
systematic inculcation of that role in females by society does
itself constitute chronic psychological abuse. *The danger is
that, precisely because this type of abuse is the norm, clinicians will fail to recognize it as abuse and thus will over-
diagnose this disorder.* Or, the category will become useless,
because it can be usually or always shown to result from
abuse.

4. The other exclusionary clause — according to which the therapist does not assign the "self-defeating personality disorder"
label if the behavior in question occurs only when the patient
is depressed — constitutes either a danger or a rendering of the
whole category useless. Nickerson, O'Laughlin, and Hirschman (1979), for example, show in their review the markedly
higher incidence of learned helplessness and depression in
contemporary American women as compared to men. Depression is thus likely to be the appropriate diagnosis, and indeed
much of the behavior described in the proposed diagnosis sig-
nifies depression, and learned helplessness keeps one from

getting out of a depressing situation or life pattern. The proposed category entails the serious danger that depression
would be missed because of the new label being applied instead.
5. It is particularly damaging that "self-defeating" should be
classified as a "personality disorder" rather than some other
kind of mental disorder, since personality disorders are notoriously difficult to change and are defined as maladaptive organizations of the entire personality, not as a limited problem.

Three sets of hearings have been held on this diagnosis, at which
feminist psychologists and psychiatrists have testified against it
with an eloquent and unified voice. As of this moment in time the
Board of Trustees of the American Psychiatric Association has
voted to relegate this diagnosis from the body of the *DSM-III* Revised to an Appendix. No matter what the outcome. two things are
now crystal clear. First, the proponents of the revisions for *DSM-
III-R* don't even feel the obligation to meet the criteria that they
themselves established in *DSM-III*. Second, in the face of powerful,
substantive arguments, only a supreme arrogance and insensitivity
to the realities of living, breathing, feeling women could have allowed these people to push ahead as far and as hard as they have.
And so, the struggle must go forward, for even if we prevail for
DSM-III-R, there soon will be *DSM-IV*.

REFERENCES

American Psychiatric Association (1980). *Diagnostic and Statistical Manual of Mental Dis-
   orders* (Third edition).
Bernardez, T. (December, 1985). Report to Committee on Women (members and Advisory
   Group) about meetings with the Ad Hoc Committee and Board of Trustees [of American
   Psychiatric Association].
Braude, Marjorie (February 27, 1986). Letter to "Editor, APA Journal."
Caplan, P. J. (1984). The myth of women's masochism. *American Psychologist, 39*, 130-
   139.
Caplan, P. J. (1985). *The Myth of Women's Masochism.* New York: E. P. Dutton.
Carmen, E. (November 7, 1985). Masochistic personality disorder *DSM-III-R:* critique.
Committee on Women, American Psychiatric Association (Autumn, 1985). Issues in the
   acceptance of masochistic personality disorder (working paper).
Fausto-Stirling, A. (1985). *Myths of Gender: Biological Theories About Women and Men.*
   New York: Basic Books.
Kass, F., MacKinnon, R. A., & Spitzer, R. L. (1986). Masochistic personality: An empirical
   study. *American Journal of Psychiatry, 143*(2), 216-218.
Leo, J. (December 2, 1985). Battling over masochism. *Time,* p. 76.

Metcalfe, R. (April 22, 1986). Personal communication.

Miller, J. B. (1976). *Toward a New Psychology of Women*. Boston: Beacon.

Miller, J. B. (May 13, 1986). Presentation in symposium-debate on controversies about DSM-III-R. American Psychiatric Association Convention, Washington, DC.

Newman, F. (April 28, 1986). Personal communication.

Nickerson, E., O'Laughlin, K. & Hirschman, L. (1979). Learned helplessness and depression in women or how to be a women without being depressed. *International Journal of Women's Studies, 3,* 340-348.

Report of the Ad Hoc Committee of the Board of Trustees and Assembly [of the American Psychiatric Association] (December 7, 1985) to Review the Draft of *DSM-III-R*.

Spitzer, R. L. (December, 1985). Defining masochism (letter to the editor). *Time.*

APPENDIX

301.89 *Self-defeating Personality Disorder* (Changed from masochistic personality disorder, draft form)

A. A pervasive pattern of self-defeating behavior beginning by early adulthood. The individual may often be drawn to situations or relationships in which he or she will suffer, avoid or undermine pleasurable experiences, and prevent others from helping him or her.

The diagnosis requires the repeated occurrence of at least (five) of the following:

1. chooses persons and situations that lead to his or her disappointment, failure or mistreatment, even when other realistic options are clearly available.

2. turns down opportunities for pleasure or is reluctant to acknowledge having enjoyed him or herself (despite having adequate social skills and the capacity for pleasure).

3. fails to accomplish tasks crucial to his or her own goals despite demonstrated ability to do so; for example, helps fellow students write papers, but is unable to write his or her own.

4. is bored with or uninterested in people who consistently treat him or her well, e.g., unattracted to caring sexual partners.

5. following positive personal events (e.g., new achievement) responds with depression, guilt or a behavior that brings about pain (e.g., car accident, loss of wallet).

6. rejects or renders ineffective the attempts of others to help him or her.

7. is surprised that his or her behavior incites angry or rejecting responses from others.

8. excessive self-sacrifice that is unsolicited or even discouraged by others.

9. feels unappreciated, even when his or her efforts for other people are clearly acknowledged.

B. The behaviors in A do not occur only in response to, or in anticipation of, being physically, sexually, or psychologically abused.

C. The behaviors in A do not occur only when the individual is feeling depressed.

Prevention of Sexual Assault Through the Resocialization of Women: Unlearning Victim Behavior

Jan Leland-Young
Joan Nelson

INTRODUCTION

Many writers have stated that growing up female in a patriarchal society is a socialization process which teaches women passive and victim-like roles and behaviors, in social, sexual and economic relationships. Narrow choices and limited options, in personal behaviors and roles, constrain women and enhance their vulnerability to all forms of exploitation. Some of us believe that one of the worst of these forms of exploitation is sexual assault victimization. According to the Federal Bureau of Investigation, at least one woman is sexually assaulted every two minutes in the United States; it is termed the most frequently committed violent crime in this country (FBI, 1973). It would be an understatement then, to say that sexual assault, or the fear of it, affects every woman's life.

In my work as a women's movement advocate, a therapist and educator over the last ten years, I have come to realize that fear is the last remaining enslaver of women. In other words, birth control technology, social values and economic necessity have opened the door for women's full and equal participation in Western society. Violence, specifically sexual assault, has increased to epidemic proportions and closed the door on women's freedom. Over the years,

Jan Leland-Young is a clinical social worker. She is an instructor at Lansing Community College Women's Resource Center and a private practitioner in Lansing, Michigan. Joan Nelson is a sexual assault and self defense educator and consultant and founder of Movement Arts in Lansing, Michigan.

whenever I would embrace a women's issue and work for equality in one sphere or another, I always came back to dealing with violence against women. No matter how many reforms were accomplished, if women were in danger and in fear of utilizing those reforms, they were useless. It seemed to me that our society, by ignoring and often condoning violence against women, had very successfully found a way to make women oppress and limit themselves. It was not necessary to forbid women to go to school or work. With the fear of rape, women would avoid certain jobs, locations, libraries, buildings, even cities.

With this awareness, in the early 1970s I turned all of my energy toward sexual assault prevention and treatment. I began by treating the trauma suffered by sexual assault victims (or what I call sexual assault "survivors," since language is a major socialization tool, which stigmatizes women into passive roles). I have practiced a wide range of traditional and non-traditional treatment modalities with different survivors: psychodynamic theory, crisis intervention, systems theory, family therapy, conjoint therapy, behavior modification, reality therapy, problem-solving therapy, biblio-therapy and so on. Using client evaluations, through peer and supervisor assessments, and based on my own evaluation of my therapeutic relationships and treatment outcomes, I can say that my use of each approach has been successful to some extent with most sexual assault survivors. Yet, as a feminist, knowing what I know about the role and socialization of women as a class, I became discontented with the commonly referred to "band-aid approach" to sexual assault treatment. I began to seek more encompassing and creative approaches to prevention as well as treatment.

BACKGROUND

There are several sources of research which significantly influenced the development of the model I will present here. Amir (1971) found that about 70 percent of all sexual assaults are planned in advance to some extent. Gebhard (1965) found that a majority of assailants have access to a willing sexual partner. Amir and Gebhard have provided a dynamic for the crime which indicates that it is not at all a sexual crime, but a crime of violence and degradation. It is an expression of hostility and rage, which is committed by sexual means toward a violence end, and is premeditated. Beyond premeditation, other researchers Selkin (1975), Javorek (1975), and Javorek and Lyon (1975), have outlined a selection process by which assailants consciously or unconsciously determine who would be a good potential victim.

This selection process includes: choosing, testing, intimidating and finally, sexual transaction or physical force. Women who behave in a non victim-like manner (unfeminine, if you will), are likely to be passed over early in the process. Later on in the process, Selkin (1975) found that women who resisted by verbal assertion or fleeing were likely to escape from assault as well. Most interesting to me as a therapist is Selkin's assertion that women who employ these non victim-like behaviors also suffer "fewer symptoms of psychological stress" and are "less anxious, less depressed after the ordeal" (p. 74).

The Queens' Bench Foundation Study (1975) found that "victim resistance is highly correlated with deterrence of sexual assault." They found that prior to nearly all assaults there is a period of interaction between the assailant and the potential victim during which the assailant may be deterred. Queens' Bench states that rapists themselves feel women should resist with verbal objection, screaming and self-defense techniques. The study concludes that "preparing women to prevent rape will require overcoming attitudes that teach women to be passive, polite and dependent. This is what I call the resocialization of women, or unlearning victim behavior.

Armed with these facts, a number of anti-rape activists and martial artists began in the mid-1970s to develop a sexual assault prevention and self-defense model to do just that: to successfully resocialize women so that, when faced with a potential sexual assault situation, they could use the period of interaction to communicate to the assailant with their behavior that they are not good victims.

MODEL

A model program has been developed and implemented by Joan Nelson, an antirape activist and martial artist, at Lansing Community College, Michigan State University and various community centers in Lansing, Michigan. The program began in 1975 and continues. Well over 5,000 women have participated in groups of 10-20 members each. The initial goal of the program was to both prevent and treat sexual assault by resocializing women in non-victim behavior. This is accomplished by informational and experiential means, on three levels.

1. The Theoretical Level

Much like the information presented here, information provides women with a framework for conceptualizing female victimization and oppression. It also involves the provision of current and accurate information to dispel popular misconceptions about sexual assault which promote victimization. For example, they learn that:

a. Sixty to 80 percent of sexual assaults are by a familiar person and they occur in the victim's home (FBI, 1973).
b. Less than four percent of all sexual assaults involve any behavior on the part of the victim which could be construed as provocation. This is the same percentage as for other violent crimes (FBI, 1973).
c. A majority of rapists are not deviant, or unique, but have normal sexual personalities (Amir, 1971).
d. Begging, pleading and verbal stalling (passivity) are correlated with extreme violence (Queens Bench Foundation, Note 3).
e. Ninety percent of all sexual assaults are between people of the same race and economic status (Amir, 1971).

2. The Strategic Level

This is an examination of the stages of victim selection mentioned earlier. It also includes situational assessments (or drills), the assessment of one's own strengths and skills in any given situation, and the interplay between these two. Components of this level are displayed in Table I.

3. Tactical Level

This involves the development of physical, verbal and psychological techniques and options to use in an assault situation and the extensive practice of these techniques with a partner. Many of these techniques are derived from martial arts, but are modified and self-defensive in nature, devised to end, not win, the encounter. Tradi-

Table I

Stage

A. Choosing a victim   accessibility - environmental
   (prior to assault)   (deadbolts, peepholes, etc.)

                                        vulnerability - persona
                                        projected

B. Testing a victim   attitude - vigilant and wary
   (period of interaction in   vs passive and deferential
   which assailant assesses the   body language - eye contact and
   potential victim)   assertive posture vs shrink-
                                           ing away
                                        clothing - restrictive vs
                                           non-restrictive

C. Force   flexible physical response as
   (escalation to physical   needed
   violence)   (blocking, striking, running,
                                        shouting, etc.)

tional martial arts training does not always take into consideration
the dynamics of sexual assault, is considerably more expensive, and
not designed for women exclusively.
   Techniques include:

   a. Identification of the vulnerable parts of an assailant's body and
      how to use them to the best advantage. Examples: eyes, nose,
      throat, solar plexus, testicles, knees.
   b. Identification of the vulnerable parts of your body and how to
      protect them. Examples: side stance, defensive guarding and
      shielding.
   c. Identification and development of the weapons which women
      have on their bodies. Examples: brain, head, arms, legs,
      voice.
   d. Use of these physical weapons in specific physical techniques.
      Examples: heel hands, blocks, punches, gouges, kicks, yells.

e. Identification of assailant's likely skill with a weapon and techniques in weapon defense.

f. Verbal confrontation and de-escalation techniques.

Beyond these components, this model offers more subtle contributions to resocialization. There is the explicit message that women are not helpless, nor are they too weak or too stupid to successfully escape assault. The model offers strong, empathic assertive female role models, with whom the participant can identify. These women offer options in such a way as to validate and respect each woman's right and ability to make her own decision as to how she responds in an assault situation.

SUCCESSFUL PREVENTION

Those of us involved with this model have found it difficult to assess scientifically as to whether it prevents sexual assault. One of the problems is that if a woman deters an assailant in the choosing or testing stage, she may never know if an assault would have occurred. We can, however, look to Selkin's research. He found that assailants had frequently passed over several potential victims (who behaved in a non-victim-like manner) prior to finally selecting a passive victim for the completed assault (Selkin).

Another study, (Smith, 1983) surveyed a group of resocialized women and a control group of women aerobic dance students. Smith conducted pre-, post- and six month follow-up surveys. She concluded that the resocialized women would be more likely to assert themselves in an assault situation, had better self-esteem and believed less in passivity than the control group. Smith found that both groups considered sexual assault a great danger, thus indicating that the resocialized women were no more likely to have a false sense of security than the control group.

Our self-defense instructors repeatedly say that students return to them and report successful deterrence from what they believed to be a potential assault, as well as actual assaults. Based on anecdotal evidence, we estimate that women trained in the self-defense model are three times less likely to be selected by an assailant than women who have not been trained.

SUCCESSFUL TREATMENT

We initially feared that sexual assault survivors who participated in this model might suffer additional trauma from the vivid similarity between the discussions/practice and their own assault experience. Due to the large numbers of survivors interested in the model, they were included with the following recommendations: (1) they could leave the session at any time; (2) they could withdraw from the entire program; (3) they knew and understood the potential risks in their participation; (4) they were encouraged to obtain therapy while participating; (5) they were encouraged to find a partner sympathetic to their feelings. Nelson estimates that of the 5,000 participants, about 1,000 were "survivors." The "survivors" have reported feeling a reduction in the terror and paralysis that resulted from the attack. In the words of one participant "survivor":

> I feel more in control of my life . . . I have fewer fears in general and my nightmares have gone away altogether . . . I think I'm happier with my personal relationships. I like myself more than I did before I was assaulted . . . I've grown from what I've learned. (Note 5)

This "survivor's" remarks indicate what we have believed to be true for many of the women who have participated in self-defense programming. Beyond our initial goal of resocializing women to be non-victim-like in potential assault situations, the model may have succeeded in helping women to change their overall view of themselves, as well as their behavior in all aspects of their lives. These women appear more assertive generally, more self-confident, less dependent and report a sense of greater control and satisfaction in their interpersonal relationships (Smith, Note 4).

CONCLUSION

Obviously, many of these findings pertaining to the degree of success in prevention and treatment of sexual assault are far from scientifically conclusive. Many of us have found it virtually impossible to obtain research funding. There is, however, at least enough indication of success, I believe, to warrant continued use of this model. We need to continue to work toward legitimacy in the research and clinical communities.

The link between violence and oppression, the sexual assault incidence rates the dynamics of assailants and characteristics of victims, the role of women in Western society and the evidence of violent oppression of women are, obviously, quite real and verifiable.

As women treating women, I believe we have a very special obligation to continue in the development and implementation of more creative and encompassing approaches to both prevention and treatment of sexual assault. Without this freedom to be physically safe, opportunities for equal participation in society are worth nothing and are merely the rhetoric of a society which has successfully threatened and frightened the majority of its population into limiting and oppressing themselves.

NOTES

1. Javorek, F. *A Multivariate Analysis of the Victim, Attacker, and Situational Factors which Discriminate between Attempted and Completed Rape Cases: A Preliminary Report.* Research Bulletin 75-1, Violence Research Unit, Denver General Hospital, unpublished manuscript, 1975.

2. Javorek, P. and L. Lyon. *California Personal Inventory Factor Structure for Targets of Rape Versus a General Population of Women,* Research Bulletin 75-3, Violence Research Unit, Denver General Hospital, unpublished manuscript, 1975.

3. Queens Bench Foundation. Rape Victimization Study. Unpublished, San Francisco, 1975.

4. Smith, D. A Program Evaluation: The Effects of Women's Self Defense Training Upon Efficacy, Expectancies, Behavior and Personality Variables. Michigan State University, unpublished manuscript, 1983.

5. Taped interviews with student participant survivors, in Self Defense Class, Movement Arts Center, Lansing, Michigan, 1984.

REFERENCES

Amir, M. (1971). *Patterns of Forcible Rape.* Chicago: University of Chicago Press.
Gebhard, P. (1965). *Sex Offenders: An Analysis by Types.* New York: Harper and Row.
Federal Bureau of Investigation (1973) *Uniform Crime Reports for the United States.* Washington, DC: U.S. Department of Justice.
Selkin, J. (1975, January). Rape, *Psychology Today,* 71-76.

The Family Intervention Program

Erica Rothman
Kit Munson

THE PROGRAM

The Family Intervention Program is a 6-week educational course for couples for whom violence is a problem. The course consists of one session per week, lasting two hours and continuing for six consecutive weeks.

The primary goal of the program is to stop the violence. Secondary goals are: (1) for each spouse to decrease his/her verbal abuse of the other, (2) to increase their communication with each other, (3) to learn communication skills for confrontation purposes, and (4) for both partners to learn how to get out of their victim and aggression roles.

The decision of whether or not the couple stays together during the process of the violence ceasing is up to each partner. Some people find new strength and can make the relationship work, while others cannot.

RATIONALE

Most mental health professionals have witnessed the impact of violence on the family. The effect on each spouse; on the observing children, family and friends; and even on succeeding generations, is enormous. Along with their concern about the prevalence of this social problem, clinicians often feel baffled about the "correct"

Erica Rothman is a psychotherapist in private practice in Chapel Hill, North Carolina. Her practice includes workshops on women's and men's issues. She is an organizational consultant. Kit Munson is an adult outpatient therapist. She does community grassroots work for services for women. She is Director of the Family Intervention Program for Orange Person Chatham Mental Health Center.

intervention. Who should be treated? What constellation of family members should be seen in what environment?

Our program is a particular approach for couples that we have developed which addresses these two questions. Also, within the context of presenting the rationale for this program, we will discuss the dynamics of spouse abuse from psychological and sociological perspectives. Our program is one answer; it is by no means totally successful but we hope it will be a springboard for new ideas.

The Family Intervention Program was conceived by two female clinicians at the local mental health center who became frustrated by the appalling number of abused women on their caseloads, and concerned that the resources did not seem effective for decreasing the numbers. The community provided services that tended to impact only half of the couple involved. Women went to shelters and contacted 24-hour emergency lines. Men, on the other hand, rarely used these services, and when in court on assault charges, were waived even court costs with the admonishment to use the saved money to buy groceries for their children. Given the high correlation between alcoholism and family violence, one doubts that many men carried out the judge's wish.

As a result of our frustrations, we began exploring various intervention strategies. From our family systems perspective, we knew that to change a dyadic interaction the most effective means is to include both participants. We also knew that men do not come voluntarily to programs attempting to reduce their violent behavior. Finally, we felt it was time the court system began taking the charge of assault on a female more seriously.

Combining these goals we decided upon a couples' program that not only would be imposed upon the man by a judge, but also would be strongly encouraged for the woman partner.

In evaluating the possibilities for a program that would address the concern of both partners, we reviewed the different possible interventions. One study (Cookerly, 1973) maintained that conjoint individual therapy was the most effective therapy for couples wishing to stay married. Conjoint group therapy was the most effective treatment for couples obtaining a divorce. For those divorcing couples, individual marital therapy was the least effective. In working with couples with marital problems both conjoint individual therapy and conjoint group therapy have been effective.

In working with couples specifically involved in violence, treating the batterer alone in therapy is the least effective method of decreasing his violence. Galles (1982) criticizes treating only the man because this approach does not take into account the context of the violent relationship, which involves another person. Conjoint therapy can address the abusive behavior, the effect of violence on both partners, and it can break the assailant-victim dyad.

Group therapy for distressed couples is a viable alternative to individual conjoint therapy (Watts & Courtois, 1981). In addition to its efficacy, group treatment is a means of addressing the great demand for marital therapy that often cannot be met for individual couples by existing personnel resources. Moreover, other advantages of group marital therapy include: modeling by other group members; feedback from peers, which may be assimilated far more easily than by receiving it from therapists; group cohesiveness which can produce an increase in self-disclosure; and the opportunities to observe change in other couples which can decrease demoralization and maintain positive expectations (Liberman, 1970; Liberman, Wheeler & Sanders, 1976).

Some may argue that expecting the woman partner to attend a 6-week group course is punishing the victim. From our experience as marriage counselors, we had begun to believe that in abuse situations the woman partner was likely to be abusive as well, verbally if not physically. Men and women often related that during arguments both partners were using aggressive behaviors. This was later substantiated by our data analysis.

Even in relationships that report no abuse on the woman's part, we feel that each partner's understanding of his and her role is crucial for change. We are not saying that she is responsible for his abusive behavior, nor is she responsible for changes in behavior. What we are saying is that the relationship has a better opportunity to be non-violent if the woman has an understanding of her role in its existence in the couple relationship. For example, in situations where the woman is extremely passive, her new understanding of her behavior may lead her to set limits with her partner, something she may not have dared to do in the past. Or she may decide to leave. As we will describe later, much of the Family Intervention Program is based on confronting sex-role socialization. For men, this may take the form of their learning new, non-macho ways of expressing their needs. For women, the program helps them to become aware that women deserve not to be beaten.

Encouraging women to participate in this program can also be justified from a psychological perspective. In incestuous families, husband and wife are often from families where they were under-nurtured as children. In adult life, the mother's intense fear of loss and separation can lead to her accepting even unreasonable demands and withdrawing from confronting her husband for fear that he will leave her. A similar dynamic may be true for abused women as well. Also, women who were abused as children may bring the rage from that experience into their current family situation in the form of abuse towards their partner and/or children.

Including a woman in a group experience and giving her tools to feel empowered can have a long-lasting benefit on her self-esteem and her interactions with others. Contrarily, excluding the woman partner from the educational group can be interpreted as reinforcing that the woman is powerless — "We'll take care of you (by taking care of him)." This unspoken condescension can also lead to her feeling that she must only continue to be attentive to his responses and it is yet another aspect of his life from which she is excluded.

Men and women in our society do not often have the opportunity to have positive group experiences. For men, the legitimate group may consist of drinking buddies or a springtime softball team. Participating in the Family Intervention Program provides a man with the opportunity to hear other men admit to some of the social stresses that he himself might have felt but had not wanted to acknowledge out loud. He can witness a couple working out their differences non-aggressively and see that the man does not become powerless as a result.

Abused women are historically known to be isolated from others by virtue of the fear of retaliation by their partners if others were to be told of his behavior. In the Family Intervention Program they can hear their husbands being told by a female role model (the group co-leader) that it is not acceptable to batter. Moreover they witness this confrontation by a woman who is not afraid, and who can deliver the message in a caring way.

For both partners the group approach is a medium for obtaining much needed nurturance. As mentioned earlier, abusive couples often come from emotionally deprived childhoods. Our evaluations consistently show that participants want a longer program. One interpretation we have concluded from this is that people experience the group as a safe place to get some of their psychological needs met. There is a strong possibility that feeling undeserving of intimacy may be a major contributing factor to the continuation of abuse in relationships.

STRUCTURE AND CONTENT

The structure of the program is such that it can be organized and run with as few staff as possible. At bare minimum, the program can be run by two staff members (one male and one female) who conduct the classes and screen the class participants, a secretary who is in charge of class materials and notification to participants of the class starting date, and one or two court counselors per county to facilitate the court referral process.

With all linkages working as they should, the court counselor preliminarily screens the couple at court, suggests the use of the program to the district attorney and the Judge, and gives them an appointment for further screening at the Mental Health Center. The clinician doing the screening will specifically screen out people who are sociopathic, have problems with alcohol (in which case they are referred to the Alcohol Program or a Detoxification Program first), or have a thought disorder or clinical depression that would require other attention first. If the couple does not show up for their screening appointment, another appointment is sent by registered mail, with the reminder that if the appointment is not responded to, the defendant's name will be returned to the district attorney's office as noncompliant.

Our program is educational in nature, as we assume that after we screen out the sociopathic personalities, most men *do* want to change their behaviors but do not know how and/or feel powerless to stop something that they think "takes them over."

We find, as with most character-disordered men, that we first need to get their attention. There are two things that acting-out people will generally respond to: (1) "muscle" — authority, power, strength, and (2) symbolic "muscle" — money. The courts provide us the muscle we need quite effectively to get the men to the classes. It is our experience that if they protest too loudly about having to attend the classes, and/or do not follow through, we tell them they can always go back to court and discuss it with the Judge. The compliance at that point is 10%. The $100 fee for the course is found by the men to be quite distasteful, but it *does* get their attention. It allows us to run the program, and hopefully, the financial consequences will make them reconsider before they strike their partners again. Scholarships are available for families in which finances are a significant pre-existing problem. Arrangements can be made to pay the fee over a period of time; however the balance must be paid at the last class session to avoid returning to court as "noncompliant."

Once we have their attention, we find that the men need to hear the message that the courts and the community will not allow men beating women. Then we use as many media as possible to get people interacting in order to cut down on denial. We use films, and a combination of groups, such as the whole group, small groups, and men's and women's groups (the latter lending safety in speaking out). We as facilitators talk about our own experiences with abuse, our own thinking and decision-making around this issue. The male co-facilitators confront tirelessly, and deflect responsibility for violent behavior back to the men. Once their denial and minimization are lowered, the work of replacing violent behavior with non-violent alternatives and picking up on cues leading to loss of control can begin. We point out the penalties for abusive behavior as deterrents, such as potential loss of status in the community and/or workplace, alienation from family and friends, severe injury, homicide, suicide, etc. Time is spent identifying and expressing other emotions than anger, and looking at society's stereotyped ideas of what "macho" is and its effects on relationships. We focus on childhood so that the men make the connection between being a past victim of abuse and their present abusive behavior.

It is our feeling that the women also have their own set of problems that they need to attend to, such as problems of falling into victim behaviors that leave them feeling powerless and rageful, the latter causing problems of cross violence. When a woman finds herself in a violent relationship, she has two choices: she can leave or she can stay. If she stays, she can either fight back, both in self-protection and out of her rage at being treated like a shock absorber for her husband's feelings, *or* she can recoil and withdraw, instead of confronting him as to his inappropriate behavior. If she does not confront him, she inadvertently gives him the message that the battering is okay and perhaps justified. Hence begins a vicious cycle where both partners lose respect for each other and fall into a very negative and destructive life together.

Hence, in our program, we address the women and their issues also. We work with them, helping them learn to empower themselves with the message that battering is wrong and will not be tolerated by the community, that their own physical striking out (except in self defense) and verbal snipping at their partners is destructive to the relationship, and that they have every right to not accept their partners' violence and verbal degradation. We feel that it is also important for the women and men to know the consequences of remaining in an abusive relationship over years, as there is denial of the long term effects of family violence. We know that women who cannot effect change in their husband's violence do sometimes join them and become as acting-out as their husbands, including participating in child abuse, drug and alcohol abuse, massing as much denial around them as their husbands. On the other hand, we know that women who take on victim stances over the years, become terribly emotionally crippled and "give up" in the most profound ways—by psychotic reactions, severe withdrawal leading into schizophrenia, manic-depressive illness, multiple hospitalizations, suicidal and homicidal thoughts and acts, all rendering them and their lives so compromised that they would rather destroy themselves, and perhaps their husbands, than leave them. We want women to be aware of the heavy emotional toll of staying in a long term violent relationship.

We, as the female co-facilitators, model for the women the empowering, non-victim-like behavior that we want to address with them. We are willing to confront their partners, we tell them again and again that no one deserves to be beaten *no matter what they did*, we model working as equal team members with our male co-facilitators, we model saying "no" and other assertive communication skills, and we show interest in them and encourage them to speak out and claim their lives. We tell them that no longer are women tolerating abuse of any kind (physical, verbal, sexual)—not to ourselves in relationships, not to our children, not to our sisters, not to our mothers (as violent teenage boys often join in beating on their mothers), and not to our elders. We also tell them that this program is a chance for them to see if their husbands *do* take the issue of their violence seriously and try to follow up on their many promises of intended change. This is perhaps the most revealing function of the program for some women.

FAMILY INTERVENTION PROGRAM
OBJECTIVE RESULTS

Over eighteen months time, the progress of 31 couples and 11 separated men who participated in the Family Intervention Program (a couples' group treatment program for court-referred couples where violence is a problem) were assessed along the dimensions of violent behavior and quality of their interpersonal relationships. The testing tools used were McIntosh and Hudson's Index of Spouse Abuse (1981) and Guerney's Inventory of Relationship Skills (1977). The tools were administered at screening, at the first class, the last class, and at the one month follow-up time.

The results indicated that while in treatment, the men's violent behavior decreased significantly ($p < .05$), that their non-physical violence decreased as well, but only to a near statistically significant degree and that the couples' level of trust, intimacy and communication increased significantly ($p < .01$). At one month follow-up, gains made during the treatment had fallen to below statistical significance, but not below the levels recorded at the beginning of treatment. This study supports the efficacy of a skills training approach to spouse abuse in reducing violent and non-violent abuse and in increasing levels of trust, intimacy and communication. In order to maintain gain beyond treatment, longer length of treatment than six weeks seems indicated.

ENDING COMMENTS

We as women who are in the forefront of mental health issues for women, helping to empower ourselves and our sisters to strive for more equal and non-abusive relationships between ourselves and our male or female partners, must link arms with others and continue to work on setting limits on what is acceptable behavior and what is not, speak out about violence that is occurring in our relationships, to our children, on school and college campuses, in our society in the forms of pornography, murder, and death penalty executions, and finally but perhaps most urgently, speak out against international abuse, more commonly called war and potential nuclear holocaust. The aggressiveness, denial and disrespect most often begins and/or is tolerated at home, can stop there with our collective voices and role-modeling.

REFERENCES

Cookerly, J. R. (1973). Outcome of 6 major forms of marriage counseling compared. *Journal of Marriage, 35*(4) 608-611.
Gelles, R. (1982). An exchange/social control approach to understanding intrafamily violence. *Behavior Therapist* (1981), *5*(1), 5-8.

Guerney, E. G. (1977). *Relationship Enhancement; Skill Training Programs for Therapy, Problem Prevention and Enrichment*. San Francisco: Jossey-Bass.

Hudson, W. W. & McIntosh, S. P. (1981). The Assessment of spouse abuse: Two quantifiable dimensions. *Journal of Marriage and the Family, 43*(4), 873-888.

Liberman, R. P., Wheeler & Sanders. (1976). Marital therapy in groups: A comparative evaluation of behavioral and interactional formats. *Acta Psychiatrica Scandinavica, Supp. 266*, 3-34.

Lieberman, M. A. (1967). The implications of total group phenomena analysis for patients and therapists. *International Journal of Group Psychotherapy, 17*(1), 71-81.

Watts, D. L. & Courtois, C. S. (1981). Trends in the treatment of men who commit violence against women. *Personal and Guidance Journal, 60*(4), 245-249.

Women to Women:
Facilitating Decision-Making
About Contraception

Martha E. Zuehlke

A clinical research project designed to address adolescent sexual
activity and contraceptive behavior taught us more than we anticipated. Partially by design and partially as an unfolding of the process of the work a number of basic feminist truths were communicated to and integrated by the adolescent girls in the project. It
seems in retrospect that this may in fact be the real value of the
experience over and above the behavioral outcome measures.

A group of women social scientists and mental health professionals formed the nucleus for our research project. The presence of
Ann Peterson, an active and prolific research psychologist whose
academic credentials lent validity to the serious study of specifically female development, was critical to our project. She was approached by the Department of Obstetrics and Gynecology for a
solution to what was perceived as inappropriate adolescent pregnancy. This triggered a gathering of people, all women but one,
who shared a concern about the consequences of adolescent pregnancy as well as a sense that many current sexual education and
contraceptive programs were not addressing the relevant issues.

Over a period of two years our research group struggled with
defining our task, our approach and our outcome instruments. We
were a group of women trying to work collaboratively, not hierar-
chically, and continuously striving to achieve consensus. This fos-

The author is a practicing child and adult psychiatrist, an assistant clinical professor of
psychiatry at the University of Chicago, and an attending psychiatrist at Michael Reese Hospital in Chicago, Illinois.

This research was supported by grants from the Michael Reese Hospital and Medical Center and from the MacArthur Foundation.

tered considerable sharing and learning from each other as our backgrounds, training and personalities varied greatly. At times the
process was exceedingly slow and laborious and the project was
nearly abandoned. I believe part of the frustration was that we were
not always conscious of our own need to avoid conflict, to minimize
hierarchical interactions nor that we were working in a way counter
to most of our training and most of our colleagues' work. Let me
elaborate more on the thinking behind the project as a preface to
what we see in retrospect.

We approached female adolescent sexual behaviors as women.
That is, we were predominantly interested in what motivates this
behavior and particularly what is involved in the pregnant outcomes—why weren't girls preventing pregnancy? Despite a considerable volume of work in this area, the general assumption remains
that girls get pregnant because they're either stupid, thoughtless or
want to be pregnant. Given an adult, social scientist perspective,
which is predominantly male identified, this conclusion leads to
interventions that try to manipulate girls into doing what they were
told to do—"don't be sexually active or if you do, contracept," the
girls remain as seemingly unable to be responsible for themselves.

Luker's book, *Taking Chances* (1975), was exceedingly helpful
in clarifying our differences with those assumptions. She studied
women seeking abortions and found that women had been balancing
a number of conflicting goals in their sexual, and specifically their
contraceptive behaviors. It should not come as a surprise to us that
women seek to balance competing needs—within themselves and
between themselves and the significant others in their lives.

Once again we are confronted with the difficult task women assume in their decision making—balancing self interests with the
need for connection (validation?) to others.

This book formed a pivotal part of our approach which assumed
that girls *were* making decisions about their sexual activity and that
perhaps they could be helped to make decisions that would be more
in line with their own interests. That is, perhaps we could increase
their sense of control over their own lives and thereby increase their
actual control and responsibility in this sphere of their lives.

To this end we attempted to design a project that would foster
better self care through its content as well as through the experiential process. We designed a program of 12 weekly meetings for
groups of 10 to 20 adolescent girls. The groups were led by 2 to 4
adolescents trained as peer leaders and assisted by one adult, female

staff member. The two hour sessions were each organized around a specific topic (see Table 1) and utilized a variety of exercises that reinforced appropriate decision making and self care related to sexuality and contraception. The inclusion of activities such as group discussions, brainstorming, handling contraceptive materials and participating in and observing role plays of relevant situations made the process an active and meaningful one. We attempted to provide an experience that would enhance the factors we felt contributed to appropriate self care in their sexual lives: a sense of one's own power to choose goals and to pursue them, a sense of connection and support from peers, an opportunity to experience conflicting needs and uncertainty without self denigration and an opportunity to experience and practice self actualizing behaviors. The curriculum was organized conceptually to move from discussions of sexual intimacy to discussions of pregnancy, the experience and the alternatives confronting a pregnant teenager. We attempted to maintain the broader context of deciding on, clarifying and acting on overall life plans and goals. For example, we would initiate a discussion about being sexually active as a teenager. We overtly supported reserving sexual activity for meaningful and mutually-gratifying relationships and using contraceptives to delay child bearing until adulthood but openly acknowledged the positive and negative consequences of these positions. We utilized techniques to foster a cost-benefit analysis of the decision to be sexually active. We would encourage active participation from all the group members, listening to the varied points of view and helping the participants grasp the range of opinions and choices that were revealed in the discussion. In this way we attempted to model and encourage conscious decision making in the context of personal values and goals.

The peer leaders were crucial elements that embodied the message that adolescent girls can think, share ideas and responsibly function in the sphere of sexual activity and in the broader context of their lives.

I should add that we were told by our colleagues and "superiors" that our target population would not participate in such an extended program. Our hospital is located in a neighborhood of low income, urban, black people with the usual multiple problems of social, racial and economic disadvantage. Not only did we consistently have good response in attendance but we found we had to expand our project's size to accommodate the numbers of girls who were invested in participating. And we found that most of the girls who

Table 1

Curriculum Outline

Week 1	Introduction, preassessments
	Videotape of peers in role play
Week 2	Making decisions, setting goals
	Film and videotape
Week 3	Birth Control - I
	Film of methods
Week 4	Birth Control - II
	Guest speaker - demonstration
Week 5	Costs and Benefits - I
	Role plays
Week 6	Abortion
	Guest speakers and role play
Week 7	Teenage Pregnancy
	Guest speaker and film
Week 8	Teenage Parenting
	Film
Week 9	Costs and Benefits - II
	Role plays
Week 10	Others' Opinions
	Members bring boyfriends to group
Week 11	Looking to the future
	Role plays
Week 12	Summary and postassessments
	Refreshments

---

wanted to be peer leaders were able to function successfully in that role.

I would like to focus on the data we collected after the intervention from the peer leaders. In addition to our written pre and post instruments, we conducted extended individual focused interviews with all the peer leaders (as well as a subsample of the girls in the intervention and control groups). The remainder of my remarks uses this interview material. We coded and analyzed transcripts to look for the girls' responses to the project experience because this was not measured by our highly structured evaluation. It was in looking at this data — the girls' own comments about their experience — that led me to be aware that we had been raising the consciousness of these young women through the process we designed to influence their sexual decision making — and that it may very well be that it is this very thing that constituted the appeal as well as the special value of the program.

The focused interviews were done individually 6 to 12 months after the intervention and were conducted by one of two staff members. All the peer leaders knew all the staff but the specific staff member who worked with a particular peer leader did not do the interviewing. Despite this and other attempts to encourage expression of dissatisfactions, the girls consistently focused almost exclusively on positive aspects. Some criticisms did emerge but the overwhelming response was intense enthusiasm.

The area most commented on had to do with the personal benefits of participating as peer leaders. All of them made mention of their increased sense of self worth and confidence subsequent to the experience. Let me give you some direct examples of this.

Yeah, it was a great experience for me, because I really learned a lot; I learned a lot about people and how to deal with people and leadership. That was good for me because it helped me a lot in school and where I go. Because I can — at school I used to be like afraid to like read out in front of everybody in class or get up and talk and read my reports and stuff, but now it's really easy, because I've been you know, talking and everything. Well, sometimes I still get the jitters but it was real good.

I got the satisfaction of knowing there might be some more girls out there who will make better decisions than what they

already make, or either at least that they know they, like they
know, they can make decisions on their own. A lot of girls out
there let society make their decisions or something like that, or
their boyfriends or something like that. It's helping them be
their own person and when I see I, you know, help them to do
that I got a lot of satisfaction out of just doing it.

It was striking to hear these girls experiencing their own strengths
in this way and to be so self aware of that strength. There were some
clear indications about the source of that increased strength in terms
of their self awareness as well as their experiencing greater sharing
and connection with their peers. As one girl expressed:

No, except for it was a lot of fun and I hope we can do the
program again. Because I know it helped, well one girl that
goes to my school . . . It helped her a lot because she said she
didn't know anything about birth control and all and after she
went through the program she understood it and she knew. It
sort of helped you make your own decisions and understand
what's right for you, what's wrong for you and understand the
world surrounding you and how your boyfriend is and things
like that. So it really did help me make a lot of my decisions
also.

The comfort and relief that so many of these girls felt as they
heard other girls' feelings and confusions reflect their own was to
me very evocative of my experiences of first sharing with other
women in the consciousness-raising groups in the '60s. The tremendous relief as well as sense of power that comes from a sense of
union and shared feelings was coming alive here for these young
women in ways they had not previously dared to explore. This way
of exploring oneself is most facilitated by a sharing kind of teaching
as compared to a didactic format.

Perhaps it should not be so surprising that the experience of leadership, having responsibility, should prove to be so strengthening
for the girls. Perhaps they are feeling relief and strength from the
sense of consensus that the group sharing facilitated more than actual connectedness to their peers. However, a large number of the
girls made observations of what styles of leadership — what types of
experience — would not have been productive. And it is here that I
see the most vivid reworking of the values we as staff must have
communicated through our styles. In investigating what techniques

and types of approaches felt least successful, 8 of the 12 girls spontaneously mentioned authoritarian styles as not working.

What is of interest to me is that in practice we as staff spent a lot of time working on ways to make the message of preventing pregnancy feel relevant to these girls and certainly we saw the connections between postponing pregnancy and having a sense of control over their lives. But I think it was primarily through the way we worked with each other and with our peer leaders that made it possible for the peer leaders to grasp the necessity and value of communicating and acknowledging the intrinsic worth of each of the girls. The enhanced respect for themselves and associated self confidence allowed a greater respect for each girl's own process of realizing her capacity to make decisions for herself. We frequently made use of the phrase "not to decide is a decision." This was an attempt to confront the girls with the unavoidable nature of choice and decision making. And it was an attempt to demystify the process of choice. Most of our techniques of teaching about contraception were attempts to make more explicit, the process of decision making, more explicit and less expert bound. At times this felt like oversimplification in an attempt to foster confidence about making an attempt to assume some control over their lives. We swung back and forth between stressing what others chose and felt and then using that knowledge to go back to focus on what each of them felt and chose. The capacity to take support and help from others without abdicating one's own strength and autonomy was being nurtured. And our peer leaders were acutely aware of the necessity and the difficulty of that task.

In looking at what it was that we did as staff that felt most useful to our peer leaders we see a continuation of this balance. Techniques mentioned as most useful to the peer leaders were the training sessions, the pre-meeting sessions with the staff, the presence of the staff member and the session outlines. We provided the leaders with an outline of each session that provided a summary of the goals for the day, suggested exercises and discussion points and a loose structuring of the meeting. Ten of the 12 leaders mentioned this as useful as a starting place or organizer. But nine mentioned the simple presence of the staff person during the sessions as fulfilling similar functions. Here are some of their observations about this.

> . . . Michelle she just sat you know, back. She wanted to see if we could handle it ourselves. She really didn't want to get involved; she wanted us to do it ourselves.

Because they were always there when we needed them, you know, and if it was something we were stuck on, you know, they were always there then.

Here I think the parallel processes of the staff's interrelationships, the staff-peer leader interrelationships and the peer leader-member interrelationships is revealed. As we struggled to work collaboratively and be mutually respectful of each other we communicated a way of working and a value system that corresponded with the content of our intervention; that to assume responsibility for parts of one's life — such as one's sexual and reproductive functioning requires not just information and access to resources but a sense of one's own value and strength. This is something that comes from being heard, being recognized, being respected and having the actual experiences of being effective and in control.

Their strength was dizzying at times — almost frightening to us even though we had struggled so to find ways to unlock it. One of the sessions was organized around a demonstration of the various contraceptive devices during which major emphasis was placed on the girls becoming comfortable with these items. Each girl learned to actively and successfully examine and handle each item. A grab bag drawing of condoms, foam and jelly was done and some of the girls left with these items. It later came up that on the way home the girls continued to play — creating condom water balloons and squirting foam at each other. We conferenced about this, concerned that we may have overly stimulated the girls and encouraged inappropriate acting out. However, further reflection suggests that perhaps it was their exceedingly casual treatment of things previously untouchable, unthinkable and certainly unsharable that was shocking to us and to the community. Having a greater sense of control over their reproductive choices also meant having to be less respectful and submissive to the devices themselves. This behavior then appears to be a step toward more real control and appropriate responsibility for their own sexuality.

It may well be that one of the sources for the relative failure of sex education and contraceptive services programs to impact on adolescent pregnancy is that the message continues to be "You women need to be managed and taken care of." To the extent that we, as therapists and interviewers, continue to believe this, we only continue the hopelessness and impotence of the women we work with. In this project we learned that our having a collective planning process enabled us to develop a format in which the girls could take leadership and assume responsibility which proved far more fruitful than we anticipated. When we gave them an opportunity to develop and use their capabilities they developed knowledge control and decision making capabilities over their reproductive lives which extended into all of their lives. I hope this project and our experiences will serve to promote an examination of the ways we work with each other and the assumptions about our patients and clients that may be undermining our collective selves, and present a model for change.

REFERENCE

Luker, K. (1975). *Taking Chances: Abortion and the Decision Not to Contracept.* Berkeley: University of California Press.

The Role of "Coming Out" by the Lesbians in the Physician-Patient Relationship

Susan R. Johnson
Susan M. Guenther

At first glance, the subject of medical care for lesbian and bisexual women seems out of place among the other papers in this collection. However, early in the process of studying the health problems of these women (Johnson, Guenther, Laube & Keettel, 1981), we discovered that many of our research subjects regarded unsatisfactory interactions with health care professionals to be more significant than concerns about specific diseases. While some of the problems were related to more generic issues such as physician behavior or sexism, the principal difficulties revolved around the issue of revealing sexual orientation ("coming out") to the physician.

Why should a lesbian want to come out, and why should her physician care if she does? In this paper, we will develop the argument that the development of a satisfactory physician-patient relationship depends on it, and then review the empirical support for this position. We will describe the barriers that appear to inhibit coming out: homophobia, prejudice, ignorance and indifference. Finally, we will suggest some ways that concerned health care professionals can create a more supportive atmosphere. We will focus primarily on lesbians, but most of the comments apply to gay men as well as bisexuals of either sex.

Susan R. Johnson is a gynecologist who is an assistant professor in the Department of Obstetrics and Gynecology, University of Iowa College of Medicine, Iowa City, Iowa. Susan M. Guenther is a psychologist who is an intensive outpatient counselor at the Midcastern Council on Chemical Abuse, Iowa City, Iowa.

For correspondence, contact Dr. Johnson at the Department of Obstetrics and Gynecology, University of Iowa Hospitals, Iowa City, IA 52242.

There are several reasons lesbian patients may choose to reveal their orientation to their physician (Johnson & Palermo, 1984). The differential diagnosis of specific symptoms can be adjusted appropriately, suggesting additional tests, or eliminating the need for others. For example, a lesbian with vaginal bleeding and pain is unlikely to have an early pregnancy complication such as spontaneous abortion or ectopic pregnancy. Certain medical disorders may result from specific sexual behaviors (e.g., sexually transmitted diseases), or may affect future sexual activity (e.g., postoperatively). The physician cannot provide appropriate educational information if he or she is not aware of the patient's particular situation. Lesbian patients who have serious or chronic illnesses require the support and care of their partner and/or close friends. The involvement of these individuals is best facilitated if they are directly included the decision-making and therapeutic process.

These reasons are all important, but they are limited in that they only apply to specific medical circumstances. We will develop the more general claim that, irrespective of the medical situation, the quality of care given and received depends on the quality of the physician-patient relationship, and that relationship in turn is dependent on the lesbian coming out. It is important to be clear that we do *not* mean that sexual orientation must be discussed in every individual medical encounter. It has little relevance in the immediate treatment of a broken ankle in the emergency room, or a blood pressure measurement in a shopping mall screening clinic. However, the broken ankle may need surgery and complicated aftercare, or the blood pressure may be elevated, requiring difficult long term treatment plans. Now the relationship between patient and physician becomes more important; complex decisions may be needed,and these can be best made in an atmosphere of honest communication.

It may still not be clear why coming out is important to this process. We will further develop the idea from two directions: first, from the point of view of the philosophy of medicine, and second, from the perspective of gay interpersonal development.

THE PHYSICIAN-PATIENT RELATIONSHIP
IN MEDICAL PHILOSOPHY

Pellegrino and Thomasma (1981) argue that a major feature distinguishing medicine from the arts and pure sciences is the clinical encounter, i.e., the coming together of a physician and a patient for the purpose of establishing a healing relationship. They go on to say that "medicine's proper motive is compassion or friendship, it's purpose is an individualized satisfactory state of well-being, and it's structure falls into a category of a relationship." This expression of the physician-patient relationship as a personal one seems to us to be the view most physicians learn during their formal education (Morgan & Engel, 1969), and despite the many problems that have arisen recently to challenge it, we believe it is the view most commonly held by practicing physicians and their patients.

Why is this the case? While it is a truism to say that doctors treat patients and not diseases, examining the several meanings of the expression will help answer the question:

1. The same disease often presents differently in different patients, due to biological variations in both individuals and pathologic processes.
2. Individuals experience each disease in unique ways, due to a variety of factors such as differing pre-disease physical conditions, pain tolerances, social support or cultural views of illness.
3. The objectives for the medical encounter vary between patients, even when the disease process is similar, depending on the individual's life goals.
4. Disease always has an impact on the patient's social system, and these systems, which include family, love relationships, friends, and career, are unique.

From examining this list, it seems obvious that the physician must be familiar with many parts of the patient's life, both to effectively diagnose the illness and offer appropriate treatment. Physicians are privileged to have access to the most intimate facets of a patient's life *because only with this information can they offer comprehensive care.* Patients, in turn, are responsible for revealing themselves honestly. Clearly the communication required for this kind of interchange will not occur unless there is trust between patient and physician.

WHAT DOES "COMING OUT" MEAN FOR GAY PEOPLE?

"Coming out" is a process that is often misunderstood by some heterosexual people who view it as "flaunting" sexual activity, imposing on the sensitivities of others, or revealing personal information inappropriately. In contrast, we will discuss three purposes of coming out which appear to have particular relevance to the physician-patient relationship.

Sexual identity is an important facet of any person's self concept; for heterosexual men and women, sexual orientation is ordinarily taken for granted since heterosexuality is considered the cultural norm. Unless there is internal conflict, the heterosexual rarely has need to discuss (or perhaps even think about) this critical matter. For gay women and men, this is obviously not the case; they are raised in a heterosexual society, which in American culture means being exposed to negative, often hostile attitudes toward homosexuality. These societal views are frequently internalized, and the struggle to overcome them can be prolonged and not always successful. One of the marks of self-acceptance is the ability to comfortably reveal oneself to others. From a developmental perspective each instance of coming out (when voluntary and intentional) could be viewed as a reflection of increased self-acceptance and enhanced self-esteem. Berzon (1979) has described a developmental model for gay people which includes a series of coming out situations, starting with the self (i.e., recognizing and accepting one's own homosexual orientation), and branching out to a progressively wider group, including friends, family, colleagues, and finally (although not inevitably), the world at large. The physician in whom one places trust for advice and care surely belongs on this list. We would argue, in fact, that a gay person will have difficulty in developing an honest relationship with any individual unless sexual orientation is revealed.

One also might take a political, rather than personal view, and say that unless lesbians come out to their physicians (and others) there is little hope that attitudes will change (Denneny, 1981). Physicians will continue to believe that there are no gay people in their practices (Good, 1976), and that there is no reason for them to consider the issue. Not every lesbian will subscribe to this view, and even if they do, may not feel safe in acting on it.

Finally, and perhaps most importantly for this discussion, coming out reveals more than ones's type of sexual behavior. Although the details are individual, the areas of disclosure may include kind of relationship, friends, ties to family, work, etc. By coming out, the lesbian does not give away the *content* of her life, but at least suggests a different context. Put another way, heterosexual patients are routinely asked about family and marital status, perhaps partly out of social convention, but also because this knowledge contributes to the physician's understanding of the richness of the patient's life. Homosexual men and women, on the other hand, rarely expect that others will know-or ask about—their orientation. When that happens. the physician loses an opportunity to know the whole person.

EMPIRICAL SUPPORT

Before continuing, it is important to acknowledge the difficulties of obtaining representative data from the gay population (Bell & Weinberg, 1979). Most investigators are forced to rely on samples of convenience; conclusions based on such samples must be considered tentative, and not necessarily generalizable.

While the data in this area is limited, three recent studies support the idea that coming out to their physician is considered important to many gay women and men. Dardick and Grady (1980) surveyed 622 gay men and lesbians about their experiences with health care professionals. The sample represented 23% of the subscribers to a Boston gay newspaper; 27% of the respondents were female, and most were white, young, urban and well-educated. Sixty three percent of the men and 49% of the women surveyed had revealed their orientation to a physician. Less than 10% of either sex reported that they would prefer to not come out to the physician under any circumstances. There was a direct association between being "out" to significant others (family, friends, etc.) and disclosure to the physician. Individuals who had come out to their physicians were much more likely to report satisfaction with their health care and to believe that the physician was competent than those who had not. Not surprisingly, those who perceived their health care professional to be supportive were more satisfied than those who thought the professional was hostile.

Our own studies were carried out in two phases. The pilot project was based on a survey of 117 women recruited by advertisement and word of mouth in Johnson County, Iowa (Johnson et al., 1981). A year later, we obtained a sample of 2,382 women from two women's music festivals in the midwest and northeast (Smith, Johnson, & Guenther, 1985). Eighty point six percent identified themselves as lesbian and the remaining 17.8% as bisexual. Gynecologic health care was our particular focus, partly because of the specialty interest of one of us, and partly because it is in this context that questions about sexual activity are most likely to arise.

The demographic description of our samples was similar to that of Dardick and Grady: young, white, urban and well-educated, although because of the large sample size, a larger absolute number of women over 40 and rural women were included than in any previous study. As part of a more comprehensive survey of health issues, we asked several questions about disclosure of sexual orientation to physicians. Because the results of the two studies were similar, we will only report data from the second larger sample. A total of 46.8% of the lesbians and 30.2% of the bisexuals had disclosed at some time to a physician; the majority had volunteered the information without being asked. An additional 36.4% and 37.2% of the lesbians and bisexuals, respectively, reported that they would like to be able to do so. Less than 1% of either group had ever refused to disclose when directly asked by a physician, although 15.5% of lesbians and 30.5% of the bisexuals said they would prefer not to disclose.

Despite the strong evidence from both Dardick and Grady's work and our own that coming out to the physician is a desirable goal, there is also evidence to suggest that such disclosure not infrequently has adverse effects. In the Boston survey, 27% felt that they had encountered a health care professional who was unsupportive or hostile, and women were more likely to report this than men. In our second study, 30% of all respondents who had come out to a physician had encountered an overtly negative response; these responses included embarrassment, "coolness," and overt rejection.

Some of the consequences of negative attitudes on the part of health care professional's attitudes were (a) seeking nontraditional sources of health care, (b) reluctance of patients to give complete medical histories, and (c) occasionally failure to obtain care at all.

Attitudes commonly expressed toward gay people in our society include homophobia, prejudice, heterosexism, and ignorance. A discussion of the reasons for these negative attitudes is beyond the scope of this paper. Scattered evidence in the literature in addition to the studies discussed above makes it clear that some physicians hold these attitudes as well. Pauly and Goldstein (1970) surveyed 937 physicians concerning their attitudes in treating gay men. Twenty seven percent reported that they seldom or never feel comfortable treating this group of patients, and a slightly smaller number said that knowledge of homosexual orientation would interfere with their ability to give appropriate care. Masters and Johnson (1979) report that in a group of 81 gay men and women who were treated at their institute for sexual dysfunction, 57 had been refused treatment by at least one primary care physician, and were not referred to any other source of care.

In addition to these examples of homophobia and prejudice, several authors have discussed the adverse effect that language reflecting heterosexist assumptions has on disclosure (Whyte & Calpadlini, 1980, Owen, 1980, Johnson & Palermo, 1984). Some comments made by two women in our study may help to illustrate this point: "the physicians I have gone to assume that I am heterosexual. There is much time wasted in discussing birth control methods. This makes me uncomfortable and it is harder for me to be open about my own concerns about my body to the physician"; and "sometimes they ask if you are sexually active—if you say yes, they assume heterosexually and if you say no, you lie . . ."

IN CONCLUSION

If we agree that trust must be established as part of the development of the physician-patient relationship, and that for gay people, "coming out" is integral to the development of trusting relationships, we are left with the conclusion that coming out is important part of the relationship between gay patients and their physicians. The data we have cited supports this view. We are unfortunately also forced to the conclude that not all health care professionals are prepared for such disclosures.

The solutions will not be easy, and at a basic level, will depend on changes in attitude at the societal level. In the meantime, we encourage medical educators to continue to include in the curriculum information about the health care needs of gay women and men (Thomas, Scott & Brooks 1980). We also hope that practicing physicians will recognize that they almost certainly have gay patients in their practices. We hope that they will carefully examine (and if necessary, revise) their own attitudes toward homosexuality as well as educate themselves about the health needs and concerns of these patients. If we believe those famous words of Peabody (1927), that "the secret of the care of the patient is in caring for the patient," the medical profession is obligated to do so.

REFERENCES

Bell, A. P. & Weinberg, M. S. (1978). *Homosexualities: A Study of Diversity Among Men and Women*. New York: Simon and Schuster.

Berzon, B. (1979). Developing a positive gay identity. *Positively Gay*. Millbrae, CA: Celestial Arts.

Dardick, L. & Grady, K. E. (1980). Openness between gay persons and health professionals. *Annals of Internal Medicine, 93*, 115-119.

Denneny, M. (1981) Gay manifesto for the 80s. *Christopher Street*, January, 13-21.

Good, R. S. (1976). The gynecologist and the lesbian. *Clinical Obstetrics and Gynecology, 19*, 473-482.

Johnson, S. R., Guenther, S. M., Laube, D. W. & Keettel, W. C. (1981). Factors influencing lesbian gynecologic care: A preliminary study. *American Journal of Obstetrics and Gynecology, 140*, 20-28.

Johnson, S. R. & Palermo, J. L. (1984). Gynecologic care for the lesbian. *Clinical Obstetrics and Gynecology, 27*, 724-731.

Masters, W. & Johnson, V. (1979). *Homosexuality in Perspective*. Boston: Little, Brown & Company.

Morgan W. L. & Engel, G. L. (1969). *The Clinical Approach to the Patient*. Philadelphia, W. B. Saunders Company.

Owen, W. F. (1980). The clinical approach to the homosexual patient. *Annals of Internal Medicine, 93*, 90-92.

Pauly, I. B. & Goldstein, S. G. (1970). Physicians attitudes in treating male homosexuals. *Medical Aspects of Human Sexuality, 4*, 27-45.

Peabody, F. W. (1927). The care of the patient. *Journal of the American Medical Association, 88*, 877.

Pellegrino, E. D. & Thomasma, D. C. (1981). *A Philosophical Basis of Medical Practice*. New York: Oxford University Press, 1981.

Smith, E. M., Johnson, S. R. & Guenther, S. M. (1985). Health care attitudes and experiences during gynecologic care among lesbians and bisexuals. *American Journal of Public Health, 75*, 1085-1087.

Thomas, J. L., Scott, L. K. & Brooks, C. M. (1980). Attitude change in a human sexuality course that de-emphasizes small group activities. *Medical Education, 14*, 254-258.

Whyte, J. & Calpaldini, L. (1980). Treating the lesbian or gay patient. *Delaware Medical Journal, 52*, 271-277.

Choice in Childbirth: Power and the Impact of the Modern Childbirth Reform Movement

Martha Livingston

This paper is about childbirth and power: the power women have to give birth; the power to control how that birth is achieved, which has been wrested from us; and the power we are struggling to win back in today's childbirth reform movement. Birth is nothing if not physiological, but like all human activity, this physical act occurs within a social context which profoundly shapes how we regard it. There are two models of birth in operation in the U.S. today—the medical model and what some have called the "midwifery" model (e.g., Nash & Nash, 1979; Rothman, 1982). One, in the medical model, views birth as an inherently dangerous and life-threatening activity, made safe only when tightly controlled by medical specialists and technology. The other, "midwifery" model, views birth as a normal, healthy activity of the human female, and as much a social and psychological as a physiological event. How these models shape the way birth is practiced in the U.S. today, and how we can regain power over the conduct of childbirth, are the subject of this paper. But we cannot understand how birth as socially defined in the U.S. got to be the way it is without looking at its history, in Western Europe and the U.S., at least in broad brush-strokes.

The author is a social psychologist, childbirth educator, and mother. Among her publications is *The Minds of the Chinese People: Mental Health in New China* (Prentice-Hall, 1983). She is currently working on a dissertation about childbirth and self-esteem.

Readers wishing to obtain reprints or a copy of the original, more historically complete version of this paper should address inquiries to the author at the Department of Psychology, State University of New York at Stony Brook, Stony Brook, NY 11794.

THE LEGACY OF BIRTH IN EUROPE

Because birth is a universal human activity, every society has its own history and culture of birth; far from there being one idealized "primitive" birth culture, birthing practices vary widely (Jordan, 1983; Stanton, 1979). One aspect of birth outside our own culture that appeals to childbirth activists, however, is that in most of the world, whatever the surrounding culture and rituals, birth seems to be understood as women's work. Throughout the Middle Ages, birthing women in Western Europe, like their sisters around the world, were attended almost exclusively by midwives, who were women past childbearing age who had assisted at numerous births and had a great store of practical knowledge about birthing.

Midwives held their own as caretakers of normal birth until the 17th century, when the advancement of organized medicine brought the first serious competition from male practitioners (Ehrenreich & English, 1973). A real advance came about with the development of the forceps, which could dislodge an impacted fetus without killing it. For a variety of reasons, midwives never took to using forceps, and consequently lost many of their most affluent clientele (Litoff, 1978; Wertz & Wertz, 1979).

BIRTH IN AMERICA

In colonial America, the midwife was a highly respected practitioner, licensed, for the first time, by civil authorities (Wertz & Wertz, 1979). Well into the 19th century, most doctors seemed to conceive their role as providers of care in abnormal birth, leaving the normal to midwives and in fact helping midwives gain access to the more advanced scientific knowledge they had obtained abroad.

But this comfortable, well-delineated relationship was not to survive the early years of the 19th century, as medical colleges were founded, medicine became organized, doctors became licensed by the states, and, perhaps most importantly, delivering babies came to be viewed as a natural way to build a medical practice. As one physician wrote in 1824 (in Arney, 1982, p. 43):

> If females can be induced to believe that their sufferings will be diminished, or shortened, and their lives and those of their offspring, be safer in the hands of the profession; there will be

no difficulty in establishing the universal practice of obstetrics.

THE TWENTIETH CENTURY:
MODERN OBSTETRICS ASSERTS ITSELF

The thrust for the establishment of a more modern obstetrics grew
more powerful in the early years of the 20th century. Leading obstetricians such as J. Whitridge Williams (of *Williams' Obstetrics*, still
a leading medical text) and Joseph B. DeLee (of forceps and episiotomy fame) urged the construction of more maternity hospitals so
that *all* births could take place in them, providing, they believed,
safer conditions, convenience for the medical specialist, and a supply of subjects for obstetrical residents. In discussing the apparent
absurdity of a pathology model of birth, DeLee wrote (in Wertz &
Wertz, 1979):

> So frequent are these bad effects, that I have often wondered
> whether Nature did not deliberately intend women to be used
> up in the process of reproduction, in a manner analogous to
> that of the salmon, which dies after spawning.

Other proposals urged by Williams and others included the stricter
regulation of medical schools and the abolition of midwives.

Although many middle class women were still having their babies at home, they began to believe the argument that the hospital
was a cleaner, safer, more "modern" place to have a baby than the
home.

The "twilight sleep" movement for painless childbirth of the
second decade of this century dovetailed nicely with the professional agenda of the modern obstetricians. The method involves (I
use the present tense because it is still in use) the use of scopolamine, an amnesic, and morphine, or, more recently, Demerol, a
painkiller. Scopolamine removes the woman's conscious memory
of the events of labor and delivery; she experiences it as though she
had had general anesthesia (which cannot be used in childbirth since
it stops uterine contractions entirely, necessitating delivery by cesarean section). In fact, women given twilight sleep lose conscious
control over their behavior, ranting and screaming and requiring
physical restraints for their own safety. Anyone who has seen labor-

ing women treated with twilight sleep can hardly imagine that
women themselves demanded the treatment, but the "modern
women" of the World War I period saw it as a modern and humane
technique for bearing children. They subscribed to the ideology that
"civilized" women could not bear children without suffering un-
speakable pain, and saw it as their right to be given the most up-to-
date, scientific treatment which would render birth painless and
even encourage more civilized women to have more babies, thus
"improving the race" (Miller, 1979). For women of this period
who sought freedom from an endless cycle of compulsory motherhood and baby-minding, this was the era of contraception, bottle-
feeding, and hospital birth supervised by the modern birth specialist, the obstetrician. So widespread did the use of twilight sleep
become that Dr. Rudolph Holmes, who helped introduce it into the
U.S., urged, at the American Medical Association's 1936 convention, that it no longer be used (in Iffy & Kaminetzky, 1981).

I was the man who brought scopolamine to America. I didn't
know what I was doing. I have found out since. We must
protest vigorously against making the human mother an ani-
mated mass without any mentality.

Twilight sleep remains in use today, fifty years after Holmes's im-
passioned speech.
    Another goal of the movement to modernize obstetrics was the
elimination of the midwife, primarily to do away with the competition. In 1910, half the women in the U.S. were still giving birth at
home, attended by midwives. Midwives were never well organized;
many worked in isolated areas, many did not speak English, and
their power was no match for that of organized medicine. By 1930,
only 15% of births in the U.S. were attended by midwives, and by
1976, over half the states had legislation prohibiting the practice of
midwifery (Litoff, 1978). In the 1920s and 1930s, two training
schools, the Frontier Nursing Service of Kentucky and the Maternity Center Association of New York City, began for the first time
to train a new kind of midwife, the nurse-midwife. These practitioners have grown in public acceptance especially since the early
1970s, but there are still very few nurse-midwifery training programs, and the profession of obstetrics welcomes this competition
as little today as it did seventy-five years ago.
    By the 1950s almost all American women were giving birth in the

hospital (Devitt, 1977), heavily medicated and presented with their babies only hours, or a day, later. Meanwhile, another vast social transformation had occurred. At the end of World War II, the "modern woman" of the 1920s and '30s, the Rosie the Riveter of the war years, found herself thrust back into the home when she had to give her job to returning veterans. Once again, in a conservative political climate, the joys of motherhood were proclaimed throughout the land. But the childbearing and childrearing methods that had been developed for the "modern" woman were still in place, and the ideal woman of the 1950s was put in a bind so contradictory that it could not last. She was supposed to rejoice in her primary role in life, but be knocked out and controlled in childbirth by a male specialist; she was supposed to be a nurturing angel to her children, but feed them from a bottle on a schedule dictated by another male specialist. Quite traditional women protested the treatment they were receiving in childbirth in such radical publications as the *Ladies' Home Journal* (Edwards & Waldorf, 1984), recounting horror stories of hostile treatment from medical staff, pain, fear, and lengthy periods of isolation. At the same time, women and professionals alike started to write about the dangers to newborns of the heavy medication their mothers were receiving, and tragedies brought about through waiting on the convenience of medical staff rather than delivering babies when they were ready to be born.

THE BIRTH OF THE MODERN
CHILDBIRTH REFORM MOVEMENT

It was in this spirit of outrage and concern that the modern childbirth reform movement was born. It did not spring up overnight, but was based on the work of a number of organizations and individuals who had been functioning outside the dominant paradigm for some years, such as the Frontier Nursing Service, the Maternity Center Association, and the Chicago Maternity Center; Doris Haire (e.g., Haire, 1972) and Lester Hazell (e.g., Hazell, 1976); Dr. Virginia Larsen of Seattle, who formed the Association for Childbirth Education (ACE) in the early 1950s; and Margaret Gamper, who founded the Midwest Parentcraft Center in Chicago just after World War II, making her perhaps the first American childbirth educator. These and other women founded the International Childbirth Education Association in 1960.

Natural Childbirth

In searching for more humane alternatives to the overmedicalized birthing model of the 1950s, childbirth reformers turned first to the work of the earliest proponent of "natural childbirth," the English doctor Grantly Dick Read (Read, 1944). Read believed that women's most important reason for being was to bear children, and saw childbearing as the highest form of love. From a religious standpoint, he could not understand why God would have made this most perfect example of his love painful. Although Read was no feminist, he approached laboring women with respect and awe, leading Rothman (1982, p. 86) to comment that "while [this view] may not do much for women's place in the larger society, it is not necessarily a bad perspective with which to approach a laboring woman."

As Read tells it, his awakening came when he attended a very poor woman in labor in her Whitechapel, London slum. When it came time for the baby to be born, he handed her a chloroform mask, which she refused. He later asked why she had refused the chloroform, and she said, "It didn't hurt. It wasn't meant to, was it, Doctor [Read, 1944, p. 2]?" This experience persuaded him that the pain of what he later called cultural childbirth was not a natural state, but was brought on by a combination of fear and tension, which were caused by ignorance of the birth process, by the isolation in which women were left during labor, and by the unsympathetic care they received in hospital labor and delivery suites. The woman who has been led to believe that childbirth is a painful experience will interpret the novel sensation of uterine contraction as pain; this interpretation will lead her to tense the round muscles in the lower uterine segment which in the "natural" state would be flaccid, allowing for the passage of the baby. This holding back of the baby contrary to the normal physiology of labor leads to real pain, which, however, was caused entirely by culturally-induced fear. Read dubbed this the fear-tension-pain syndrome. Unlike some later proponents of various forms of natural and prepared childbirth, Read did not blame the victim: he saw the culture in general as responsible for the fears of laboring women, not the women themselves.

Read's natural childbirth method consisted of educating women and their partners about the anatomy and physiology of labor, and training them in progressive relaxation techniques. Relaxation, as he saw it, would lessen both the tension that gave rise to pain in labor and would reduce fatigue, which magnified the subjective experience of the pain of labor. Read was also well aware of other psychological principles and their relation to pregnancy and childbirth, writing about autosuggestion, imagery, and the conditioned reflex. Read's method asked both more (patience) and less (intervention) of obstetricians and medical attendants, and was not well received. The Read method was imported into the United States in the 1940s, but was never widely used. Those women who tried to use it here were confronted with trying to accomplish natural childbirth amidst hostile hospital environments, often rooming with women who had been given twilight sleep and were out of their minds and screaming, and with little or no encouragement from labor and delivery room staff. One widely-held misinterpretation of Read's method, which he stoutly refuted, was that he withheld pain medication from women who wanted it. Though the Read method did not catch on here, recent work in the childbirth field supports many of Read's findings. For example, recent studies show that higher circulating levels of catecholamines (adrenaline and noradrenaline, the "fight or flight" hormones) in anxious laboring women render their uterine contractions less effective, leading to prolongation of labor and a reduced supply of oxygen to the fetus (e.g., Levinson & Shnider, 1979). Their description of anxiety leading to less effective uterine contractions exactly parallels Read's work of nearly forty years earlier. And all of the later methods of prepared childbirth have built on Read's understanding of education, relaxation and support during labor as major components of uncomplicated, unmedicated birth. Since that time, however, there have been two major directions in the childbirth preparation movement, one which followed on Read's work, and one which has become the major form in use in this country, the Lamaze method. They are not diametrically opposed; although they are based on a number of different assumptions, all childbirth preparation contains many similar elements, including education about the anatomy and physiology of pregnancy and birth, to reduce fear of the unknown; relaxation, including breathing techniques; prenatal exercise; and training a support person.

Husband-Coached Childbirth

One early and enthusiastic supporter of Read's method of natural childbirth, Dr. Robert Bradley, an American obstetrician, modestly attributes his adopting natural childbirth to his wife's influence; just as he was finishing his obstetrical training, "and knew just about everything [Bradley, 1965, p. 9]," she was reading Read. Bradley started to use Read's natural childbirth techniques in 1947, and evolved a popular new form of childbirth preparation, called "husband-coached childbirth," from it. Making the husband the major supplier of comfort and support, Bradley exhorts him to "play the lover role during the glorious climax to your act of love — the birth of your baby" (Bradley, 1965).

Arms (1975) feels that the success of the Bradley method lies in the fact that, with the husband running interference with hospital personnel and providing the kind of support necessary to keep the woman calm, she can achieve something like natural childbirth in a U.S. hospital.

The Psychoprophylactic ("Lamaze") Method

The psychoprophylactic method, or PPM, of "painless" childbirth, has been far more positively received than Read's or Bradley's method both in this country and around the world. Its theoretical foundation differs from Read's; it postulates that childbirth is by nature a painful event, but that there are psychological, or psychosomatic, ways of overcoming that pain to achieve a painless birth without resorting to the use of drugs.

The psychoprophylactic method was developed in 1949 in the Soviet Union by a team of Kharkov medical researchers including two neuropsychiatrists, I. Velvovsky and K. Platonov, and two obstetricians, V. Ploticher and E. Shugom (Chertok, 1959). For a great many years before this, many Russian researchers had been studying the use of hypnosis in producing "painless" childbirth, but they had not achieved widespread success using hypnotism.

Russian workers shared with Read the understanding that fear and tension lead to pain, and believed that education, exercise and relaxation techniques, and a sympathetic hospital environment, could do a great deal to reduce the pain of labor (Velvovsky, Platonov, Ploticher & Shugom, 1960). But they were critical of Read's encouraging what they viewed as a passive role for the laboring woman. Several breathing techniques were developed to distract women from the pain of the uterine contractions; in addition, women were trained to massage their tummies ("effleurage") during the later stages of labor. The woman using PPM is trained to *do* something, working on a task which will take her mind away from the activity of the uterus (Vellay, 1960). For the second stage of labor, the PPM teaches what it considers a more efficient kind of pushing in which the woman's breath is held (Velvovsky, Platonov, Ploticher & Shugom, 1960).

The psychoprophylactic method of childbirth was publicized and adopted nationwide in the Soviet Union in 1951 (Chertok, 1959).

In that same year the Soviets held an international symposium on the method, and a French obstetrician, Fernand Lamaze, head of the maternity hospital of the metallurgists' union, was invited. Lamaze determined to bring the method to France on a large scale, and when he returned to the Soviet Union in 1955, his former teachers congratulated him on having actually established the method in France (Vellay, 1960). The second country outside the Soviet Union to adopt the psychoprophylactic method was China; a large 1957 study (Ch'en, 1957) reports the successful use of the method in a Beijing hospital.

Lamaze had little success in trying to introduce the method in the United States in the early 1950s. Arms (1975) attributes this poor reception to the political climate of the McCarthy period, in which Lamaze was seen as a foreigner who worked at a "communist" union hospital and had adopted a Russian childbirth method. When the method was praised by Pope Pius XII in 1956 as a "benefit for the mother in childbirth" which "fully conforms to the will of the Creator (Karmel, 1965; Vellay, 1960)," some of the political stigma previously attached to it was removed. In 1959 the method was introduced into the United States by an American woman, Marjorie Karmel, who had given birth to her first child at Lamaze's hospital in France, and wanted to repeat the experience in the United States for the birth of her second child. Her book (Karmel, 1965), in which she described her two childbirth experiences, was the first work published in this country about the method, which Karmel referred to as the "Pavlov method" (Karmel, 1965).

With Elisabeth Bing, Karmel founded the American Society for Psychoprophylaxis in Obstetrics, and the method rapidly gained popularity—to some extent because the founders of ASPO worked very hard to involve obstetricians in their organization, going to great lengths to reassure them that their authority was in no way being challenged. Though its proponents take great pains to explain that the psychoprophylactic method is not "natural" at all, but a method of careful preparation for childbirth (e.g., Tanzer, 1976; Bing, 1979), it is nonetheless spoken of by the general public as "natural" childbirth; this much, at least, remains of Read's legacy!

The experience of being present at the birth of one's child makes an enormous psychological difference to women. This writer, in conversations with many women whose children were born before 1960, has found a long-term feeling among them of having missed out on the birth of their children. They express envy of the younger generation of women, who now get to "be there" when their babies are born. Another profound change brought about with the institution of the Lamaze method in American hospitals is the acceptance of the presence and active participation of the father, which has coincided perfectly with the increased emphasis given shared parenting by the women's movement in recent years. The image of the father-to-be pacing the floor nervously outside the labor and delivery suite has been supplanted by the image of father-as-coach (and indeed, some Lamaze-trained men wear "coach" t-shirts to the hospital).

Of course, there are also great advantages for babies whose mothers have taken less medication during labor and delivery. So great has the impact of "awake and aware" childbirth been that nowadays women who *haven't* taken childbirth preparation classes are given smaller doses of medication than women who *had* taken Lamaze classes 25 years ago were given (Charles et al., 1978)!

In recent years, there has been much criticism of the Lamaze method as it is currently practiced in American hospitals. Many feel (e.g., Rothman, 1982) that the method has become so popular from the standpoint of doctors and hospital staff because the Lamaze-trained laboring woman is in fact in control only of her own behavior, not of the situation and the medical decisions that are being made about how to conduct her labor. Instead of grunting, crying, hollering or otherwise making a nuisance of herself, the Lamaze-trained woman pants and puffs politely with each contraction, saying in effect, "I'll behave myself if you'll please let me stay awake and watch the birth of my baby." Hospital staff are trained to do something for women who make noise, as they are for patients whose illnesses cause them to be in pain; if the women keep quiet, and do something, like breathing, to control their own discomfort, the hospital staff will not intervene. Thus the Lamaze method, with its interventionist philosophy, more easily meshes with American medicine's own interventionism than does a relaxation method such as Read's, in which women aren't *doing* anything – except having babies. Many childbirth professionals see the process of birth as one of the woman's letting go of the baby, allowing her body to open up and let the baby be born. The psychoprophylactic method, with its focus on *control* of the birth process, interfering with uterine sensations by using artificial breathing techniques, is viewed by many critics as actually impeding the progress of labor. In addition, the use of the Valsalva breath-holding maneuver for the expulsion of the baby has been seen as injurious both to the perineal tissue of the mother and to the oxygen supply to the fetus (e.g., Barnett & Humenick, 1982; Noble, 1981). Many Lamaze instructors have been adjusting their teaching of pushing in line with these principles.

The Lamaze, or psychoprophylactic, method, had as its original intention the achievement of pain-free childbirth through control mechanisms designed to reduce pain messages from the uterus of the laboring woman to her cortex. Whether or not its model of labor control rather than relaxation made it an ideal candidate for cooptation into the American medical system, it has clearly become so coopted to a large degree. Most childbirth classes given today are given by hospital nurses in the hospitals at which they work; they teach not only Lamaze breathing techniques, but "preparation" for the particular procedures and interventions practiced at their hospital. These teachers are proud that they are training women for a "realistic," "controllable" experience, in which the physician is the authority (Sandlin et al., 1975).

CHILDBIRTH EDUCATION: CURRENT THEORIES AND TRENDS

The astute reader will by now doubtless have observed a shortage of women's names among the theoreticians who developed the various childbirth preparation methods; this weakness will soon be corrected, as we examine the major methods in use today. Part of the problem, of course, is the alacrity with which medicine attaches a doctor's name to the technique, or disease, s/he reports on. Read never talked about the "Read Method"; in fact, Kitzinger (1978a) points out the debt Read owed a number of English women physiologists of his time. Nor did Lamaze talk about a "Lamaze Method." Indeed, the Lamaze Method as practiced in the U.S. today owes as much to the work of Elisabeth Bing as to Lamaze.

The Psychosexual Method: Kitzinger

Sheila Kitzinger, an English anthropologist and childbirth educator, has contributed a wealth of research on childbirth, mothering, breastfeeding and women's sexuality (e.g., Kitzinger, 1978a, 1978b, 1979, 1981, 1985). The mother of five daughters herself, Kitzinger is as good a writer as we have on the role of birthing as part of the sexual cycle of women. Her method relies principally, as do those of a number of writers who follow in Read's tradition, on training women how to relax and respond to their bodies in labor, including "allowing" women to make the noises women make in labor. She is one of the first to write convincingly of the "birth climax," the intense sexual feeling produced by the crowning of the baby's head when the woman is unmedicated (Kitzinger, 1978a). She is both a researcher and activist for change in birthing practices, writing extensively, for example, on episiotomy (e.g., Kitzinger, 1981).

Noble: Physiological Pushing

Elizabeth Noble, a physiotherapist and childbirth educator, is best known for her efforts to replace the forceful Valsalva breathholding pushing most women are trained to use in the U.S. today. She has demonstrated (e.g., Noble, 1981) that physiological (sometimes mis-named "gentle") pushing safeguards both the maternal perineum and the fetal head, and does not deprive the baby of oxygen, as Valsalva pushing can.

Nutrition: The Brewers

The role of nutrition in sustaining a healthy pregnancy and enabling women to give birth naturally has nowhere been better articulated than in the work of Gail Brewer, a childbirth educator, and her husband, obstetrician Tom Brewer (e.g., Brewer, T. H., 1982;

Brewer & Brewer, 1983). Their work is helping to eliminate the practice of restricting weight gain in pregnancy, which has been shown to produce fragile, low-birthweight babies. In addition, Gail Brewer has written a handbook for expectant parents (Brewer, G. S., 1983) utilizing a method called cooperative childbirth.

Active Birth

Janet and Arthur Balaskas and Meloma Huxley, working out of the Active Birth Centre in London, are among many who are demonstrating the importance of an upright position in aiding labor, making it both shorter and less painful (Balaskas & Balaskas, 1983). Most women in the U.S. labor in bed on their backs and give birth in what Sheila Kitzinger calls the "stranded beetle position," legs up in stirrups.

Gentle Birth: Leboyer

The Leboyer method of delivery (Leboyer, 1976) is a gentler method of bringing babies into the world. Instead of bright lights and a lot of noise in the delivery room, the lights are dim, voices hushed. Instead of turning the baby upside down and spanking it, it is gently placed on the mother's abdomen. Instead of clamping the umbilical cord immediately, the cord is allowed to stop pulsating, which takes a couple of minutes, before it is clamped, allowing a small additional volume of blood into the baby. The best-known element of a Leboyer-style delivery is the bath. The newborn is soon immersed in a body-temperature bath. Babies whose bodies have been tense relax in this more familiar medium, unscrew their faces, open their eyes and begin to look around. Depending on whose book you read (Berezin, 1980; Leboyer, 1976; Odent, 1984a, 1984b), either the obstetrician, the father, or the mother holds the baby while it is in the bath. In this country, the father is the most likely candidate for the job, and many observers see the function of the bath as a beautiful way to involve the father right at the beginning in behavior that is likely to increase attachment to the newborn. One observer, however, has remarked that "the symbolic reemergence from the amniotic fluid and the rebirthing by the father's hands is the male improvement over the female's birthing (Rothman, 1982)."

De-Medicalization: Odent

A major contribution in showing how untampered with and "natural" birth in the hospital can be is that of Michel Odent (1984a, 1984b), director of the maternity unit at Pithiviers Hospital in France. One innovation for which the unit has become known is that women are permitted to labor in water, which is enormously relaxing. Some women have even given birth while sitting in the pool, though this was not Odent's original intention. (Some work is currently being done in the Soviet Union on underwater birth, and some small groups in the U.S. are trying it, but there is no published information about this method here yet. From newspaper accounts, it appears that the Soviets are finding what women at Pithiviers have found: that labor contractions don't hurt as much under water.) What is important to Odent is not that any particular technique be used, but that a philosophy of respect and non-intervention be adopted.

THE CURRENT SITUATION
IN CHILDBIRTH REFORM

Much research has been done in the last twenty-five years; working from a holistic "midwifery" model, we have developed a body of knowledge about what works best in normal childbirth for the mother, the baby, and their family. We know, for example, that just having a support person can so relieve a laboring woman's anxiety that the length of her labor is shortened dramatically (Sosa et al., 1980). We know that Read was right in describing how fear inhibits labor's progress and how relaxation enhances it, and we can describe these processes in terms of body chemistry (e.g., Levinson & Shnider, 1979). We know that ambulation in labor both shortens labor and makes it more comfortable, without the discomforts and side effects associated with chemical stimulation (e.g., Caldeyro-Barcia, 1979; Flynn et al., 1979; Read, Miller & Paul, 1981). We know that allowing women to eat and drink during labor preserves their strength and prevents the maternal exhaustion which often leads to cesarean section (e.g., Brewer & Greene, 1981). We know that an upright position during delivery is mechanically more efficient than the lithotomy (or "stranded beetles") position, reducing the incidence of tears and the rate of episiotomy (e.g., Odent, 1984b; Kitzinger, 1981).

But what we know, and what is routinely done to laboring women giving birth in hospitals in this country, are two quite different things, and studies, as one author put it, don't make change by themselves (Cassidy-Brinn, Downer & Hornstein, 1984). Standard birthing practice in this country involves a woman coming into the hospital at some time during active labor, at which time she will probably be temporarily separated from her partner, examined internally by a resident, given a shave and an enema. She will be escorted to a labor room, where she will change into a hospital gown, be rejoined by her partner, be given an intravenous glucose drip since she will not be allowed to have any food or drink, and be put to bed with an electronic fetal monitor attached either around her belly or internally, to the baby's head. Her bag of waters will probably be artificially ruptured, if it hasn't already broken, either to attach the internal monitor's electrode to the baby's scalp, or just to speed up the labor. If her labor does not progress according to the Friedman curve, which describes time parameters for cervical dilatation, the woman will be given pitocin to stimulate her contractions. Since artificially-stimulated contractions are more painful than naturally-occurring labor contractions, the woman may need to use pain medication, most often Demerol; but Demerol may slow the labor. During this time, the woman will be examined internally at least several times. For the second stage, pushing out the baby, the woman will be transferred to a table in the delivery room, where her feet will be placed in stirrups, and she will be covered with drapes. For the delivery, the woman will probably be offered epidural anesthesia, which numbs all sensation below the waist and makes it impossible for the woman to feel her contractions. She may still be able to push her baby out by responding to her doctor's instructions, but she may require a forceps delivery, which would entail her having a large episiotomy. In any case, depending on what hospital she is delivering in, the woman will have a one-and-a-half or two-hour limit, after which time the doctor will have to intervene in some way to get the baby delivered by the deadline. This scenario is the most common birth scenario in the U.S. today, and apart from the use of forceps, is considered an "uncomplicated" vaginal delivery. What's wrong with it is that none of it is necessary for an "uncomplicated" delivery; much of it is at least uncomfortable; many of the interventions mentioned lead to, and necessitate, the others; even the most innocuous of the interventions is not without risk; and some carry quite substantial risks with them. Childbirth activists know less invasive alternatives to virtually every one of the pharmacological and technological interventions catalogued above. As Marshall Klaus said about a study in which he had participated (Sosa et al., 1980), if the discovery they had made which dramatically shortened women's labors had been a new drug, or a new machine, every maternity unit in the country would have rushed out to buy it. But the discovery was that having a support person made the dramatic difference, and there is no money or glory to be made from this finding. (A more detailed description of standard birthing practice, contrasted with a home birth, may be found in Feinbloom & Forman, 1985, Ch. 1.)

The impact of the childbirth reform movement has been great. In the past twenty-five years, we have progressed from being asleep to being awake for the birth of our babies. Our partners are now allowed to be with us, to comfort and support us during labor. Elective inductions are no longer performed in this country. Mothers are routinely exposed to far less medication than they were 25 years ago (Charles et al., 1978), producing more alert babies, whom they are allowed to interact with immediately. More women are at least starting breastfeeding, and hospital schedules are more flexible so as to accommodate nursing couples. Nurse-midwives are in practice in many areas; some out-of-hospital birthing centers exist; and many hospitals, competing for the obstetric trade, have refurbished their maternity suites and set up "birthing rooms." These changes are significant, and came about when consumers—birthing couples—voted with their feet.

But in spite of the progress we have made, the medical model continues to function as the guiding model in current U.S. obstetrics. Birth is always a risky business, and paradoxically, because of the strength of the childbirth reform movement and the resulting desire of most birthing couples to have what they call a "natural" birth, the profession has responded by creating a new label of "high-risk," and a new subspecialty called "high-risk obstetrics," and has defined up to 70% of birthing women into that category. Before about ten years ago, this label did not exist. Women with serious pre-existing medical conditions such as diabetes or heart disease were called "at risk," and a woman so labelled was considered "at risk" *for* something, such as diabetes-related complications or pregnancy. Now, apart from true pre-existing medical conditions and pregnancy-related conditions such as toxemia of pregnancy, women are labelled "high risk" because of socioeconomic status (poor women are automatically "high-risk"); ethnic group (most nonwhite women are considered "high risk"); age (under 21 and over 35 are automatically "high risk"); breech presentation; multiple gestation; and previous cesarean section (in a country in which the cesarean rate was 20.3% in 1983 [Taffel, Placek, & Moien, 1985]). The high-risk label serves not to describe a specific medical problem which is being forestalled for the woman so labelled by unusual interventions; rather, it serves to define women *out* of the category of low-risk, and consequently out of being able to make choices about the way their births will be conducted.

Most of the childbirth reform movement has utilized a consumer model of change, as exemplified by ICEA's motto, "Freedom of choice based on knowledge of alternatives." Given the composition of the childbirth education and reform movement, this model comes as no surprise; the movement is a delightful mixture of feminists who come out of the women's health care movement, and traditional, family-oriented women who see birth as women's most important role and therefore want to make birthing a more fulfilling, "family-centered" experience. Thousands of teachers have taught tens of thousands of pregnant couples how to negotiate with their medical caregivers to get the birth they want. Although much change has occurred through the power of the purse, sending couples in one by one to do battle with the medical model, the institution of the hospital, and the fee-for-service medical reimbursement system which encourages maximum intervention and use of technology to amortize the expensive equipment is simply not an effective political strategy. In human terms, it results in thousands of women "trying for a natural," as they phrase it, and winding up with a birth much like the typical one described above. The movement itself gets decimated as teachers burn out after years of doing their best to educate individuals and watching those well-intentioned individuals go like lambs to the slaughter of high-tech medicalized hospital births.

New technologies for birth are being developed all the time, and their use within the context of a for-profit health care system follows an inexorable pattern. A piece of equipment which was invented to solve a specific problem — ultrasonic imaging of the fetus to diagnose twins, or locate the fetus for amniocentesis, say — then has to pay for itself, in the doctor's office or hospital. And doctors need to learn how to use the equipment. What started out as a piece of equipment with great potential for saving life, albeit with some attendant risks, now gets used on all pregnant or laboring women — in the case of ultrasonic imaging of the fetus, to "confirm a woman's dates," for example. And the ratio of risk to benefit now changes dramatically; when there is no benefit to the patient, any risk whatever is intolerable. However, as new technologies are introduced, we soon lose the right to refuse them, not only because institutions need to pay for the equipment, but also because of what is called the medical "standard of care." In any given locality, there is a set of practices generally accepted by the local medical profession as the right way to do things. When a practitioner's work is called into question, as in a malpractice case, the "standard of care" is the yardstick by which the parties determine whether proper care was given. An individual woman who doesn't want to be immobilized in labor by an electronic fetal monitor doesn't stand a chance against an individual obstetrician's need to demonstrate that the standard of care is being upheld; the individual doctor also loses freedom to practice in a less interventive way in this context.

A major limitation of the "choice" model of childbirth reform is that you can't have the choice if it isn't on the menu (Richards, 1982). The consumer model assumes that smart shopping will turn up just that array of options one has selected for one's birth experience, but this model does not take into account the power of organized medicine to challenge consumer demand by claiming professional expertise, and to resist the economic and professional threat posed by alternative health care providers. Even in the largest of cities, midwives may not be legally available; lay midwives are still outlawed in at least half the states (Litoff, 1978); nurse-midwives have a hard time obtaining hospital privileges, physician backup, and malpractice insurance in an area of the insurance industry at least partly controlled by doctors. As an advocacy group for midwives, The American College of Nurse-Midwives has not been politically active, but a new group, the Midwives' Association of North America (MANA), composed of both nurse- and lay midwives, was formed in 1983 to unite both kinds of midwives organizationally. In 1985, a crisis in malpractice insurance temporarily drove many nurse-midwives out of business; the ACNM eventually was able to secure coverage, at least temporarily, but the problem of malpractice insurance for midwives remains serious. And in other than the largest cities, women may have little choice of birth attendant. The most recalcitrant, interventionist obstetrician can do a booming business if there is no competition.

With little power to change the way hospital labor is conducted, some birthing women have exercised their one remaining freedom, the freedom to leave. Out-of-hospital births now account for one or two percent of all births in the U.S. There are now a few dozen out-of-hospital birth centers around the country. These centers also operate within state licensing laws and local standard-of-care parameters, and cannot accept women defined as "high-risk." When they first open, such centers have difficulty getting licensed, getting third-party reimbursement for the women who use them, getting insurance, and finding a hospital to provide emergency backup. In 1985, a number of birthing centers which had weathered the storms of their first few years in existence had to close because of an insurance crisis. These centers have organized into a National Association of Childbearing Centers to help each other stay alive.

Some women choose to birth at home, a choice made more difficult by the array of legal restrictions on home birth. It takes a good deal of courage to opt for a home birth knowing that if a problem arises one may have to be separated from one's caregiver in order to get hospital care. But lay midwives never have hospital privileges, and nurse-midwives generally function with physician backup for emergencies. Most doctors will not attend home births; even those few who are philosophically committed to it find it too threatening to put their medical licenses on the line. While it is unrealistic as a political strategy to expect the majority of American women to vote with their feet and stay home to birth their babies, the home birth movement provides both a humane alternative and a potentially powerful challenge to the medical model of birth.

The rise of cesarean section rates to epidemic proportions in this country—from just over five percent in 1970 to one in every five births at last count, and rising yearly (e.g., Taffel, Placek, & Moien, 1985; Young, 1982)—has led to the establishment of several organizations formed to educate women to avoid unnecessary cesareans and to work for change in the current medical practice (e.g., Cohen & Estner, 1983). The best known of these are Cesarean/Support, Education and Concern (C/SEC) and the Cesarean Prevention Movement (CPM). The work of groups such as these as well as individual lobbyists such as Doris Haire and Diony Young effected a change in the former obstetric practice of "once a cesarean, always a cesarean"; in 1980, the American College of Obstetrician-Gynecologists (ACOG) put forward a new official position allowing many women who had had previous cesareans at least to try to deliver subsequent babies vaginally. While the new policy is a powerful tool for change, it does not carry any legal weight, and most obstetricians still perform automatic repeat cesareans. As long as cesarean section is both faster to perform and reimbursed at a far higher rate than uncomplicated vaginal delivery, there is little incentive for physicians to change.

And as long as the medical model dominates birth, problems will keep springing up. Obstetricians are highly-trained medical specialists who are not, however, well skilled in the conduct of normal, uncomplicated labor; as one so gracefully put it, he wasn't trained to sit around all day "watching a hole [Ehrenreich & English, 1978]." Recently, one obstetrician published a position paper advocating (in selected cases, he hastened to add) *prophylactic* cesarean section at term— that is, cesarean section not as a response to a problem, but in order to head off a possible future problem (Feldman & Freiman, 1985).

WHERE DO WE GO FROM HERE?

One area in which those of us who are health care providers and mental health professionals can contend is in challenging the medical model, in which mortality and morbidity are the only outcome measures considered for childbirth. It is time we started seriously examining psychosocial morbidity, as one researcher has put it (Oakley, 1983), for as Rothman (1985, pp. 92-93) has said,

> If birth is defined in other than narrow medical terms, other outcome measures would be perceived as equally appropriate. If we see birth as an event in the lives of women, families, and communities, new outcome measures are generated. To take the extremes: . . . A birth which leaves wives angry at husbands and husbands feeling that they have failed their wives is *not* the same as a birth experience that draws the two closer together. A birth that leaves the woman unsure of her mothering abilities and unable to comfort her crying baby is *not* the same as a birth experience that leaves her feeling competent. A birth which leaves the woman fearful of her body functioning, unsure of just what was cut "down there" or why, is *not*

the same as a birth which leaves the woman feeling strong and positive about herself, and more rather than less comfortable with her body.

The childbirth education and reform movement is composed largely of women who are health care professionals and mothers. They are caring and hardworking, and certainly not in this line of work for the money; most make little money indeed. Some, who are nurses and identify as part of the health care profession rather than as advocates for birthing women, teach classes which prepare women only for the birthing practices in place in their institutions, rather than the full range of possible options.

Though there are feminists who work within this movement, the movement as a whole has not been organized politically in the same way that we have organized for other women's health issues, such as the struggle for legal, safe, available abortions. There is little communication and unity of action between childbirth reformers and other women's health activists. Many feminists outside the childbirth movement seem not to understand its importance as a women's health care issue, perhaps because childbearing has not been on their agendas, perhaps because they are ceding hegemony over this womanly function to traditional "family-oriented" women. At the 1985 ICEA regional conference, there was for the first time a session about the childbearing needs and concerns of lesbian women, building new bridges between women whose concerns have sometimes seemed very different.

The movement has done as much as it can do to wage the struggle individual birthing woman by individual birthing woman. We need organized political action. We have some good lobbyists in the movement, and they have had an important impact. We have the support of the World Health Organization, whose 1985 position paper on standards of obstetric care calls for a utilization of the midwifery model and an abandonment of overly interventive obstetrics (World Health Organization, 1985).

In London, in April, 1982, a small group of childbirth activists called a "Birthrights Rally." Expecting a fairly small turnout, they got a crowd of 5000 women, pushing prams and demanding the right to birth their babies in the position of their choosing, carrying such picket signs as "Stand and Deliver!" It's high time for American women to unite, use the political knowhow we have gained in other women's rights battles, and win our own birthrights.

REFERENCES

Arms, S. (1975). *Immaculate Deception: A New Look at Women and Childbirth.* New York: Bantam Books.

Arney, W. R. (1982). *Power and the Profession of Obstetrics.* Chicago/London: University of Chicago Press.

Balaskas, J. & Balaskas, A. (1983). *Active Birth.* New York: McGraw-Hill.

Barnett, M. M. & Humenick, S. S. (1982). Infant outcome in relation to second stage labor pushing method. *Birth, 9,* 221-229.

Berezin, N. (1980). *The Gentle Birth Book.* New York: Simon & Schuster.

Bing, E. (1979). *Six Practical Lessons for an Easier Childbirth.* New York: Bantam.

Bradley, R. A. (1965). *Husband-Coached Childbirth.* New York: Harper & Row.

Brewer, G. S. (1983). *Nine Months, Nine Lessons: A Practical Guide to Managing the Stress of Labor and Childbirth.* New York: Simon & Schuster.

Brewer, G. S. & Brewer, T. H. (1983). *The Brewer Medical Diet for Normal and High-Risk Pregnancy.* New York: Simon & Schuster.

Brewer, T. H. (1982). *Metabolic Toxemia of Late Pregnancy: A Disease of Malnutrition.* New Canaan, CT: Keats Publishing Co.

Brewer, G. S. & Greene, J. P. (1981). *Right from the Start: Meeting the Challenge of Mothering Your Unborn and Newborn Baby.* Emmaus, PA: Rodale Press.

Caldeyro-Barcia, R. (1979). The influence of maternal position on time of spontaneous rupture of the membranes, progress of labor, and fetal head compression. *Birth and the Family Journal, 6,* 10-18.

Cassidy-Brinn, G., Hornstein, F. & Downer, C. (1984). *Woman-Centered Pregnancy and Birth.* Pittsburgh, PA: Cleis Press.

Charles, A. G., Norr, K. L., Block, C. R., Meyering, S. & Meyers, E. (1978). Obstetric and psychological effects of psychoprophylactic preparation for childbirth. *American Journal of Obstetrics and Gynecology, 131,* 44-52.

Ch'en Wen-chan. (1957). A clinical analysis of 8063 cases of painless labor by the psychoprophylactic method. *Chinese Medical Journal, 75,* 337-343.

Chertok, L. (1959). *Psychosomatic Methods in Painless Childbirth: History, Theory and Practice.* London/New York: Pergamon Press.

Cohen, N. W., & Estner, L. J. (1983). *Silent Knife: Cesarean Prevention and Vaginal Birth after Cesarean.* South Hadley, MA: Bergin & Garvey.

Devitt, N. (1977). The transition from home to hospital birth in the United States, 1930-1960. *Birth and the Family Journal, 4,* 47-58.

Edwards, M. & Waldorf, M. (1984). *Reclaiming Birth: History and Heroines of American Childbirth Reform.* Trumansburg, NY: The Crossing Press.

Ehrenreich, B. & English, D. (1973). Witches, midwives and nurses. *Monthly Review,* 25-40.

Ehrenreich, B. & English, D. (1978). *For Her Own Good: 150 Years of the Experts' Advice to Women.* Garden City, NY: Anchor Press/Doubleday.

Feinbloom, R. I. & Forman, B. (1985). *Pregnancy, Birth and the Early Months.* Reading, MA: Addison Wesley.

Feldman, G. B. & Freiman, J. A. (1985). Prophylactic cesarean section at term. *New England Journal of Medicine, 312,* 1264-1267.

Flynn, A. M., Kelly, J., Hollins, G. & Lynch, P. F. (1978). Ambulation in labour. *British Medical Journal, 2,* 591-593.

Haire, D. (1972). *The Cultural Warping of Childbirth.* Minneapolis, MN: International Childbirth Education Association Special Report.

Hazell, L. (1976). *Commonsense Childbirth.* New York: Berkeley Press.

Iffy, L. & Kaminetzky, H. A. (Eds.). (1981). *Principles and Practice of Obstetrics and Perinatology.* New York: John Wiley & Sons. 2 vols.

Jordan, B. (1983). *Birth in Four Cultures.* Montreal/London: Eden Press.

Karmel, M. (1965). *Thank You, Dr. Lamaze.* Garden City, NY: Dolphin Books, Doubleday.

Kitzinger, S. (1978a). *The Experience of Childbirth.* New York: Penguin Books.

Kitzinger, S. (1978b). *Women as Mothers.* Glasgow: Fontana/Collins.

Kitzinger, S. (1979). *Birth at Home.* Oxford: Oxford University Press.

Kitzinger, S. (Ed.). (1981). *Episiotomy: Physical and Emotional Aspects.* London: National Childbirth Trust.

Kitzinger, S. (1985). *Woman's Experience of Sex.* New York: Penguin Books.

Leboyer, F. (1976). *Birth without Violence.* New York: Alfred A. Knopf.

Levinson, G. & Shnider, S. M. (1979). Catecholamines: The effects of maternal fear and its treatment on uterine function and circulation. *Birth and the Family Journal, 6,* 167-178.

Litoff, J. (1978). *American Midwives: 1860 to the Present.* Westport, CN: Greenwood Press.

Miller, L. G. (1979). Pain, parturition, and the profession: Twilight sleep in America. In S. Reverby & D. Rosner (Eds.), *Health Care in America: Essays in Social History.* Philadelphia: Temple University Press.

Nash, A. & Nash, J. E. (1979). Conflicting interpretations of childbirth: The medical and natural perspectives. *Urban Life, 7,* 493-512.

Noble, E. (1981). Controversies in maternal effort during labor and delivery. *Journal of Nurse-Midwifery, 26,* 13-22.

Oakley, A. (1983). Social consequences of obstetric technology: The importance of measuring "soft" outcomes. *Birth, 10,* 99-108.

Odent, M. (1984a). *Entering the World: The De-Medicalization of Childbirth.* New York: Marion Boyars, Inc.

Odent, M. (1984b). *Birth Reborn.* New York: Pantheon.

Read, G. D. (1944). *Childbirth without Fear.* New York/London: Harper and Brothers.

Read, J. A., Miller, F. C. & Paul, R. H. (1981). Randomized trial of ambulation versus oxytocin for labor enhancement: A preliminary report. *American Journal of Obstetrics and Gynecology, 139,* 669-672.

Richard, M. P. M. (1982). The trouble with "choice" in childbirth. *Birth, 9,* 253-260.

Rothman, B. K. (1982). *In Labor: Women and Power in the Birthplace.* New York/London: W. W. Norton & Co.

Rothman, B. K. (1985). Beyond risks and rates in obstetric care. *Birth, 12,* 91-94.

Sandlin, C., Whitley, N., Kenney, P. M., Hommel, F., Johnston, R. D. & Knauth, D. (1975). Whatever happened to choice in childbirth? – Readers respond. *JOGN Nursing,* May-June, 57-61.

Sosa, R., Kennell, J., Klaus, M., Robertson, S. & Urrutia, J. (1980). The effect of a supportive companion on perinatal problems, length of labor, and mother-infant interaction. *New England Journal of Medicine, 303,* 597-600.

Stanton, M. E. (1979). The myth of "natural" childbirth. *Journal of Nurse-Midwifery, 24,* 25-29.

Taffel, S. M., Placek, P. J. & Moien, M. (1985). One-fifth of 1983 US births by cesarean section. *American Journal of Public Health, 75,* 190.

Tanzer, D. (1976). *Why Natural Childbirth?* New York: Schocken Books.

Vellay, P. (1960). *Childbirth without Pain.* New York: E. P. Dutton & Co.

Velvovsky, I., Platonov, K., Ploticher, V. & Shugom, E. (1960). *Painless Childbirth through Psychoprophylaxis.* Moscow: Foreign Languages Publishing House.

Wertz, R. W. & Wertz, D. C. (1979). *Lying-In: A History of Childbirth in America.* New York: Schocken Books.

World Health Organization. (1985). Appropriate technology for birth. *The Lancet,* August 24, 1985, 436-437.

Young, D. (1982). *Changing Childbirth: Family Birth in the Hospital.* Rochester, NY: Childbirth Graphics, Ltd.

Single Mothers by Choice: A Family Alternative

Ruth Mechaneck
Elizabeth Klein
Judith Kuppersmith

In recent years, we have witnessed a major change in the traditional family structure (Macklin & Rubin, 1983). The rising divorce rate has created many single parent families, almost all of which are headed by women (Gongla, 1982; Ross & Sawhill, 1975; Stein, 1983; Thompson & Gongla, 1983). One emerging alternative is that of unmarried women in their late 20s, 30s and early 40s who are choosing to bear and rear children on their own (Klemesrud, 1983; Morrisoe, 1983). These women, whom we will call "single mothers," are educated and economically independent, and represent a new and separate phenomenon from the classic unwed mother who was generally poor, a teenager, unprepared for motherhood and socially ostracized (Bowerman, Irish & Hallowell, 1966; Hartley, 1975; Sauber & Rubenstein, 1965; Vincent, 1961). The number of single mothers is growing and a recent book (Merritt & Steiner, 1984) states that as many as 300,000 women have made this choice in the last 5 years.

Parenting can be separated from marriage, as the rising divorce rate and the increase in single parent families has shown us. While the life of the divorced single parent has been well-documented, as

---

Ruth Mechaneck is a clinical psychologist in private practice in New York. Elizabeth Klein is a clinical psychologist in private practice in New York. Judith Kuppersmith is a clinical psychologist in private practice and an assistant professor at College of Staten Island, New York.

© 1987 by The Haworth Press, Inc. All rights reserved.

has the experience of the classic unwed mother, a profile of the single mother by choice is just beginning to emerge. The present study represents an attempt to understand this new phenomenon in terms of the experience of these mothers and to examine society's attitude toward this lifestyle. The group of women we have focussed on is an older, better educated, financially stable group. Many planned their pregnancies, and others found themselves pregnant and decided to continue the pregnancy and raise the child on their own. There has been almost no formal study of this group, neither of the mothers and the children involved, nor of the psychological and social issues which they are going to encounter.

Under prevailing social mores, women can be educated and have successful careers, their own homes and extensive social networks, but until recent years, single motherhood was not considered an available option. Single motherhood has become a viable choice due to the general influence of the women's movement, the delaying of marriage and family due to career building, changing societal mores (Yankelovich, 1981), the rapidly growing advances in reproductive technology (Andrews, 1984; Goodman, 1984), and the fact that there are significantly fewer single men compared to single women in the 20-40 year-old age group (Guttentag & Secord, 1983; Novak, 1983). The results of a 1984 Yale-Harvard study analyzing census data from 1982 (Bennett, Craig & Bloom, 1986) presented the remarkable findings that women who have not yet married by 25 years of age have only a 50% chance of marrying. The percentages of those marrying rapidly decline thereafter: 20% for women 30 years old, 5% for those who reach 35, and only 1% beyond 40. It is not inconsistent with this data that in 1984, 27.1% of babies in New York State were born out of wedlock. *The New York Times* reported in March, 1986 that the greatest increase in out-of-wedlock births from 1983 to 1984 occurred among women 35-39 years of age, an increase of 10.1%.

Our study of single mothers focussed on two primary issues: (1) the attitudinal context in which the decision to become a single mother is made, and (2) the experience of these women. We will begin by presenting the results of an attitude survey which we administered in an attempt to explore societal attitudes toward single motherhood. Findings related to the single mothers' experience will then be discussed, followed by our own work on this topic, including 3 case studies of single mothers.

ATTITUDE SURVEY

Background

In the past, attitudes toward illegitimacy carried severe social stigma which affected both mother and child. The unwed mother was viewed as promiscuous, psychologically deviant, and a social problem. Until recently, these mothers were under tremendous pressure to relinquish their children at birth. The child of the unwed mother was considered an outcast, with limited legal rights to support and protection (Bremner, 1974). Children with absent fathers were discovered to have irremediable psychological deficits in areas of moral development, academic achievement and sex-role identification. These conclusions have been seriously challenged by studies and changing practices in the fields of law, sociology, psychology and medicine (Adams, Milner & Schrepf, 1984; Golombok, Spence & Rutter, 1983; Herzog & Sudia, 1968; McGuire & Alexander, 1985). Attitude surveys have shown significant changes over the past 30 years toward unmarried mothers. There has been an increasing acceptance of the notion of a woman having a child and raising it on her own (Yankelovitch, 1981).

Our attitude survey addressed questions relating to (1) the single woman's chosen method of conception: adoption, artificial insemination by donor (AID), coitus with a known man who consented to father a child, and coitus with an unknown man who did not consent; (2) perceived differences between single mothers who are divorced and those who have never been married, and (3) the potential effects of such lifestyle choices on the children of these women. We speculated that the more closely the method of conception approximated the traditional one, the less social disapproval there would be.

METHODS

Attitude questionnaires were distributed to 151 Ss: 59 high school students from a suburban Long Island community and 92 adults from Staten Island, N.Y. There were 56 men and 95 women ranging in age from 14-71 years. Subjects were predominantly white and middle class. Single and married males and females were equally represented. Three broad categories were established for purposes of scoring: (1) societal concerns, such as ostracism due to illegitimacy or deviance; (2) the significance of the father; and (3) the life situation and personal characteristics of the mother.

RESULTS

Respondents showed a wide range in attitude toward the method of conception chosen by a single woman as shown in Table 1. Significant differences existed between categories, with adoption receiving the most favorable ratings and an unknown man without consent (the "stud") the least favorable. Insemination and conception with a known man who consented fell in between, and did not differ significantly from one another. These ratings were consistent by age and sex of subjects. These findings tended to confirm the hypothesis that the more traditional the method, the less social disapproval there would be. Adoption has a long history, and is often considered an act of altruism. Ethical and moral considerations toward sexuality, deception, and lack of commitment undoubtedly play a part in the condemnation of a "stud" in fathering a child. People appeared to be less certain about artificial insemination as an option, as indicated by the finding that 40% of all the "not sure" responses were in this category.

The life situation of the single mothers was perceived as significantly different than that of the divorced mothers by the majority of respondents (75% men, 69% women). Children of the single mother were seen at a disadvantage compared to the children of the divorced mother by a minority of the women (39%) and slightly less than half of the men (47%).

Different reasons were invoked for differentiating these two groups of women, and they appeared to reflect differences between the perceptions of men and women. Men tended to emphasize to a greater degree the negative consequences for the child of not having a man in the role of father, whereas women placed more emphasis on the situational and personal context and characteristics of the mother in question. There appeared to be minimal concern about social stigma, although women tended to show more concern about the child being stigmatized than did men. Advantages and disadvantages of the life situation of both single and divorced mothers were cited. The potential presence of the father was seen as a plus for the

Table 1

Attitudes Toward the Method of Conception Chosen by Single Mothers[a,b,c]

METHOD OF CONCEPTION

Subjects	Adoption	Insemination	Known man who consented	Unknown man who did not consent
Males (N=56)	3.86	2.96	2.73	1.96
Females (N=95)	4.29	3.04	3.07	1.81

a. Mean attitude rating scores are given

b. Attitudes were rated on a 5 point scale: 1=disagree strongly, 2=disagree, 3= not sure, 4= agree, 5=agree strongly

c. Sign tests indicated the following differences between categories: Adoption > Insemination = Known man who consented > Unknown man who did not consent All differences were significant at p < .005.

child of the divorced mother, whereas the trauma of divorce for the child was considered devastating. The divorced mother was considered to be less prepared for the responsibilities and hardships entailed in being a single mother. Respondents who felt that the situation of the two types of mothers were not essentially different focussed on the fact that they both had to cope with being alone, and the conviction that a "good mother": who genuinely wanted and cared for her child could manage well despite all odds. General comments showed an even greater differentiation between the attitudes of men and women. Men's comments, on the whole, were critical. Women, on the other hand, were more supportive, expressed a greater diversity of opinions, were more uncertain and torn by the complexities of the issue, and indicated genuine empathy with the woman's situation, although a few were condemning. Both men and women, however, often qualified their statements with the assertion that a child still needs two parents.

The high school students appeared unfamiliar with the single adult woman's situation and seemed detached from the issue. It may have been an alien consideration for them, at a time in their lives when they were just beginning to explore the possibility of love relationships. They were much more emotional, however, about the issue of divorce and the traumatic consequences for the child.

Only 18% of the adult males knew of a woman who was, or was thinking of becoming a single mother, whereas 40% of the women had some familiarity with a woman in this situation.

In summary, attitudes toward single unmarried mothers reflected in this sample were diversified, broke down according to male-female lines, and supported certain traditional values connected with the family. Attitudes were not, however, rigidly fixed. One factor of importance for attitude change in the future would seem to be the outcome of research on single mothers and their children.

THE EXPERIENCE OF THE SINGLE MOTHER

Background

A review of the existing literature provides very little data on the experience of the single mother. The overall impression which has been borne out by our own research is that many of these women are faring much better than might be expected. They are hampered financially by not being part of a couple where one if not both partners work, and many miss the emotional support of a full-time coparent, but most of these women appear to be satisfied with their lives and seem to have adapted well to the maternal role.

Three studies addressed this subject directly: Goldsmith (1975) compared 13 unmarried mothers with 5 divorced or separated mothers, all over the age of 21; Rexford (1976) compared 10 married and 10 unmarried mothers aged 25-42; and Fox (1979) studied factors predictive of maternal role adaptation in 20 single mothers over age 22 from late pregnancy to 2 months postpartum. Using a larger sample of 50 unmarried mothers, the UCLA Family Styles project (Alexander & Kornfein, 1983; Berlin, 1983; Eiduson, 1983; Zimmerman & Bernstein, 1983) examined the effects of alternative family styles, one of which was motherhood without marriage, on child development from the mother's third trimester of pregnancy until the child reached age 6. Two recent books (Merritt & Steiner, 1984; Renvoise, 1985) have attempted to document the experience of the single mother through the use of direct interviews of 100 women throughout the U.S. and 20 women from the U.S., Britain, and Holland, respectively.

The vast majority of women in all these investigations were white and college educated and came from middle class backgrounds. Most had had previous relationships with men. One of the questions that concerned all the researchers on this subject was whether there are distinguishing differences demographically and/or psychologically between those women choosing to become single mothers, and those women who follow a more traditional path. Of the studies that did direct comparisons of these two groups, both the Rexford and the Family Styles studies found significant differences in the single mothers' relationships to their families of origin. Traditional married mothers were found to have maintained better relationships with their own mothers throughout childhood and adolescence than did mothers who chose alternative life styles. Rexford found a significant difference between married and single mothers' descriptions of their relationships with their fathers. Single mothers were considerably more negative, perceiving their fathers as "unrelating and/or angry most of the time." Renvoise reports that many of the women had "very uneasy" relationships with their own fathers. However, there was conflicting data on the relationships of these women to their families of origin, with Merritt and Steiner claiming that most of the women they interviewed had been raised in warm, loving families.

The decision to become a single mother is one that has involved considerable reflection by the women in these studies. Rexford found that the single mothers appeared to have put much more thought into their decision to become mothers than did the married mothers, many of whom acted out of social expectation rather than personal desire. She reports that several of the single mothers felt that the passing of their 30th birthday was a motivating force. Others indicated that motherhood meant a greater sense of stability and rootedness in their lives, which was something that they were looking for. These findings were corroborated by Merritt and Steiner and Renvoise. Goldsmith suggested that for many of her subjects the choice of unwed motherhood may have been directly influenced by previous pregnancies which were terminated by abortion.

The decision of how to become a single mother was invariably a complex one. The method of conception employed by many of the women studied was often not the original one desired. Various obstacles led women to try a number of strategies for conception before finally reaching their goal. These included an inability to find a willing partner, resistance by doctors to using artificial insemination with single women, difficulty conceiving, concerns about the use of a "stud" and difficulties in arranging for adoption. Renvoise spoke to a number of women who chose adoption because they feared the social stigma of an unmarried pregnancy.

Once the child was born, a number of factors began to influence the experience of the single mother. Living arrangement was found by Fox to be a significant factor in maternal adaptation. She found that mothers living alone with their children showed greater maternal adaptation and less postpartum depression than mothers living with other adults, or with the baby's father. In fact few of the biological fathers tended to remain in the picture after the baby was born, and women who conceived with the hope of having the father participate were often embittered and disappointed (Merritt & Steiner, 1984; Renvoise, 1985).

The family headed by the single mother experiences a number of difficulties, especially during the first year after the child is born. Economic, occupational and overload problems are all reported to be major stresses. The single mother appears to be most vulnerable in the area of parental psychological stress; isolation, financial problems and the lack of consistent satisfying interpersonal relationships are cited as major contributors (Eiduson, 1983).

Although the women interviewed felt that marriage would not guarantee the optimal growth and development of their children and themselves as parents, many of the women expressed hope for finding a future father for their children, which would increase their socioeconomic security and provide for shared parenthood responsibilities.

INTERVIEWS WITH SINGLE MOTHERS

Method

The subjects for the study were obtained in two ways: through a New York based organization called Single Mothers by Choice, and through an informal network of single mothers. Each woman was called on the telephone and asked if she would like to participate in the study. An appointment was then made for the interview. Once the interview process began. there were no dropouts. Eighteen of the women live in New York City, with the remaining two living in rural areas on the East Coast.

Twenty single mothers were interviewed in depth by the authors of this study. The interviews, which ranged in length from one hour to two and a half hours, and took place in one, two, or three sessions, followed a questionnaire designed by the authors. The questionnaire was created and refined during a one-year period from 1982 to 1983, and interviews were conducted from 1983 to 1985.

Five central issues emerged in the interview construction process: (1) Who are these women? Cultural stereotypes, reinforced by the media, depicted them as lesbians, feminists, women incapable of forming relationships with men, emotionally disturbed or selfish women who fostered symbiotic relationships without concern for the child's ultimate welfare. These stereotypes, as we discovered, were incorrect. (2) What were the contributing factors that led to the decision to become single mothers? (3) What form of conception did they use and why? (4) How were the women and children faring, and what did they see as the unique issues in their lives? (5) How do these mothers deal with the issue of the absent father?

The questions selected were based on the authors' interests, questions raised in related research, and issues that emerged during the first few pilot interviews. The questionnaire consisted of 38 items divided into 5 sections: (1) demographic data; (2) attitudes; (3) family and relationship history; (4) absent father issues; and (5) single motherhood.

FINDINGS

All of the women were white, were from middle class backgrounds, and represented a variety of ethnic and religious backgrounds. Their average age was 39 and their average income was $39,000. One woman was a high school graduate, while all the others were college graduates. Six had Masters degrees plus additional professional training, three had Ph.D.'s, two were lawyers and one was an M.D. Nineteen of the 20 women were heterosexual. Eleven of the women stated that they were influenced in their life choices by the women's movement. Nine of the mothers were not interested in the women's movement and felt that they were not influenced by it.

All 20 of the women were *intensely* interested in becoming mothers and the majority of them felt that they desired motherhood at the time of their decision more than they desired marriage, if they desired marriage at all. Eighteen women expressed a desire to marry in the future. The decision-making process was often prolonged, lasting an average of 4 years. One woman reported that she had actively considered becoming a single mother for as long as ten years. Twelve of the 20 women had previously been pregnant. Only one had given birth: the others had either miscarried or had opted for abortion (53% of the women, in fact, had had an abortion prior to their becoming single mothers). This is in keeping with findings of Goldsmith (1975). Virtually all of our subjects had had a previous relationship with a man, with 1/3 or the women citing previous marriages, all of which were terminated prior to conception.

As to method of insemination, 10 of the 20 women chose intercourse, most of them with men they knew to some degree. Four of the women chose artificial insemination and 6 women adopted their children. These decisions were not easily arrived at, as the following quotes illustrate:

K.P.: Perhaps it was the 36-year-old crisis. I didn't want to let my body cease to be able to have a child by default. I had thought about it for years, but my 36th birthday was the turning point. Even if Prince Charming had come along then, it would have taken too long before we would have, in the natural course of things, had a child. It wasn't something outside of my control, the way marriage was. When I was 24, a friend became pregnant, and came to live with me. I helped to take care of her child. I liked to fantasize that she was mine. It helped me in feeling that it could work. Not having a child was not an option, since children have always been so important to me.

At first I decided to go for AID. However, I was also seeing someone at the time and asked him if he'd be willing to father the child and he agreed. So, for awhile. I ran parallel tracks. After 6 months my boyfriend ran away. I kept trying insemination but didn't conceive. I went through all the tests, a laparoscopy, and even now I'm taking drugs to see whether I'll be able to conceive in the future. It seemed very important to me to be pregnant, but I was also concerned about the genetic aspects, particularly about having an intelligent child. However, when I decided to adopt it was a relief compared to what I'd been through before. I could use all my skills in helping bring it about.

M.V.: I was 40 years old, starting to feel secure, and in a relationship with another woman. We both wanted to have a child together and since she was afraid of the process of being pregnant, and I had a positive sense of it, the decision emerged. We both went to therapy together for awhile, which helped us reach the decision. The choice of method was an issue. We both had some concerns about our child not knowing the other parent and could imagine the child saying "you're a real shit." We decided against a man for legal reasons, so we arranged for an anonymous donor with no way of finding out who it was. My lover had many more fantasies about the father than I did. I used to look at my brothers and think my son has some of their genes. It doesn't seem relevant now.

M.J.: I devoted my time—three years—before I was 36, to looking for a man. It was a project. I finally decided that I could live without a man but not a baby. I was discouraged

about finding a mate and was afraid I would miss out biologi-
cally on having a baby.

   I had started to work on adoption. I was close to having an
Indian baby arrive, the week before I had conceived. I had
intercourse with a man I knew sort of. He and I even talked
about adoption that evening. I didn't think I could use AID. I
really needed to know who the person was and not have to deal
with the fantasy. I didn't feel good about using a man. It was
out of character. I'm not sneaky and unfair. I felt he could
handle it and that he would be minimally involved.

   Most of the children in the sample are still quite young. Their
average age was 4-1/2 years at the time of the interview. Of the 21
children, 12 were male and 9 were female. Only one mother decided to have two children. Many others stated that they would like
to have more children, but felt they could not because of financial
reasons. Fifteen mothers were living alone with their children, 3
had live-in help and 2 mothers shared communal living arrangements. The average amount of outside child care was 37 hours per
week. Eight had babysitters at home, 8 children were in school, 3
were in day care, and one was at home with the mother full-time.

   Of the 20 women interviewed, 15 of them bring men into their
children's lives in active and intentional ways—for example, godfa-
thers, grandfathers, uncles, cousins, babysitters, male friends, and
the biological fathers. The other mothers had not yet planned how
they might bring men into their children's lives because the children
were still quite young. Four of the mothers and their children see the
biological father on some regular basis. Ten of the children have no
identifiable father, 4 of those due to artificial insemination. Three
fathers saw their children occasionally as infants but "dropped out"
gradually, and one father pays support although he does not see his
child. With one exception, the women interviewed expressed varying degrees of concern at the absence of a consistent male figure in
their children's lives.

   M.J.: My impression is you can't create a father substitute.
You can only expose your child to men. I introduced his god-
father when he was 10 months old. We hardly knew each
other. He was married to my best friend and they decided to be
the godparents. They see each other alone some of the time
and with me for dinner at least once a week. They have taken

him on weekends too. I have a strong feeling that my attitude toward men is more important than the physical presence. I tell him that it is great to grow up to be a man.

J.F.: I live communally for several reasons. My kids can have intimate contact with men, that is, day to day. It takes some of the minute-to-minute stress off me and it gives me more freedom of movement. During the time I was alone with them there was isolation. It was hard for me to take on babysitters when I wanted to play, not when I wanted to work. There would have been nobody really to call if I needed help except a paid sitter. Now I would turn to R.

Few of the women experienced social ostracism, although some did cite instances of disapproval from parents and co-workers. Grandparents eventually accepted the children, except for one woman who feels that her family rejected her child because she was racially mixed. Many of these women included among their closest friends other single mothers, and cited organizations such as Single Mothers by Choice (SMC) as a major source of support. Several women reported that the people in their lives that seemed the most uncomfortable with their decision were male friends. However, a number of men were supportive and became actively involved with the children on a consistent basis from birth.

Fifteen of the 20 women had told or were planning to tell their children the whole truth of their parentage. Three women were telling some truth—one woman, for example, was withholding information about the violent personality of the biological father. Two of the women, those with the youngest children, did not yet know what and how they would tell their children about their origins. The artificially inseminated women were often searching for what to tell their children and had some concern about the effect of their story on their children, and even on their future relationships with their children.

C.J.: I'll tell her the exact truth when it's age appropriate. She has asked "where's my daddy?" and I tell her she doesn't have one. I'll explain the whole process to her when she's old enough. I'm concerned about whether she'll be able to establish close relationships with men. I think she's going to suffer less than my son who's been through 2 divorces. She doesn't feel rejected or abandoned. She'll feel angry at me, but I hope it won't affect her feelings of desirability.

Several of the women who had chosen intercourse felt that perhaps they should have used AID because of problems of disappointments with the biological father. These women reported the greatest sense of dissatisfaction.

S.S.: I'm concerned that she'll resent me for not giving her a father, especially with AID. Right now there is no male figure at all. I haven't thought about it a lot because of her age. I date men; I'm seeing someone now. I do see it as a drawback for her because she doesn't have a complete set of parents. Fathers do provide certain things for daughters. It's not a complete picture.

F.S.: I'm not concerned about the father issue. He sees a lot of men. Men in the street, men in the world. One of my best friends is a kind of surrogate father. He sees him once a month, but is on the phone daily. We'll go to the park or zoo. My feeling is that a daddy is not a necessity in life; it may be a hindrance. I've taken on both roles. A lot of men I know think I'm too rough. I throw him up in the air and tickle him. My role is a parent more than a mother.

M.P.: The birth father is there. He was very unhappy about the pregnancy and birth of our child. We had been married, and then divorced and having a sexual affair after the marriage ended. He kept away from us for the first one and a half years. At that time he had a change of heart and went into analysis and decided he wanted to co-parent. His daughter is the most important person in his life.

Nine of the women were actively dating men and 11 were not. The difficulties in dating were described as primarily a function of lack of time, lack of resources, and occasionally lack of energy or sexual desire. Sixteen of the women were socially active and involved between 2 and 3 times a week. Only four of the women were rather isolated.

R.E.: I have about 8 good women friends in New York, and lots of acquaintances. I get together once or twice a week with female friends, date on the average of once every two weeks. I socialize a lot less than I used to. I have contact with Single Mothers by Choice, and friends through them. I used to seek out men more aggressively. I feel I'm always choosing between my child and a man. I don't want a strange man coming into bed with us, though I don't mind his father doing so.

K.C.: I'm pretty isolated. I have a friend who works nights. I speak to one woman every day on the phone. I don't get a chance to see people now, but I didn't before either.

It is interesting to note that women who were conceived by AID and who are now in their late 20s, when interviewed on a popular television show (Phil Donahue, Transcript #08033, 1983). expressed great anger at the destruction of records as to who their biological father was, thus preventing them from ever finding out about their origin. They did not blame their mother, however, for having opted for AID.

All of the children who had reached three years of age had asked about Daddy. There seems to be considerable variation as to how often they asked, how interested they appeared to be, and the kinds of reactions they had to the information offered. None of the children, as reported by the mothers, seemed to be distraught about the absent father. Most of the mothers, however, did appear concerned over the issue of the absent father, though to varying degrees.

M.V.: In the last year he's invented a father. His father is in Africa, has a dog, lets him eat ice cream. He's said to us "where's my daddy?" I told him he doesn't have a daddy, but he has two mommies who love him. Certain men respond to a kid who doesn't have a father. He seems to be starting to understand. He seems to be aware he's telling stories. He has another thing: a physical contact thing with men. It seems as if he's absorbing an identification, a real physical connection.

K.C.: She calls every man "daddy." I told her she doesn't have a daddy. But she only calls people daddy a lot when another kid in the park calls out daddy. She has no concept of what a daddy is. Her doll play has no daddies in it.

J.F.: They are minimally concerned with who their father is. They have not pushed me. At 4 or 5 they asked me a couple of

times but they never pursued it. I thought there might be more
concern on their part. It worried me that they would pursue it
but it doesn't seem to be a problem for them. They never came
back to tell me anything about how the world viewed them as
fatherless. I have not told them the identity. I have said yes,
there was someone but he doesn't know and until I ask him I
can't tell them.

When we inquired about their family histories, 15 of the 20
women reported negative feelings about their own parents' marriage, with only two reporting positive feelings. This did not appear
related, however, to specifically negative feelings about their fathers since half the women felt either negative or ambivalent, and
half felt positively toward their fathers.

Given the young age of the children, the mothers seemed to be
coping fairly well. The two most difficult issues seemed to be wor-
ries over finances regardless of income, and the amount of time they
can and do devote to socializing. Some reasons why the single
mothers we studied seem to be faring better than the UCLA sample
is that we studied an older, better educated, financially more stable
group, most of whom have an established ongoing social network.
Our findings, on the whole, tend to be consistent with the studies
reported previously. These are white middle class women, living in
an urban environment who have experienced little perceptible discrimination from others. All of the women we interviewed had an
enormous interest and investment in being mothers and parenting
their children well. Many of them seemed very determined to educate themselves in parenting skills. Most of the women were very
positive about their experience of motherhood and they presented a
fairly balanced view of their roles as single mothers. A recurrent
theme among the women was how happy they were to have pursued
motherhood on their own rather than to have waited for a man who
might not have arrived, and taken the risk of being childless.

SUMMARY AND CONCLUSION

This study presents a picture of the new single mother that differs
in many ways from the stereotyped image of the unwed mother
which has dominated the literature. These single mothers are successfully raising children on their own. They are an older, educated,

financially stable group who actively chose to become mothers outside of marriage. All of them had a strong desire to become mothers, regardless of the consequences.

Our data suggest that their chosen method of conception influences the way in which they are viewed by society. Adoptive mothers are regarded favorably, whereas the use of a "stud" meets with general disapproval. People appear to be uncertain about the ramifications of artificial insemination with single women; this includes members of the medical profession who are, at present, debating the issue in medical journals.

All of the women interviewed reported that they were happy with their decision, and they appeared to be concerned and supportive mothers. However, those women who were involved with men at the time of conception and expected them to share parenthood responsibilities expressed the most dissatisfaction when their expectations were not met. Relatively little sustained negative societal reaction was encountered. These women experienced several common concerns: what and how to tell their children about their origin; the issue of father absence; social isolation; and financial difficulties. Many also missed the experience of sharing their child's accomplishments with someone else. Many of them had expended considerable energy in bringing a consistent man into their children's lives. Most women still desired marriage, but found little time for dating. Formal support groups, such as Single Mothers by Choice were utilized by some, while others created their own social networks. Limited financial resources was the most frequently cited reason for not having a second child.

Important questions for further study concern the consequences of single motherhood on the psychological development of the child: the effects on the child's ability to form relationships with the opposite sex; the consequences of no identifiable father on the child's sense of identity; the effect on the child's ability to individuate in adolescence; and the development of the child of the single lesbian mother.

Our data suggests that single motherhood is a viable option for many women, although the long-term effects on the child's development remains uncertain. Whether this is a phenomenon that will continue to grow at its present rate or is a passing demographic trend, it has become a solution for many single women who would otherwise remain childless.

REFERENCES

Adams, P. L., Milner, J. R. & Schrepf, N. A. (1984). *Fatherless Children*. New York: John Wiley & Sons.

Alexander, J. & Kornfein, M. (1983). Changes in family functioning amongst non-conventional families. *American Journal of Orthopsychiatry, 53*(3), 408-417.

Andrews, L. (1984, December). Yours, mine and theirs. *Psychology Today*, 20-29.

Bennett, N., Craig, P. H. & Bloom, D. (1986). Marriage patterns in the United States. Yale University, Unpublished study.

Berlin, I. N. (1983). On conflict in non-traditional families: A clinical perspective. *American Journal of Orthopsychiatry, 53*(3), 436-438.

Bowerman, C. E., Irish, D. P. & Hallowell, P. (1966). *Unwed Motherhood: Personal and Social Consequences*. Chapel Hill: Institute for Research in Social Science.

Bremner, R. H. (Ed.) (1974). *Children and Youth in America: A Documentary History*. Cambridge, MA: Harvard University Press, Vol. III, 796-864.

Eiduson, B. T. (1983). Conflict and stress in non-traditional families: Impact on children. *American Journal of Orthopsychiatry, 53*(3), 426-435.

Fox, M. L. (1979). Unmarried adult mothers: A study of parenthood transition from late pregnancy to two months postpartum. Boston University School of Education, Unpublished Dissertation.

Goldsmith, J. (1975). A child of one's own: Unmarried women who choose motherhood. California School of Professional Psychology, Unpublished Dissertation.

Golombok, S., Spencer, A. & Rutter, M. (1983). Children in lesbian and single-parent households: Psychosexual and psychiatric appraisal. *Journal of Child Psychology and Psychiatry, 24*, 551-572.

Gongla, P. (1982). Single parent families: A look at families of mothers and children. *Marriage and Family Review, 5*, 5-27.

Goodman, W. (1984, February 27th). New reproduction techniques redefine parenthood. *New York Times*, 21.

Guttentag, M. & Secord, P. (1983). *Too Many Women? The Sex Ratio Question*. Beverly Hills: Sage Publications.

Hartley, S. F. (1975). *Illegitimacy*. Berkeley: University of California Press.

Herzog, E. & Sudia, C. E. (1968). Fatherless homes: A review of research. *Children, 15*(5), 177-182.

Klemesrud, J. (1983, May 2nd). Single mothers by choice: perils and joys. *New York Times*, B-5.

Macklin, E. D. & Rubin, R. H. (Eds.). (1983). *Contemporary Families and Alternative Lifestyles*. Beverly Hills: Sage Publications.

McGuire, M. & Alexander, N. J. (1985). Artificial insemination of single women. *Fertility and Sterility, 43*(2), 182-184.

Merritt, S. & Steiner, L. (1984). *And Baby Makes Two. Motherhood Without Marriage*. New York: Franklin Watts.

Morrisoe, P. (1983, June). Mommy only. *New York Magazine*, 21-29.

Novak, W. (1983, September 12th). Where have all the men gone? *New York Post*, 32-33.

Rains, P. M. (1971). *Becoming an Unwed Mother. A Sociological Account*. Chicago: Aldine Atherton.

Renvoise, J. (1985). *Going Solo. Single Mothers by Choice*. London: Routledge & Kegan Paul.

Rexford, M. T. (1976). Single mothers by choice: An exploratory study. California School of Professional Psychology, Unpublished Dissertation.

Ross, H. L. & Sawhill, I. V. (1975). *Time of Transition. The Growth of Families Headed by Women*. Washington, DC: The Urban Institute.

Sauber, M. & Rubinstein, E. (1965). *Experiences of the Unmarried Mother as a Parent*. New York: Community Council of Greater New York.

Stein, P. (1983). Singlehood. In E. D. Macklin & R. Y. Rubin (Eds.), *Contemporary Families and Alternative Lifestyles*. Beverly Hills: Sage Publications, 27-45.

Thompson, E. H. & Gongla, P. A. (1983). Single-parent families in the mainstream of American society. In: E. D. Macklin & R. M. Rubin (Eds.), *Contemporary Families and Alternative Lifestyles*. Beverly Hills: Sage Publications.

Vincent, C. E. (1961). *Unmarried Mothers*. Glencoe, IL: The Free Press.

Yankelovich, D. (1981). A world turned upside down. *Psychology Today, 15*(4), 35-91.

Zimmerman, I. L. & Bernstein, M. (1983). Parental work patterns in alternative families: Influence on child development. *American Journal of Orthopsychiatry, 53*(3), 418-425.

SECTION III

New Models

The obvious consequence of our moving ahead in knowledge, vision, and power is that we women develop and bring into reality models to meet our needs. The following papers describe a series of such models developed by women that utilize our new theoretical knowledge. These models focus attention on health education, the importance given to relationships, and the more egalitarian orientations crucial to women. The models serve as prototypes that could be implemented in similar ways elsewhere, or could be used as transitions to future models.

It is critical that we construct and adhere to good models because we women form a major market place, and many profit making purveyors of health services are trying to tap this market place with services purported to meet our needs. We need to have criteria by which to examine these to determine whether they truly meet our needs. These criteria include the degree to which the model adheres to the principles stated in the preface of this volume.

What we have been taught about our bodies, minds, and selves is sometimes at considerable variance with our own experience. Judy Norsigian and Wendy Sanford are two of eleven lay women who formed a collective that analyzed the health information available and combined it with their personal experience. They have become an international clearing house and publisher of women's health, sexual, and psychological information. In addition to maintaining an egalitarian organization in their own work, they have cut through the mystique which states that only a professional can be knowledgeable about health and illness, and have demonstrated the value of good information about our bodies in enabling us to obtain health care in a much more egalitarian way.

Jackie Yeomans describes a model for information and referral which empowers women in two ways. First, referrals are made only to therapists screened for their adherence to feminist principles and acceptable practice, and second, the woman making the choice is enabled to make her choice in a powerful and knowledgeable way.

In Karen Johnson's model for a woman's health center, many feminist principles are put into practice. A separate woman's center combines a health education program with the provision of health services. Through its hospital affiliation it provides a full range of services when needed. It is successful in today's marketplace.

The theory and treatment of alcohol abuse is an area where most of the research included only men, and treatment programs were framed around the needs of men. Little attention was paid to the needs of women and sometimes programs condoned abusive sexual practices toward women. Perhaps it was no accident that Marjorie Moyar and others initiated a woman's treatment program in Cleveland Women's General Hospital. This was one of the hospitals developed in the nineteenth century by women physicians who were denied training and practice elsewhere. While the Women's General hospital has now closed its doors, women's alcoholism program goes on. It utilizes women's relationship skills in a mature way, and has an outstanding success rate for its women clients.

Women have defined both residential and outpatient psychiatric treatment programs for women. Ann Beckert describes a five month residential rehabilitation model for a woman and her children that offers a radically different program from psychiatric hospitals or halfway houses. It addresses the needs of severely disabled women many of whom are poor, victims of violence, users of psychoactive medications, and have serious psychiatric diagnoses. The program offers them an opportunity to develop self esteem and independence. The women are not separated from their children. This provides a vision of a different kind of care and the potential of substantial change for the woman with many serious problems.

Women have often questioned our existing acute care psychiatric hospitals. To what extent do they meet women's needs and to what extent do they reinforce low self esteem and realistic helplessness? Can we design special units or special programs for women that would improve them for women? A first model for change has been developed by Jean Baker Miller and Nicolena Feldene in a program for women at the Charles River Hospital, a private psychiatric hospital in which the theme of self-in-relationship is developed both in the therapeutic program for patients and in focusing on relationships between staff members.

Elaine Borins has used her feminist knowledge in the development of a psychiatric outpatient service for women in which their problems can be attentively heard. In addition to their interview information, they have developed forms for acquiring relevant and important information from women which is frequently not asked for in conventional case histories. They are developing new information about the kinds of problems which bring women to seek help.

As we develop models for service, it is inevitable that conflicts arise. Some of these center around the woman physician, who is now entering practice in greater numbers. Is she a natural leader for women? Some women entering medicine have a strong intent to make change to benefit all women, others are simply pleased to be allowed to enter the male hierarchy, and passively obey the rules.

The questions are not simple and many kinds and combinations of answers are possible. Our tradition of medical care emphasizes the personal doctor-patient relationship. The personal aspect certainly fits our sense of the importance of relationship, and many of us have felt the pleasure of having an empathic woman surgeon, gynecologist, internist or psychiatrist. However, all of us are caught in the hierarchial aspects of the system. We need the ability of a highly competent person to handle emergencies and situations which require much technical knowledge and yet we need the ability to exercise a reasonable amount of freedom and equality with that person. How do we maintain both of these values?

One part of the women's movement, feminist health centers, have gone to an extreme of simply hiring the physician on an hourly basis to perform services, without any ongoing relationship to the person served or voice in the management of the clinic. They also provide a limited range of services so that the woman who has more serious illness is referred back into traditional medicine at a time when she needs her feminist health advocacy the most.

Conflicts present opportunities for new growth and ideas. The challenge of our future is to continue to develop new models which utilize and combine our feminist values in new and creative ways until these become norms for our society.

Ten Years in the "Our Bodies, Ourselves" Collective

Judy Norsigian
Wendy Coppedge Sanford

The *Our Bodies, Ourselves* Collective began as a one-afternoon discussion group on health at a large women's conference in Boston in 1969. We found ourselves unable to put together a list of "good" ob-gyns in our area—that is, doctors who listened to what a patient had to say; respected her opinions; explained choices, procedures, and medications; treated her as a partner in her health care rather than as a dependent child. We began to realize that doctors knew and had not shared with us a lot of information about our bodies' functioning, birth control methods, childbirth, sexuality, and more information that would help us to take better care of ourselves and to be more in control of our lives. Also, we were aware that as women we had much special information which, however, we hadn't considered legitimate because it wasn't "expert."

So we decided to keep meeting and to put together some of this information for ourselves. Each of us did research on a topic that was personally important to us, interviewing doctors and nurses willing to meet with us, and ploughing through medical texts and journals with the help of a dictionary. When we brought the factual information back to the group, we discussed the topics out of our own experiences of them in our lives. In this way, the textbook view of childbirth or miscarriage or menstruation or lovemaking, for instance, nearly always written by men, would become expanded and enriched by the truth of our actual experiences. The process was an exciting one, especially since most of us had been

The authors are members of the Women's Health Book Collective, Boston, Massachusetts.
© Radcliffe College, 1979. Reprinted with the permission of the Radcliffe Quarterly.

brought up to view other women as rivals and had not shared so honestly with each other before.

We saw quickly the power of this kind of health and sex education. The weaving together of facts and feelings made the information useful to us in a new way, and putting our stories together helped us see ways we were *all* receiving inadequate treatment, allowed us to begin to build up an effective critique of a medical system that had heretofore kept us isolated from each other.

Since that first year we have taught without charge many "Know Your Body" courses for women; participated in activist health-care consumer movements to demedicalize childbirth, legalize induced abortion, get improved medical care for poorer women and so on; and written a women's health and sex education book originally called *Our Bodies, Ourselves*. Printed in 1970 by the New England Free Press and now published by Simon and Schuster (1973, 1976, 1979), over three million copies of this book in its various editions have been sold worldwide. It exists in English and eleven other languages, with more translations now in progress. This book was totally rewritten and published in early 1985 as *The New Our Bodies, Ourselves*. Our second book, *Ourselves and Our Children* (Random House, 1978) is about the needs and experiences of women and men as parents.

OUR PROJECTS

Over the past fourteen years the work of our now 12-woman collective (funded primarily by income from royalties) has expanded in focus to include more women's health issues such as occupational and environmental health, new reproductive technologies (such as in-vitro fertilization), all aspects of violence against women, and numerous international concerns. Through discussion groups, speaking engagements, both formal and informal consulting, media interviews, and distribution of literature, we have worked with a wide range or organizations, including high schools and colleges, libraries, family planning agencies, local and national health and women's organizations, medical schools and residency programs, and, of course, other women's health groups. Some of our current projects include

— our Women's Health Information Center, which each month answers hundreds of requests for information by phone, mail and in person. The Center's resources are often used by college students preparing term papers, women researching treatment options for a particular disease or medical condition, and media representatives working of articles and news items.

— the publication and distribution of a U.S.-Spanish edition of *OUR BODIES, OURSELVES* (50,000 copies now in print). Several thousand of these books have been delivered to Latin America as well. For example, in 1984 and 1985, U.S. physicians and nurses who attended conferences with Nicaraguan health workers took down several hundred eagerly received copies.

— the Women's Health and Learning Center, a unique program for women in Massachusetts prisons, many of whom face problems of violence, substance abuse, poor health and parenting. This project receives both public (state) and private funding.

— the tampon project, which is educating women about the health risks associated with tampons and calling for proper absorbency labeling of tampons through FDA regulation.

— expanded international outreach and contact with women's groups in other countries. In 1980 we wrote and published, in collaboration with ISIS (an international women's information, communication and exchange program), the first International Women and Health Resource Guide. In 1985 a Collective member attended the UN's NGO Women's Conference in Nairobi where she led several workshops.

— Amigas Latinas En Accion Pro Salud ("ALAS"), a group of Latina women who conduct bilingual discussion groups and workshops on women's health and are working on innovative bilingual women's health literature.

— various initiatives which would expand midwifery options for women (e.g., through helping nurse-midwives to secure malpractice insurance coverage and supporting efforts to legitimize lay midwifery and the option of home birth in Massachusetts.

In addition, we have worked on several joint projects with other women's health groups. These include:

— the establishment of *Health-Right*, a women's health movement quarterly, published by HealthRight, Inc. (New York
City) between 1975 and 1979.

— the Rising Sun Feminist Health Alliance, established to increase mutual support, information-sharing, and overall communication among women-controlled health centers and
health advocacy groups in the northeast.

— the production, in Spanish, of simple, comic-book-like pam-
phlets on several different women's health issues (with
CIDHAL, a Mexican women's organization).

BACKLASH

As our books become more widely distributed (*Our Bodies, Ourselves* was on the bestseller list for more than two years) and as the
media more frequently contact us about women's health issues considered to be "hot topics," our visibility inevitably has increased.
One unfortunate dimension of this public exposure has been the
backlash to *Our Bodies, Ourselves*. In dozens of communities
around the country, both rural and urban, there have been fervent
attempts to ban *Our Bodies, Ourselves* from library and/or school
bookshelves. Despite the fact that *Our Bodies, Ourselves* was chosen by the Young Adult Services Division of the American Library
Association as a Young Adult Best Book of 1976 (and also a Young
Adult Best Book of the decade), it continues to be the object of
attack by right-wing groups such as the Eagle Forum (started by
Phyllis Schlafly). For over two years, the collective had to offer
assistance to teenagers, parents, and community groups who were
fighting attempts to censor *Our Bodies, Ourselves*. We have com-
piled supportive reviews, articles, and letters from educators, parents, physicians, and other health providers. We view the attack on
Our Bodies, Ourselves as part of the larger attack on women's
rights in general, most notably in the form of anti-ERA, anti-child
care, and anti-abortion activity. Though this activity may represent
the viewpoint of a minority, it has been well financed, has had an
alarming influence on policy makers, and represents a major challenge to the women's movement in this country.

THE WOMEN'S MOVEMENT

In both our work and our way of working, we see our group as part of the larger women's movement. By feminism (a media-distorted word) we mean, most simply, a way of looking at the world that takes women seriously as full human beings with a right to a full share in all kinds of work and creative enterprise, another word for self-respect, a habit of being identified primarily as women. We see the empowerment of women to control our bodies, especially our reproduction, seeing this empowerment as a fundamental means to control our lives and participate in the world. Of the different groups working for change in women's position in this country, we find ourselves less comfortable with those who assert women's right to move into the society's corporate structure and power elites as the primary expression of feminist goals. Instead, we are among the women who want to let our longtime experience of being the ones *without* power shape a vision that challenges the existing power structures themselves. Instead of our own piece of the pie, in other words, we want to change the recipe. Running through our work on health and parenting issues is a wider vision of social change – a dream of eliminating the exploitation and suffering that result from racism, sexism, classism, and oppressive economic and political systems. We see, for instance, that the proliferation of nuclear power and violence against women in media, street, and home are spawned by the same mind set and political systems that have denied women control over their bodies.

Given this larger vision, we believe our approach to change is more consonant with certain voices in the women's movement than with others. In our small discussion groups of women beginning to talk openly with one another about our lives, we learned that our best contribution to larger social change was to start at a personal level. What we do best is to help women look more critically at the particulars of their own health care and personal lives, to start to name the changes they want to make, and to see that they can and, in fact, have to work with others to try to effect those changes. We believe that starting at this personal level generates the motivation, energy, and skills for larger political movements; it certainly has been the source of our group's continuing and energetic public presence in the struggle for women against the organized sources of oppression. Many women who wouldn't call themselves feminists have read *Our Bodies, Ourselves* or *Ourselves and Our Children* and have begun to look more critically at their health care, at society's attitudes towards sexuality, at the ways society shapes the parenting experience. They have used the books as tools for making changes, both small and large. This is what, if you'd asked us fifteen years ago, we would perhaps most have hoped for.

Getting There and Hanging In: The Story of WCREC, A Women's Service Collective

Jackie Yeomans

This is a story about a group of women; an evolving group that struggled and changed and sacrificed, and hung on to an idea over a thirteen year period. They took that idea through a highly creative process and founded and operate the Women's Counseling, Referral and Education Center. It functions today as a unique mental-health service for women.

It is also a story about empowerment, because empowerment is the *need* that gives us our mandate. It is the constant reminder of *how* that mandate must be implemented in our work with clients. And it is a *way* of operating internally at WCREC (our Collective Structure) that is in harmony with that mandate.

THE VISION

Empowerment was clearly the issue thirteen years ago when WCREC's history began. At that time a group of Toronto women began meeting to discuss concerns about the lack of adequate mental health resources for women. It included feminists, mental health professionals and other committed individuals who were alarmed about the over-prescription of psycho-tropic drugs. They saw the widespread use of the medical model in treating life problems and they were concerned about the dearth of alternative resources for women.

The author is Direct Service Coordinator of the Women's Counseling Referral and Education Center, Toronto, Ontario, Canada. Her interests are in women and mental health issues.

They envisioned a centralized referral service; a creative alternative, where women would be helped to assess their needs; where they would be given information about the various therapies and other available community resources; and where they would then be encouraged to make their own choices.

Women using the service would not be discounted by a process of professional diagnosis and labelling nor would they be subjected to any procedure that would negate their considerable self-knowledge and decision-making abilities. Center staff would interview potential referent therapists to ensure a basic sensitivity to the special needs of women in therapy.

The group met over a two year period. They assessed the needs and designed an essential service including a therapist questionnaire and evaluation procedure. In 1975 (International Women's Year) a proposal submitted by the group to Health and Welfare Canada was approved for funding. Some of those original women stayed on to become WCREC's first Board of Directors. They set about hiring staff, finding a suitable location for the Center and in February 1976 the doors to the Women's Counseling, Referral and Education Center opened to the public.

Three years of financial security were followed by another five of funding crisis. There were times when programming was cut to a "bare bones" referral component and staff reduced by two thirds. Today the referral component of our service enjoys secure funding provided by the Ontario Ministry of Health.

WHAT WE DO

The key word again is empowerment. It forms the basis for our work with clients. When a woman calls for assistance (95% of our clients are women), we assume that she lacks power in some way and at WCREC we seek to "re-empower" in whatever ways possible. Essentially we have three kinds of callers at WCREC. The first kind approach us with a good deal of personal power. They require very little from us in the way of assistance. For example:

> . . . We're doing a lot of shouting at each other . . . just being very verbally abusive at this point. We've talked it over and I think what we want is a mediator — someone who can help us diffuse the situation and then get us looking at ways to com-

municate better in the future. We'd prefer to work with a woman . . . someone our age or older who has a lot of experience and skill in relationship work . . . at this point we'd like verbal therapy — maybe someone who uses a communications model.

This woman is very clear about what she wants from us. She gives us the information and we try to match her request with three appropriate therapists from our resource file. We would also ask her what kind of person she'd like to work with. She has told us the preferred age and sex of the therapist but she may also have a preference in terms of "personal type." Some clients say,

> I want someone who is warm and motherly because I'm feeling fragile right now. I don't want anyone who is very confrontive in approach.

or

> I don't need a mother . . . I tend to play games and I know it . . . I want someone who will confront me when I do . . . someone who won't be intimidated by me.

Similar life experiences are important to some clients. A single parent who was struggling with three teenagers said,

> I want someone who has raised kids . . . someone who's been through it and will know what I'm talking about.

We get many calls like this each day from a diversity of people wanting a whole assortment of choices. They know what they want and they have the ability to act. All that is needed from us are some names and addresses.

The second kind of caller has less personal power available to her. She may be confused about what she wants to deal with in therapy or what she hopes to get out of it. Clarity is empowering. She may want information about the different types of therapy and other resources that are available to her. Information is power. We would suggest that such a woman come in for an Educational/Referral session. The one hour appointment would include helping her to assess her needs and goals. We would provide her with information about resources and then we would encourage her to make her own choices.

> — What kind of person would you like to work with?
> — I haven't thought about that . . . I really don't know.
> — Well, you said you liked the psychologist in Montreal. What was she like?

or

> — Was there a particular type of therapy that appealed to you more than the others?
> — Umm . . . I liked what you said about Gestalt . . . was that the one where they do the "empty chair" work? . . . Yeah . . . that one appealed to me and I know I need to get more in touch with my feelings. Is it only done in groups?
> — No you could see someone individually. Would you prefer that?

The third kind of caller has even less personal power. She requires much more from us in order to act on her needs. It could be that she is in crisis and overwhelmed by feelings. We would spend some time talking with her . . . allowing her to vent . . . helping her to calm down enough to participate in the assessment process. We would probably do much more work here than with the other two kinds of clients . . . sorting out the issues, helping her to decide on goals, offering suggestions — but always giving back to her the power of final decision making.

One of our procedures is to give a client the names of three therapists so that she has some choice. We encourage a consumer approach, suggesting that she see all three before making a final decision about with whom she wants to work. We stress the importance of finding a therapist that she would be comfortable with . . . that she could trust and open up to. Sometimes clients take this consumer approach for granted; they have every intention of "shopping" when they first contact WCREC. Others are delighted by the suggestion. It hasn't occurred to them that they have the right to some choices when it comes to their therapy. The "permission to choose" is very liberating to these women. Occasionally some women choose not to shop. The very depressed client or the one in crisis may not want, or be able, to go through that kind of procedure. Still, the option is there for her and simply knowing that she does have rights in the therapy process is empowering even if she chooses not to exercise those rights.

The concept of empowerment is focal to our Direct Service. This is in contrast to many other institutional assessment procedures based on the medical model. All clients are often put through the same process regardless of their ability to assess themselves and their needs. A professional makes a diagnosis, labels the client, and determines the type of treatment s/he thinks is most appropriate. Once *in* treatment the client has very little control over her therapy. Some institutions conduct "team meetings" from which the client is excluded, where the "case" is discussed. What WCREC offers is an alternative to this kind of approach. And our hundreds of callers testify to the growing demand for just such a consumer oriented alternative.

THERAPIST SELECTION PROCESS

Since its inception in 1975 WCREC has interviewed over 400 therapists in the Toronto area. At the present time we have approximately 200 active therapists on our referral file. They include Social Workers, Psychologists, Counselors, Psychiatrists and MD General Practitioners who do supportive counseling. Their modes of therapy cover a wide spectrum from verbal-insight, to experiential to holistic, to eclectic approaches and their fees for service range from free to $75 per hour.

People often ask how we get our therapists. Do we have an active outreach program or do they approach us to be listed? The answer is "both." We are constantly looking for therapists who can work with low income women. This usually means Medical Doctors and Psychiatrists whose services are covered under the Ontario Health Insurance Plan, or therapists working within Social Service Agencies who can see low income women at no cost. Although we have a long waiting list of private practice therapists who have approached us to be interviewed our priority at this time is to interview only those therapists who can handle our increasing numbers of low income clients.

One goal of therapist selection is to gather information that will enhance the matching process. When someone is about to make a major purchase she will usually try to get as much information as possible before making a choice. If the purchase is therapy (an often costly and significant venture), the same sort of consideration should surely be given.

At WCREC we compile data for our clients on each therapist listed with us.

- We know the type of therapy practiced (Gestalt, Cooperative Problem Solving, Psychoanalysis, etc.)
- any specializations (relationship work, additions, battered women, etc.)
- the personal presentation (warm/friendly/energetic, serious/thoughtful)
- the office environment (private home/pillows on carpet, medical building/chairs/desk/plants)

And so on. Each client has a different set of preferences.

Another goal is to determine the beliefs and attitudes of the therapist on a number of issues related to women and therapy. Feminism and Feminist Therapy are the philosophy and theory which underlie our Therapist Questionnaire. Much has already been written on each but for us a feminist orientation means that the therapist holds certain attitudes and beliefs about women in society and incorporates these into her practice (90% of our therapists are women). She knows the effects of the social, political and economic structures on women and that women hold less power than men in all three areas. A feminist therapist shares her awareness with clients and works on breaking down the power imbalance by being human with them (she will share personal feelings and experiences with them when relevant). Compare this:

A woman approached a large psychiatric facility. She had been raped a year before and was just beginning to feel strong enough to deal with all the horror of the attack. She was confronted by a male psychiatrist (and two male residents) who spent an hour questioning her about her childhood and, in particular, her feelings towards her father. When she called us a day later she was feeling depersonalized and humiliated.

With this:

> Another woman, a single mother on welfare, told her therapist that she had been "sick" (depressed) for years. She was feeling powerless in her situation — tired, discouraged and a failure as a parent. She was in a great deal of emotional pain and highly critical of herself. The therapist refuted her "sick" label, told her it would be surprising if she weren't depressed considering the circumstances of her life. She told her about the very real ways that she was being oppressed (inadequate funds and housing, and lack of practical and emotional support in raising her children — a difficult task even for two parents). She also showed the woman how she had been taught to collude in her own oppression by blaming herself and thus escalating the depression. The therapist gave her encouragement, did problem solving with her, allowed her to vent her anger and frustration, and hooked her up with a community program where she was able to connect with other single mothers in a supportive environment.

A feminist orientation means a commitment to change rather than adjustment. It means looking at real needs rather than preserving institutions. The family is one institution that is often viewed as sacred . . . to be kept intact at all costs. Yet it is within the family unit that thousands of women are assaulted each year and increasing numbers of defenseless children (usually female) are subjected to incest. The feminist view holds that it is individuals who are in need of empowerment — not institutions.

The first section of our therapist questionnaire is related to this issue of power. We see the role of therapist as highly powerful. The more invested are therapists in their authority, the less likely are they to be empowering to their clients. (We hold that personal empowerment is a fundamental goal of therapy.) We want to know if therapists are aware of the strength of their influence and how they deal with that issue. We want to know if they have ever had therapy themselves and, if so, how it has affected their role as practitioner. If they have never been in the position of client how can they know what their clients are experiencing.

How do they feel about paraprofessional agencies and are they aware of those kinds of resources (hostels, rape crisis center, legal clinics, etc.) for their clients?

We have sections on feminism and political change; on violence against women; on sexuality and reproductive rights; on ethnicity and class issues.

Some of our therapists are very strong feminists. They are politically active and highly articulate on the issues. Others are less so. We don't have a "Party Line" to which everyone must adhere. We do have a bottom line and sometimes feel the differences between our philosophy and the therapist's are too great to allow for a good working relationship.

Again, what we are trying to do in determining attitudes is to facilitate a good match between client and therapist.

- A client might say "I want a therapist who is a strong feminist — that's a priority! I'm really angry right now about women's position in society and these feelings are going to come up in therapy. I don't need someone I'm going to have to fight with . . . who is going to be defensive about the status quo."
- We have some excellent therapists listed who work for Catholic Agencies and who are not permitted to do abortion counseling. Although our position is pro-choice we maintain a good relationship with these agencies. We simply wouldn't send a woman who needed to make a decision about whether or not to have an abortion.
- We live in a diverse society and it's important for therapists working with people of different racial, cultural or class backgrounds to be aware of those differences. The first step is self-awareness; becoming aware of your own background and of what beliefs and attitudes you have incorporated from it into your present value system.
- We once interviewed an MD who said that he had been reading over the questionnaire at breakfast that morning before we arrived for the interview. When he came to the section on "Race, Culture and Class" he mused to his wife "They're going to ask me about my class bias . . . and I don't think I have a class bias." He told us that his wife peered at him from behind her newspaper and said "Bull Shit . . . You're a WASP." Smart woman. We all have biases; and they are most dangerous when we remain unaware of them.

Therapists as well as clients have been impressed by our matching process. It saves a lot of time when we do a prescreening and send only appropriate clients to them. They have often been pleased with the interview session as well, saying that they found it informative and in some cases "eye opening" and that it had started them thinking about some of the issues for the first time.

OTHER COMMITMENTS

WCREC is strongly committed to the area of self-help. Often women don't need therapy. What they need is to connect with others who share similar feelings and experiences. A self-help group provides women with a place to exchange ideas, do problem solving together and give one another support and validation.

Self-help projects have been on the go at WCREC whenever funding has allowed. We have started self-help groups, trained staff of other services to facilitate self-help groups and last year we published a handbook called *Helping Ourselves* (1985) to assist women in starting their own self-help groups.

We are also involved in Networking and Community Education at WCREC. Networking because it's important for us to be connected with other organizations that share similar views and goals. For the past four years WCREC has met with other members of the Toronto Women's Services Network to exchange information about what is happening in the community and to work collectively as advocates for women's rights.

And Community Education is important to us as well. Often a group will call, say they've heard about us but don't know exactly what we do . . . could we send a speaker? And we are pleased to do that because it's important for us to meet with new groups to find out who they are—and to share with them what we have learned about women and mental-health over the past 10 years.

Energy is also directed into social action and lobbying at WCREC. It is not enough to tell women that they have the right to make choices, and it's not enough to give them the support, clarification and information that will enable them to make choices. Those choices have to be there. And within the referral component at WCREC the choices are very limited for low income women. Half of our clients cannot afford to pay more than what is covered by the Ontario Health Insurance Plan for their health care needs. We feel a responsibility, as a publicly funded group, to lobby for the needs of our clients who are also members of that public. To that end we support the activities of the Medical Reform Group and Ontario Health Coalition, whose member groups are addressing the Canada Health Act and trying to ensure that quality health care be available to all.

Economic disadvantage is not the only problem facing women today. Pornography, rape, incest and abortion are all issues which reflect women's lack of power and personal control. And as a community organization we again try to act for our callers within this larger social context. We write letters, attend rallies and participate on committees like the Metropolitan Toronto Task Force On Public Violence Against Women.

THE COLLECTIVE

All of WCREC's activities are carried on today by an active group of highly committed and often irreverent women. (And a sense of humor is important within Women's Services where the needs are enormous and the funding minimal!)

We operate as a Collective of four staff, a dozen or so volunteers and, this year, six students on placement with us from local universities and community colleges. All attend weekly business meetings and participate in the activities and decisions of the organization. Everyone is heard. Our students are women who come to us to learn something . . . and they learn a lot at WCREC. But as mature women they also contribute enormously to do our service. They contribute their time, knowledge, life experience and considerable personal skills. So we view students not just as students, but as full members of our Collective. We choose to operate this way because we believe in the principles of cooperation and shared decision making. We find it more satisfying and productive than a hierarchical structure where the power of decision making rests with a few at the top.

I think that empowerment really is the issue for women today. We are not taking enough control personally, socially or politically and we need to do more of that. So we have to increase our self-confidence. We have to be clearer about what we need and want and about how to get those things for ourselves. We also need legislation to protect our needs and rights. And while we are working on these empowerment issues, we want to be with people who are also aware and who will challenge and support us. We want this from our friends, our families, our co-workers and our therapists.

Within WCREC we are also women struggling with these issues. So we try to work together in ways that are respectful, supportive and challenging. And when we do work together in those ways we know that we are also more useful to our clients . . . women very much like ourselves who come to WCREC for this kind of assistance.

WCREC has celebrated it's 10th year of operation with a conference and party. The event was called:

Getting There and Hanging In: Celebrating 10 Years of Women Helping Women

Happy Birthday, WCREC.

REFERENCES

Women's Counseling Referral and Education Center (1985). *Helping Ourselves*. Toronto: Women's Press.

Women's Health Care:
An Innovative Model

Karen Johnson

THE WOMEN'S HEALTH MOVEMENT

During the mid-1960s the health care consumer and reform movements were expanding in several directions. Liberals were concerned with decreasing the cost of health care and increasing accessibility of services across socio-economic groups. Radicals argued for low-cost or free care as a consumer right and visionaries favored cooperative care based on self-help and patient participation. Women's health activists were one sub-group of this movement and encompassed, not always comfortably, liberals, radicals, and visionaries (Ruzek, 1979). These activists were disenchanted with the health care system. In their opinion, services cost too much, were maldistributed, and the quality ranged from ineffective to dangerous. Some physicians attempted to respond to the complaints with an increase in family centered medicine emphasizing personal contact and empathy, but the majority continued in the direction of increasing specialization with reliance on sophisticated medical technologies.

About the same time, the female culture was being rediscovered. Women's values and self-concepts were changing as they participated in the women's movement. Health care became a key feminist issue challenging the traditional authoritarian medical-professional model, particularly obstetrics and gynecology. The question became: who controls women's bodies? Feminist health activists

The author is a psychiatrist who is Coordinator of Psychological Services, Healthworks for Women, Mount Zion Medical Center, San Francisco, California.

The author is indebted to Alice Cottingham for her critical review of an earlier version of this paper.

worked to shift control from professionals and put women in charge
of their own health care. Initially the emphasis was on a woman's
right to contraception and abortion, access to information, and par-
ticipatory decision making in health matters.

At a Boston Women's Conference in the spring of 1969 several
women decided to meet to explore health issues. Their group developed a pamphlet which ultimately became one of the best selling
and most widely distributed books on women's health, *Our Bodies,
Ourselves* (1984). Nineteen-seventy-one marked the first Women's
Health Conference in New York, attended by over 800 women, and
in the same year Carol Downer began self-help gynecology in Los
Angeles by demonstrating how a woman could examine her own
cervix. Feminists also began re-asserting control over the childbirth
experience, supporting lay and nurse midwifery and expressing distrust of the male-dominated medical system.

Over the next several years, women opened their own health centers. Often the basic goal of these centers was to guarantee women
the right to control their fertility. Women were establishing female
worlds largely excluding men and male authority. This exclusionary
policy contributed to the establishment of a positive sense of self as
competent, knowledgeable, and powerful women. At the same
time, for most centers survival was chronically in question. Centers
were low-budget operations staffed exclusively or primarily by volunteers. Additionally, staff had certain expectations about how organizations should function. A collective form of organization in
which power was shared equally was the aim. Striving for consensus, the process of decision making was laborious and time-con-
suming, often exhausting even the most enthusiastic supporters.
Struggles for financial survival taxed organizational energy. Conflicts in these and other arenas often resulted in hostility among
members and not infrequently the collapse of the organization.
Those centers that have survived to the 1980s have generally done
so by altering some of their original plans so that they could obtain
funds to sustain the organization and by evolving a more hierarchical organizational structure (Riger, 1981).

SEPARATISM VERSUS INTEGRATION

The marginality of women's health centers to mainstream American medicine results in certain disadvantages as well as advantages.

For years, women's health activists have focused on the advantages, of which there are many. Women helping other women understand and care for their own bodies has been an empowering process that has had widespread consequences for women even beyond the women's health movement and the larger feminist movement. However, as "burn-out" takes its toll on the staff at women's health centers, unpaid volunteers or those on minimal subsistence salaries move elsewhere. If an entire center disbands, as too often happens, there are fewer organizations to serve women.

Understandably, early women's health activists resisted affiliation with mainstream American medicine. Originally, personal expertise and knowledge by virtue of being female were highly valued. Formal certification was not. The services of physicians when they were used at women's health centers were closely monitored by lay women. Most professional services were accepted only on a volunteer basis or at a low hourly salary. Professionals, especially physicians, were suspect, and much energy went into discussions about how to "manage" them. The relationships with women physicians were often particularly conflictual because they were viewed as potential "sisters" while at the same time "honorary men" (Ruzek, 1979).

Nonetheless, the activists' public complaints were not falling upon deaf ears within mainstream medicine. By 1982 the American Medical Women's Association had taken a strong pro-women's health position and annual medical conferences were being held in Boston co-sponsored by them and the Massachusetts Medical Society. Feminists were climbing the ranks in various medical disciplines and they along with a more vocal and assertive public were making mainstream medicine pay attention to women's health concerns.

Ironically, the medical profession's increasing responsiveness to women's health concerns caused concern among lay leaders that professionals, especially professional women, would usurp control. They envisioned doctors setting up their own women's clinics that would superficially adopt feminist forms such as emphasizing education, providing an informal atmosphere, and using paramedics, without placing real control in the hands of the women themselves. Yet, even activists recognize that feminist health centers have historically been organized to meet the needs of "well," not "sick" women. Self-help groups eliminate professionals, and non-physician, women-controlled health care addresses issues of cost, maldistribution, and control, but neither establishes female authority within medicine nor transforms health care for ill women who must use the services of the more conventional health system.

Initially women health professionals, especially physicians, were reluctant to acknowledge alliance with feminism, but increasingly women already committed to feminism have pursued training in the health professions. As the feminist health movement has placed increasing emphasis on organized lobbying and influencing social policy, credentials and expertise are valued and valuable. Collaboration between academic and professional women and lay activists, as feminists dedicated to improving health care for women, provides the opportunity for expanding the goals of the women's health movement beyond the limitations of either group alone. While activists may believe that pressure must come from outside the establishment, "insiders" are often effective change agents. Mutual interdependence permits the radicals to press for change from the outside while professionals, appearing more conservative by comparison, press for change within the system (Walsh, 1979).

WOMEN'S HEALTH RESOURCES

In 1980 Patricia Read, Associate Administrator for Ambulatory Care at Illinois Masonic Medical Center, proposed the establishment of a Women's Center run by an all woman staff. The hospital had prided itself on providing high quality, cost effective care through innovative programs and it had paid attention to what were historically considered the health concerns of women. Thus, it was proud of its excellent nurse midwifery program, its abortion unit, and the Rape Advocate Program, but like most health care facilities, it believed women's health care needs were best addressed through their reproductive systems. Ms. Read was shifting the concept of women's health care to a primary care orientation with an additional emphasis on health education and promotion and patient participation. She completed a marketing survey, the results of which were persuasive enough to gain administrative support for a center that would grow in phases (Read, 1980).

Phase I opened in April, 1982, in a renovated apartment building just south of the hospital. It was led by feminist Sally Rynne, previously a consumer health activist. There was a telephone referral service for women interested in linking up with one or more services and/or pro-women clinicians. The women answering the phones were knowledgeable in women's health and could answer many of the callers' questions or refer them to appropriate resources. Also during this phase, the staff began building a resource center for health care consumers desiring women's health information. A library with a vast collection of periodicals and books related to women's health was built. Consumers were invited to use the material on a drop-in basis or educational packets could be sent to women at longer distances for a nominal fee to cover costs. Evening educational programs were offered on a regular basis and were so well-attended and received that Women's Health Resources quickly gained a reputation in Chicago as the place to go for women's health care programs.

Phase II, providing direct health care services to community women, began in September, 1982. Both obstetrics-gynecology and alternative women's health centers have encouraged women to enter the health care system through their reproductive organs. Certainly such care has its place in women's health, but it is not all there is to a woman and her health needs. Women's Health Resources is designed to provide comprehensive care with an emphasis on collaborative decision making between a patient and her clinician. To enact a primary vs reproductive care orientation, among the first providers hired were an internist and family nurse practitioner. Attending to the mental health concerns was also a priority as a goal to discourage the mind-body dichotomy so problematic in medicine. A feminist psychiatrist with practical experience in medical self-care and consumer education was hired. Months later, a nutritionist and, one year later, a feminist ob-gyn physician joined the group. All clinicians are salaried and physicians have staff appointments in their respective hospital departments.

While the center had money from the hospital to start, long-term survival would depend upon eventually breaking into the black and repaying the loan from the hospital for their initial investment. We had to prove that there was a market for collaborative women's health care associated with a traditional medical hospital. Administrative decisions were made with this in mind. The center is modeled after a group practice, including fees, and educational programs pay their own way. Modifications in conventional practice include a minimum appointment time of thirty minutes, evening hours for working women, and open medical charts. Responsibility for weekly staff educational programs rotates among members;

these meetings keep staff informed of the latest in women's health across disciplines. Weekly provider meetings permit interdisciplinary collaboration among clinicians for comprehensive health care of individual women. An advisory board including consumers and prominent Chicago feminists outside of medicine advises the director in the areas of policy and planning, and patients are encouraged to complete evaluation forms following every education and clinical encounter. As clinicians and educators, we view ourselves as specialists in women's health, taking their concerns seriously and treating the women with respect. We encourage self-care, continuing education, and collaborative participation. Unlike most alternative women's health centers, we have the back-up of a major medical center.

VISIONS FOR THE FUTURE

The future can be planned for, but never completely predicted. Growing pains at the center have resulted in casualties as well as benefits. Ideological divisions among staff members erupt periodically into open conflict, changing informal alliances, and power struggles. No one knows how to run a feminist health center affiliated with a major medical center and we learn as much from our mistakes as our successes. If anything, we have discovered that it is easier to have innovative ideas than to find the woman power and time to implement all of them. Priorities must be set and reasonable expectations defined. The institution must be, and by and large Women's Health Resources is, responsive to the lives of the staff as well as the patients. No one balks at the women who prefer part-time positions and they need not have children to "legitimize" this preference. Simply wanting to limit the time devoted to paid work at Women's Health Resources is reason enough. Flexible work schedules allow single parents time to pick up children at day care; youngsters often roam the halls under the watchful eyes of their mothers or another staff member as parents do their jobs at the center, and pregnancies are taken in stride by the director who has mothered six children herself.

Future goals include hiring more clinicians, especially in ob-gyn and mental health, expanding the self-care program, and developing patient education materials from a feminist perspective for women's common health concerns. Many of the staff members also volunteer their time to other activities that ultimately benefit women. One is a political activist, another provides free care at an alternative women's health center, and another is a women's health writer. Fantasies of the future include a feminist in-patient unit and the emergence of women's health as a formal primary health care specialty (Johnson, 1986). We are doing what we can to encourage these, and the continuing collaboration between lay women health activists and feminist health care professionals.

REFERENCES

The Boston Women's Health Book Collective (1984). *The new our bodies, ourselves* (2nd ed.). New York: Simon and Schuster.

Johnson, K. (1986). Women's health: An emerging primary health care speciality. Unpublished manuscript.

Read, P. (1980). Women's center. Illinois Masonic Medical Center. (Unpublished report).

Rigor, S. (1981). The life and death of feminist movement organizations: A research agenda. Los Angeles, California. (Paper presented at the annual meeting of the American Psychological Association.)

Ruzek, S. B. (1979). *The women's health movement: Feminist alternatives to medical control.* New York: Praeger.

Walsh, M. R. (1979, November). The rediscovery of the need for a feminist medical education. *Harvard Educational Review, 49,* No. 4.

Female Alcoholism
and Affiliation Needs

Marjorie Moyar

THE PROGRAM

Merrick Hall for women was the first hospital-based alcoholism/
chemical dependency treatment program for women in the country.
The program is designed to meet the special needs of women and
address their unique problems. This fourteen bed unit was originally
developed at Woman's General Hospital in Cleveland, Ohio and
opened in 1975. Ten years later, it was relocated at Huron Road
Hospital.

The in-patient program at Merrick Hall consists of two phases.
The first phase is the medically supervised phase, where a complete
physical assessment is conducted, detoxification needs evaluated,
and a complete alcohol and drug history recorded. This phase is
designed to eliminate D.T.s and any other serious life threatening
complications of withdrawal.

Once the evaluation phase is completed, the clinical staff formu-
lates an individual treatment program for the patient. Entering the
second phase of the program, the patient participates in group meetings, lectures and teaching sessions conducted by the Merrick Hall
for Women staff. Volunteer members of the recovering alcoholic
community share their experience, strength, and hope with patients.
The recovery program is wholistic: the physical, spiritual, and emotional needs of the women are sensitively approached by the multi-
disciplinary staff. Majorie Moyar, PhD is the staff psychologist for
the Merrick Hall women. One of the several issues she addresses

---

The author is a psychologist in private practice and a staff psychologist at Merrick Hall for
Women, Huron Road Hospital, Cleveland, Ohio. Her specializations are in chemical dependency and depression.

313

both in group and individual therapy is the significance of affiliation needs in recovery.

As women are successfully treated in this program important discoveries are being made about the recovery process for women.

THE PROBLEM

First we will examine alcoholism, its effect on affiliation needs and the ways in which women are likely to experience alcoholism differently than men. Next, we will examine the dimensions of the problem's resolution and treatment: (a) who comes to treatment, (b) a study of social role adjustment, and (c) changing social roles.

What is alcoholism? Today alcoholism is considered an illness, a disease. The World Health Organization defines alcoholism in terms of the effect of alcohol on the user:

> Alcoholics are those excessive drinkers whose dependence upon alcohol has attained such a degree that it results in noticeable mental disturbance, or in interference with their bodily and mental health, their interpersonal relationships, their smooth social and economic functioning. . . . (Pittman, 1967, p. 4)

Some of the dramatic and concerns that lead patients to admission to the in-patient female alcoholism program are:

1. an enlarged liver
2. acute jaundice
3. a threat of employment termination for excessive absence
4. loss of a driver's license for multiple D.W.I.'s
5. loss of custody of children
6. suicide thoughts or suicidal behavior
7. fear of mental breakdown.

The moderate and severe cases of alcohol addiction that hopefully find their way to a treatment facility are easy for a health care provider to recognize. For example, Marilyn, a nurse and physician's wife came to treatment when she realized that if she drank she could not safely drive, and if she went to the beauty shop without a drink, she would continue shaking violently, a frequent withdrawal symptom. In no way was willpower an issue. This woman was both physically and psychologically addicted.

Whatever affiliations or social connections existed for a woman at the onset of her chemical dependency, they are either weakened drastically or literally disappear. By the time most women come to treatment, they are unlikely to feel positive about their social relationships. Quite often social interaction bounces back and forth between intense arguing and angry withdrawals. Concerns about others fade in importance.

The relationships that are likely to endure the assault of drug abuse are what Eric Fromm labels symbiotic, or maternal. Maternal love is defined by Fromm as the love of the helpless: it is unconditional. Those individuals who continue to support and sustain the alcoholic are likely to take on a maternal role: they judge the female alcoholic as incapable, in need of protection. The motherly love that is most appropriate for children, becomes an enabling factor for the alcoholic, facilitating the denial that a problem does exist.

What many alcoholics cannot enjoy while in the midst of their active chemical dependency is the type of love that is the prerequisite to mature brotherly, or sisterly love; that is, the love between equals. This prerequisite to wholesome adult affiliations is self-love. The female alcoholic is deeply stigmatized. While she is drinking, she is likely to feel both guilty and ashamed about her inability to quit, and also aware of the guilt and shame others place on inebriated women. There are many jokes about drunken sailors, drunken uncles, but none about drunken aunts or sisters. Her self-disgust makes self-love, a sense of integrity, seem almost impossible. How could she love herself, let alone want to care for someone like her?

The absence of sisterly or brotherly love creates two problems. Without an adult-like affiliation, the alcoholic woman is not able to give love. Her attention is away from people and on the substance. Secondly, without the ability to interact, she is removed from the great reward of sisterly or brotherly love, a sense of intimacy, a closeness.

Harry S. Sullivan describes interpersonal intimacy as a situation involving two people which permits validation of all components of personal worth. Each shares in the other's success in maintaining prestige, status, and other forms of integrity (Sullivan, 1953). The alcoholic woman most often comes to treatment with her needs for social intimacy both unrecognized and unfulfilled.

Quite often, she will bring two very potent negative feelings:

1. extreme anger toward the "mothering" caretaker, be it mother, spouse, or child for taking away her sense of freedom; and quite often her former responsibilities;
2. acute loneliness with a sense of not being understood or of being alone, not really close to anyone.

DIFFERENCES BETWEEN MEN AND WOMEN

Early work on alcoholism focused on men. They were more visible, and when a small number of female subjects participated, their responses were often discarded either because they were not in keeping with the male responses or their number was not considered significant (James, 1975).

Only in the past 10-15 years have female alcoholics been studied as a distinct population. Many of the first studies on alcoholism and women contrasted male and female. Cahalan's extremely scholarly work, *American Drinking Practices*, indicated that women generally come into problem drinking at a later age than men (Cahalan et al., 1970). Other studies suggested that women alcoholics are more likely to be depressed, more likely to be dually addicted (Schuckit, 1971). Women are more likely to associate the onset of their dramatic increase in drinking, or loss of control with a specific event, such as a health problem or a domestic situation (Curlee, 1970). Female alcoholism shows a somewhat more telescoped development, the time between regular and problem drinking is shorter (Curlee, 1970). Women are more likely to drink alone at home (Corrigan, 1980) underlining why loneliness is likely to be a greater issue for recovering females.

Women even differ in their physiological response to alcohol: a *British Medical Journal* article offered data supporting the clinical observation that women do develop alcoholic liver disease more readily than men (Saunders et al., 1981). And lastly, and most importantly, while alcoholic men have been studied in terms of their greater need for power, women have been viewed in terms of their affiliation needs and their social roles (Beckman, 1978; Durand, 1975). These many differences in the literature clearly suggest that alcoholic women need to be both studied and treated as a distinct population.

THE RECOVERY PROCESS

Who are the women who find themselves in alcoholism treatment centers? At Merrick Hall we have all economic classes. The average Merrick Hall patient is a woman 42 years of age, the mother of two children, working full time out of the home and earning about $19,000 per year. She graduated from high school. To more precisely understand these figures, it is very important to acknowledge the size of the standard deviation, keeping in mind that one *SD* includes only 66% of the sample. In 35 patients in a study at Merrick that included only women between the ages of 21 and 65, the mean was 41.2, but the *SD* was 10.2. In one typical week, the youngest patient was 15 and the oldest 80. In that same study, the mean household income was $26,652, but once again the *SD* was large ($21,031). Fifty-four percent were married, 8% widowed, 23% divorced, 8% separated and 11% had never been married. They range from women who are illiterate to women with college degrees. There is truly no typical female alcoholic at Merrick Hall.

How do alcoholic women who abstain from alcohol differ significantly from those women who continue their alcoholic drinking? Is the successfully recovered alcoholic female better able to meet her affiliation needs, to feel closely connected to others?

In a recent research project at Merrick Hall, this aspect of recovery was examined using Myrna Weissman's Social Role Adjustment Inventory:

> Social adjustment is broadly defined as the interplay between the individual and the environment. . . . In general terms, social adjustment concerns the individual's ability to function in roles. (Weissman & Paykel, 1974).

This inventory contains 42 questions that measure eight roles: functioning as (1) a worker, (2) housewife, (3) student, (4) social and leisure activities, (5) relationships with extended family, (6) marital roles as a spouse, (7) a parent, and as (8) a member of the family unit. What makes this a particularly powerful instrument in terms of the social role construct, is that both cognitive and behavioral aspects of role performance are addressed.

The research design called for comparing two groups of alcoholic women. Group I were those females between the ages of 21 and 65, just completing their first week of in-patient treatment at Merrick

Hall, Group II women aged 21 to 65 when they participated in the same program one to two years previously. Group II was also presently abstinent and had been successfully recovering. This design was based on the principle of a times-series experiment, more specifically the "simulated before and after design" (Campbell & Stanley, 1963). Using multiple regression analyses and controlling for age, it was predicted that Group II would be significantly better adjusted to their social roles than Group I.

Overall social role adjustment scores differed significantly in the predicted directions. The abstinent recovering group were functioning more successfully in their social roles. *T*-tests on the subscales on the particular roles indicated that four role areas where the differences were significant were: (1) homemaker, (2) social and leisure time, (3) extended family, and (4) family unit. Marital adjustment is conspicuously absent. Quite often a shaky marriage falls apart after recovery begins. At times the husband retreats because he no longer has a totally dependent, helpless wife, and is confused by her new sober self. Often the husband is alcoholic and not interested in his own abstinence, and the wife feels she must choose between marriage and recovery. Of course, some marriages endure and improve with recovery.

Quite often it is the improvement or creation of healthy female relationships that is the foundation of solid recovery. This is suggested by the Social Role Adjustment Inventory categories of extended family and spare time and leisure. The recovery expectation is not to make women less concerned with men, but rather to recognize and enjoy wholesome interdependency with women, as a prophylactic for unwholesome overdependency on men.

A case study that nicely illustrates this issue is Ellen. Following her hospitalization, she came with her husband for a counseling session. She complained of loneliness. Her husband strongly disagreed.

> It was impossible for his 52 year old wife to be lonely. She had a son in Boston, a daughter in an Ohio college, and of course he was living with her and he did indeed love her. "You can't be lonely," he declared. With several well-phrased questions, he did acknowledge his affiliation needs for men were met through his employment.
>
> If this patient, Ellen, is to maintain her sobriety, she will probably maintain her 30 year marriage, but just as impor-

tantly, she will have to move away from all of her friends, to only a few special friends with whom she can develop that sense of intimacy and closeness that will reinforce her self-love and give her a positive sense of herself that only relation-ships, not alcohol, can do.

This case illustrates that male relationships may be of great sig-nificance, but without healthy female affiliations, women may be-come first totally dependent, then terribly resentful toward the men who care for rather than respect them. Female affiliations are likely to offer women a sense of dignity that is essential to an alcohol-free maturity.

This is a new social model for recovery that hopefully accommo-dates the changing social roles women are experiencing. Today the average woman spends 41% of her adult life without children at home, and 23% of her adulthood without either children or a hus-band living with her.

The old model of adjusting to wife and mother roles is incomplete (Frieze et al., 1978). Many women in treatment are:

1. changing from being married and being at home to becoming divorced and unemployed;
2. changing from having no children at home to having children returning in their mid to late twenties;
3. changing from being a traditional homemaker to becoming a widow;
4. changing from low stress, routine work to an exciting, high pressure career.

In these times, women are being encouraged to expand their role options, to move beyond the home to academic, business, and in-dustrial settings. While this may be a positive step to help redefine values, life-styles, and self-images, it may also place the patient in limbo while she is facing some indecisions.

The alcohol beverage industry obviously recognizes the potential for increased sales brought about by this very role change. High power advertising is geared toward the young, upwardly mobile woman (Corrigan, 1980; Sandmaier, 1980). Increased alcohol con-sumption is certainly more likely by the young, ambitious females of the '80s. One might argue that Grandma was just more subtle and used alcoholic patent medicines, but Grandma was not as vulnerable. She was probably not medicating an identity crisis, an impending divorce, or a career change.

Therefore, changing social roles present both an aspect of recovery and a threat to conventional treatment approaches. Getting better does not mean being more conventional or being more radical, it does mean being more realistic about where a woman has been and where she would like to go. It is an approach rooted to understanding a woman as she is today.

Treatment does not simply mean rehabilitation, restoring to a former state of well-being. Rather, the social rehabilitation model for problem drinkers stresses attaining a state of mental and physical health not previously experienced. This "better than before" approach includes more meaningful relationships. The improved existing relationships are often with family members, fellow employees, neighbors. The new affiliations are likely to begin with members of the treatment staff, A.A. sponsors, A.A. members, and then others in the broader community. The female alcoholic who manages to abstain for several years and fulfills her affiliation needs becomes a bright ray of hope for those who have worried and wondered, is recovery truly possible? Yes, it is.

In conclusion, the components of female alcoholism are related to affiliation needs in a dramatic way: the woman who is rapidly moving through the phases of addiction loses both a sense of herself and her sense of being related to others. The treatment process must and can directly address this critical problem.

REFERENCES

Beckman, L. J. (1978). Sex role conflict in alcoholic women: myth or reality. *Journal of Abnormal Psychology, 87*, 408-417.

Cahalan, D., Cisin, R. & Crossley, H. (1970). *American drinking practice.* New Haven, CT: College and University Press.

Campbell, D. & Stanely, J. C. (1963). *Experimental and quasi-experimental designs for research.* Chicago: Rand McNally.

Corrigan, E. (1980). *Alcoholic women in treatment.* New York: Oxford University Press.

Curlee, J. (1970). A comparison of male and female patients at an alcoholism treatment center. *Journal of Psychology, 74*, 239-247.

Durand, D. E. (1975). Effects of drinking on the power and affiliation needs of middle-aged females. *Journal of Clinical Psychology, 3*, 549-553.

Frieze, E., Parsons, J., Johnson, R., Ruble, D. & Zellman, G. (1978). *Women and sex roles: A social psychological perspective.* New York: W. W. Norton.

James, J. E. (1975). Symptoms of alcoholism in women: A preliminary survey of A.A. members. *Journal of Studies on Alcohol, 36,* 1564-1569.

Pittman, D. (Ed.) (1967). *Alcoholism.* New York: Harper & Row.

Sandmaier, M. (1980). *The invisible alcoholics: women and alcohol abuse in America.* New York: McGraw-Hill.

Saunders, J. B., Davis, M. & Williams, R. (1981). Do women develop alcoholic liver disease more readily than men? *British Medical Journal, 282,* 1140-1143.

Schuckit, M. (1971). Depression and alcoholism in women. *Proceedings of the First Annual Alcoholism Conference of the National Institute of Alcohol Abuse and Alcoholism.* Washington, DC.

Sullivan, H. S. (1953). *The interpersonal theory of psychiatry.* New York: W. W. Norton.

Weissman, M. & Paykel, E.(1974). *The depressed woman.* Chicago: University of Chicago Press.

Mental Health:
The Elizabeth Stone
House Alternative

Ann Beckert

Women have not been effectively served by the mental health system. Despite the hard work of individual psychiatrists, psychologists, and social workers, the needs of many women in emotional distress are not always met by traditional mental health services. Most theories of mental health and methods of achieving this health have been developed by men. While women have been involved in this still developing field, our involvement has been disproportionately small, particularly when one considers that the majority of mental health consumers are women. Because psychiatry is based upon a patriarchal definition of the healthy adult, it is virtually impossible for a woman to live her life as a woman and be viewed as healthy. Affordable alternatives like the Elizabeth Stone House must be created which recognize the stresses women face and which help them overcome their feelings of isolation. In addition to therapy, women need to establish support systems through the accomplishment of practical goals. For the past twelve years, the Elizabeth Stone House has been run by women to provide women in emotional distress with a Therapeutic Community, a structured peer support system which helps to alleviate societal factors causing or contributing to a woman's distress. Such a community can complement and enhance other therapeutic systems and relationships. With the primary goal of preventing institutionalization, the program's success is evidenced by its low rate of recidivism. At a time when

The author is Coordinator of Direct Services, Stone House, since 1982 and Program Administrator, Stone House, since 1983. Her special interests are alternative approaches to mental health.

323

affordable and effective mental health services are becoming increasingly difficult to find, all of us must work together to establish and support such alternatives.

A woman's mental health can be directly related to the amount of stress with which she must cope solely because she is a woman. Sexism, racism, classism, and homophobia are often manifested against women in violent forms, such as rape, incest, child abuse, and battering. Additional stress occurs for single mothers and for poor women who are unable to financially provide for themselves and for their families. This stress is compounded by the fact that supportive, therapeutic services are not accessible to women without money. Historically, women have been "treated" for their poverty and abuse rather than provided with support, solutions, and the reassurance that they are not to blame. Child welfare agencies become involved when the children are seen as "at risk" because of the mother's poverty and craziness. Many of these agencies do little to actually alleviate the stressors in the woman's life.

Twelve years ago, poor women looking for alternatives to these traditional settings had no options. Admittance into hospitals and half-way houses meant loss of control over their own lives. Additionally, mothers had to find other homes for their children or had to relinquish custody of their children to child welfare and state agencies. Once involved with these systems, mothers found that they had little control over their children's lives as well and, in fact, had difficulty getting that control back. This situation added further stress to a woman's life. exacerbating her own level of distress.

In 1974, a group of former mental patients and mental health professionals met at the "Women and Madness" Conference held in Cambridge, Massachusetts. These women recognized a need to provide an alternative mode of treatment for women in emotional distress. Led by Mary Rafini, these women founded the Elizabeth Stone House, a Therapeutic Community which recognized the correlation between the amount of stress in a woman's life and the amount of distress she experienced. The program was founded and continues to operate today with the primary goal of preventing institutionalization. In an atmosphere of peer support, women were able to work towards the accomplishment of practical goals while increasing their support networks, improving their self esteem, and regaining their dignity. Societal causes of distress were absent in the Community setting. The program was named for Elizabeth Stone, a 19th century woman who was unjustly committed to an institution by her family because of her desire to change her religious denomination.

Today, the Elizabeth Stone House operates a five month residential, feminist, mental health alternative for women in emotional distress and their children. The program operates with the same founding goal of preventing institutionalization and with the same founding principle of self-help in an atmosphere of peer support. During a woman's stay, she outlines and works towards the achievement of her own goals which may include establishing financial resources, pursuing vocational and or educational degrees, developing parenting skills, and locating safe and affordable housing. The program is not staffed twenty-four hours a day in order to ensure that program residents will turn to one another for support and in order to place primary responsibility for a woman's life onto the woman herself. Direct service staff work as advocates, not therapists, helping women cope with the societal systems which often add to their level of distress. These advocates help women outline goals and develop plans to achieve these goals. Staff will not complete these tasks however, and in actuality, will offer only the minimum amount of assistance needed. Mothers may bring their children with them, keeping the family together, thereby minimizing the amount of trauma both mother and child experience with forced separation. The program fee is modest, making it affordable to poor women. All staff and volunteers are women. These factors make the Elizabeth Stone House the only program like it in the country.

For some women, the treatments received in the traditional mental health system are a necessary step towards emotional stability, providing these women with the needed structure and supervision. For others, however, these programs exacerbate the woman's level of distress as mental health is still defined in patriarchal terms. The woman receives a psychiatric label which does not take into account the specific experiences she may have suffered. Because treatment plans are based upon these labels, treatment plans often ignore the very issues which created the distress. The diagnostic label, by its nature, views distress as internally oriented rather than created by external circumstances, reinforcing the viewpoint that the victim is somehow the problem. It does not address the reality that the woman may be reacting very normally to situations brutally thrust upon her. As the mental health professional and the patient are encouraged by the system to think of the woman as her label, the image of Individual Identity begins to diminish. The patient is no longer held accountable for irrational or inappropriate behavior. Acting out behaviors, depressions, mood swings, and hallucinations are treated with medication. The patient is informed that her continued treatment will depend upon this medication and little time is spent exploring other options or discussing the effects of the medication. Because the woman is now labeled as crazy, it is assumed that she is unable to make decisions about treatment and need not be informed about treatment side effects. The woman is no longer treated with dignity. Upon discharge, many women find that they have lost their families, friends, and their homes. They have nowhere to go and no money. The safety and security that they may have found in the hospital setting is gone as the patient is forced to terminate with therapists and leave other patients who were able to be empathetic and supportive.

The failure of the mental health system to adequately provide for women, particularly poor women, is not due to the total absence of caring and competent professionals. Many of these individuals are overworked and underpaid. State hospitals are overcrowded. Forced medication and the use of restraints are often hastily employed to guarantee the safety of the problematic, acting out patients or the other patients on the unit. The lack of time and resources make it virtually impossible for mental health professionals to adequately address the needs of women in emotional distress. Additionally, these professionals have been trained to deal with pathologies. They look to correct what they perceive as psychological weaknesses. This viewpoint only reinforces the concept that the woman is somehow at fault; that if she did not have this weakness, she would cope better.

The fifty women who come to the Elizabeth Stone House yearly are looking for an alternative to a hospital or a half-way house. Many of the women have already been hospitalized several times. Some are homeless or are living in temporary shelters. All are looking for more support than independent living can provide. Other common characteristics include feelings of depression, helplessness, and hopelessness with little hope for the future and no self esteem. Almost 90% of the women are living below poverty level and almost 95% have been victims of violence. More than half are taking psychoactive medications and many have been diagnosed with chronic and severe psychiatric disorders. Most of the program mothers have lost custody, at least temporarily, of their children.

Many have been involved in a variety of therapies with a variety of mental health professionals.

The women who apply to the Elizabeth Stone House are looking to regain control over their own lives. Acceptance into the program is contingent upon a woman's ability to identify goals and to make a commitment to work towards the completion of those goals. Because of the lack of constant supervision, women who are actively suicidal or prone to violence, women who cannot self medicate, and active substance abusers are not eligible for acceptance. In 1985, over half the women entering Stone House had histories of suicide attempts, 50% were on psychiatric medication, and almost 25% had histories of substance abuse. In order to be accepted into the program, however, women need to make a commitment to maintain a violence-free (including self inflicted) and drug-free atmosphere. Women who have been suicidal, therefore, need to be able to verbalize a viable plan to prevent future suicide attempts. Alcohol and drug abusers are required to attend community support groups which specifically address these issues. Most importantly, women are encouraged to make educated decisions about their involvement in therapy and their use of medication.

Intake into the Stone House is a three step procedure. Interested women call to place their names on a waiting list. Staff and volunteers discuss the program directly with the caller and conduct a very basic phone screening. Because the wait period is usually six to eight weeks, prospective residents must call back weekly in order to keep their names on the list. This system allows intake staff to assess a woman's level of motivation while it places the responsibility of acceptance onto the applicant herself, the beginning of self help. When a woman's name reaches the top of list, an interview with two intake staff is scheduled. It is during this interview that the woman will discuss in more detail her own history and goals. Staff acceptance depends upon an assessment of how well the applicant will be able to benefit from Stone House and upon the need to create a community among the residents. The key to the Therapeutic Community's success is that no one individual is isolated because of who she is or because of her problems. Conversely, diversifying the types of women and their problems and patterns of coping helps to combat internalized racism, classism, and homophobia by exposing residents to others different from themselves. Additionally, it helps to prevent the reinforcement of destructive patterns of coping. In order to heal, a woman needs to have the support of others who have experienced the same event or feeling. Women who have been labeled as crazy are able to be supportive and to learn from honest and direct feedback. This process enables them to take control over their own lives. No woman is accepted into the Stone House Therapeutic Community without the knowledge that this acceptance will demand that she treats all other residents, volunteers, and staff respectfully. Final acceptance into the program depends upon an interview with program residents. Current residents are asked to assess an applicant's willingness to live in the community setting. This process also allows the applicant to get a sense of the existing community and to make an educated decision about whether or not she wants to be part of the program.

Once accepted, a woman meets with her staff advocate to outline, in more detail, her goals. A budget is devised and women with no income are helped to develop legitimate means of getting one. Referrals are made. Residents continue to meet with their advocates weekly to evaluate their own progress towards their own goals. Additionally, all residents attend two housemeetings per week where chores are assigned, announcements are made, and issues or topics of general interest are discussed. A "Mothers' Meeting" is held one afternoon per week which deals with parenting issues and skills and is mandatory for all women who have custody or are working to regain custody of their children.

All policies and rules have been established to guarantee that the Therapeutic Community remain a safe and supportive environment for all of its residents. While living in the Stone House, no one is allowed to drink or to use any drugs other than those individually prescribed. Residents are expected to behave respectfully and responsibly. For example, although there is a midnight curfew, residents may be late provided that they call to prevent other residents from worrying needlessly. Overnights out on weekends are allowed, again provided that other residents have been informed. Residents are expected to keep current with program fees and to do assigned chores daily. Everyone must be working towards the accomplishment of their goals and mothers are expected to care for their children without the use of physical punishment. Any serious infraction of program policies may result in a resident being asked to leave. No one is allowed to remain in the program if she is at risk to herself or to others.

The children who enter the Stone House have experienced or witnessed some familial turmoil or trauma. Upon intake, direct service staff work with mothers, asses the child's needs, and to devise a goal plan. Often, the child's primary need is a stable living situation. Referrals are made to local pediatricians, day care centers, and school programs. Children are also referred to child therapists for testing and counseling, when appropriate. Because children do not always move into the program at the same time as their mothers or because they have experienced periods of separation, staff work with both mother and child to help them adjust to being together again. Mothers sometimes are in need of developing their parenting skills and referrals are thus made to local parenting groups. Because the parent-child interaction can be observed on a daily basis, staff can work effectively with resident mothers to assist them in understanding issues that effect their style of parenting and in improving skills as needed.

On a daily basis, individual schedules can vary greatly. While some of the mothers remain home with their children, other residents attend vocational or educational programs, hold part time or full time jobs, or attend day treatment programs. Appointments with therapists, doctors, or dentists are scheduled around these other daily routines. While group dinners are planned four nights per week, attendance is strongly encouraged but is not mandatory due to the varying schedules. Attendance at the Mother's Meeting and at the two housemeetings is mandatory, however. Much time and energy is spent looking for and securing adequate housing. Unfortunately, this task is taking more and more time as the availability of safe and affordable housing becomes increasingly scarce. For this reason, women are encouraged to look for or to create group living situations. Many residents look for housing together.

It is important to emphasize that each resident is responsible for the completion of her own goals. For example, staff will not locate an apartment for an exiting resident. Rather, staff will work with the resident to help her secure her apartment by keeping her informed about the location of subsidized housing, by teaching her how to read the apartment classifieds, and by role playing with her the interview with the landloard. This emphasis on self help strengthens the woman by giving her power and control over her own life. Her level of confidence and her self esteem improve. Goals that require work to achieve are ones that the woman will have a vested interest in maintaining.

The Therapeutic Community is not immune to crises. Children do get sick, accidents do happen, and policies are broken. Self de-

structive patterns cannot always be altered in a few short months.
Residents are taught to deal with these crisis situations, stressing
that if they were living independently of a program, they would
have to take the responsibility of handling difficult situations. Residents, therefore, call ambulances or taxis when sick or injured residents have to get immediate medical care. The police are called
when necessary. Only after this first step has been completed or is
ruled out as a necessary action is staff called through an on-call
beeper system. The staff will then assess and follow through with
whatever steps are needed to guarantee the safety and security of the
program and all of its residents. Common actions may include a few
words of encouragement to the depressed and potentially suicidal
resident or it may include helping a resident relocate to another
program or setting.

The success of the program is evidenced in its statistics. Data is
collected on each resident four times throughout an eleven month
period, beginning at intake and ending at a point six months following her exit. Situations and goals are noted as is the progress towards these goals. Additionally, less scientific but equally as important is a woman's evaluation of her own level of confidence, self
esteem, and motivation and an assessment of her support network.
Improvements in all of these areas is obvious. The rate of recidivism is extremely low.

As mentioned earlier, one reason for the success of the program is
the emphasis on self help. Goals one personally achieves are usually
maintained before goals accomplished by others. Additionally, by
living in the Therapeutic Community, women can establish real
friendships. Feelings of isolation dissipate as experiences of poverty, abuse, and hospitalization are shared. For women who are in
therapy, success can also be correlated to the complimentary relationship between the Stone House and the services provided by the
mental health system. Women in therapy return home to a supportive environment which helps them to process without judgement
insights they might have had. While understanding the reasons behind certain defenses and behaviors, they can turn to their peers to
assess how their behaviors effect others. This honest feedback is
particularly crucial when one is deciding upon the uses of medication. Experiences repressed for years, such as incest, can surface in
an environment where others are sharing similar horrors and learning that they are not to blame. While therapy can aid the woman in
understanding her feelings and reactions, the woman can be assured

that she will not be alone in her anger and her grief when she leaves her therapist's office. Conversely, unlike a hospital or halfway house, the woman is able to physically remove herself from the therapist and from the immediacy of feelings evoked by the therapeutic process. These factors allow for more healing to occur in a shorter period of time.

The Elizabeth Stone House helps women to see that the roots of their distress are not internal. Additionally, the immediate feedback a resident is given for her behavior helps her to see the consequences of her actions. Behavior is seen as personal, not theoretical. For example, residents are helped to see that they cannot behave in a racist or homophobic manner because it is hurtful, not because they are judged for feeling racist or homophobic. By living within the diverse community, these women are helped to see that their prejudices are often rooted in ignorance through lack of exposure or through generalized experiences. Feedback for crazy behavior can also help the resident understand the effects of her behavior on those around her. Such feedback can help the woman function more effectively and thus cope better with daily tasks and with her own craziness.

At any given time, the Stone House houses eight to ten women and three to six children. There are nine staff, five full time and four part time. Of these, three full time and two part time are direct service staff. Although all direct service staff and volunteers advocate for program residents, each staff member also has a specific function built into her job description. Of the three full-time direct service staff, one is specifically responsible for training and supervising the twelve volunteers, one is responsible for assisting program residents with parenting, and one is responsible for providing housing advocacy to all program residents. The two part time positions are for a general direct service advocate and for a worker who is responsible for assessing the resident children's needs. The other four staff positions include a full-time fundraiser, a full-time administrator, a part-time bookkeeper, and a part-time outreach worker.

The Elizabeth Stone House is run under a shared administrative model. The full-time staff are ultimately responsible for the administrative and fiscal management of the program. All policy and programatic decisions are made by a consensus decision-making process which includes all staff who work at least half-time. Unlike a collective, each staff member has very clear job responsibilities and carries out those tasks within the framework of the program's per-

sonnel policies and objectives. Staff are hired to reflect the target
population; therefore life experiences are considered to be as valuable as professional training.

The Elizabeth Stone House is not perfect. Intake workers may
incorrectly assess a woman's level of depression and tendencies towards suicide. One serious suicide attempt may trigger several others, particularly if the Therapeutic Community is "weighted" with
depressed women. One alcoholic who may be unable to stay sober
without more supervision may influence another to drink as well.
Programmatically, decisions are sometimes difficult to make when
six or seven strong minded women sit down to express their opinions. While staff benefits are excellent, salaries are below what human service professionals should be paid.

The Elizabeth Stone House survives its imperfections. Its survival is largely due to the commitment of its Board and staff and to
the continual support and encouragement of former staff and residents. The indisputable recognition that the program provides a
valuable service keeps it solvent and prosperous. It is absolutely
crucial that others recognize a need for alternatives and recognize
that any service provided to any target population cannot truly succeed if it disempowers that population. The Stone House works by
recognizing that societal stressors leave women more vulnerable to
distress. By removing the blame and isolation, women are able to
heal and to regain control over their own lives. The cycle of craziness could happen to anyone. Over the past twelve years, the Elizabeth Stone House has provided 1200 women and children with a
means to break that cycle.

The Women's Clinic:
A Viable Psychiatric Clinic
in the Canadian Context

Elaine Borins

Established in 1980, the Women's Clinic is the first women's psychiatric clinic to be incorporated within a general teaching hospital in Canada and the first to be staffed entirely by women. Although the notion of women providing health care treatment for women is as old as recorded history, in today's predominantly patriarchal and hierarchal society, where women function as a disadvantaged majority, conceptual and practical changes were necessary in order to make possible the development of the Women's Clinic, which is one of several specialized divisions of the department of psychiatry at the Toronto Western Hospital (Ehrenreich & English, 1973).

THE HOSPITAL

The Toronto Western Hospital is one of the large (650 beds) teaching hospitals affiliated with the University of Toronto. Twenty-eight (28) beds in the hospital are assigned to the department of psychiatry, and there are six full time and eight part time

The author is a psychiatrist who is Director of the Women's Clinic, Department of Psychiatry, University of Toronto, Toronto Western Hospital.

The Women's Clinic uses intake, family history and information forms which elicit important information from women which is not always elicited by interviewers. For copies of the forms, please write to Elaine Borins, MD, Women's Clinic, Edith Cavell Wing Floor 1B, Toronto Western Hospital, 399 Bathurst Street, Toronto, Canada M5T 2S8.

The author wishes to thank Dr. Harvey Moldofsky for support and encouragement, Ms. Jennifer Borins and Ms. Dianne Srutwa for assistance with the manuscript.

Preparation of this article was supported by a Clarke Research Foundation Grant.

psychiatric staff. The department of psychiatry also includes seven psychiatric residents and participants in a rotational program for family practice residents, interns and clinical clerks. Also, educational programs are provided through the department of psychiatry to undergraduate nurses, occupational therapists, medical students and postgraduate research fellows (Kline & Moldofsky, 1986).

Approximately 80 percent of income supporting the department of psychiatry's medical staff at the Toronto Western Hospital is derived from Ontario Provincial Health Insurance Plan reimbursement. As well, about 20 percent of the department of psychiatry's general income is derived from the University of Toronto. The Toronto Western Hospital pays for the services of nurses, psychologists and social workers, through provincial and federal funding to the hospital (Kline & Moldofsky, 1986).

The fact that the services of non medically trained health care professionals are not covered under the health insurance plan in Ontario makes it extremely difficult financially to develop psychiatric clinics with interdisciplinary staff outside the hospital setting. The experience of the Women's Clinic has shown that the effective operation of a psychiatric clinic for women depends on the collaboration of professionals such as psychiatrists, psychologists, psychiatric nurse clinicians and social workers.

THE CLINIC

The Women's Clinic was formed in 1980 in the ambulatory area of the Toronto Western Hospital. The clinic is a product of the growth in the past thirty years of general hospital psychiatry (Lipowski, 1967). Specifically, the clinic is a product of the development in 1979 of specialized services within the department of psychiatry.

Like each specialized division of the department of psychiatry at the Toronto Western Hospital, the Women's Clinic was given seed money by the department in its first year of operation. Thereafter, however, the Clinic assumed fiscal responsibility for its own growth and expansion. While the clinic is responsible to the department of psychiatry as a whole, and while it is subject to a system of evaluation, it has been given free range to develop its own policy with respect to service and research.

The Clinic also has the freedom to develop its own policy concerning education and academic links. In this regard, the association of the Toronto Western Hospital with the University of Toronto has had advantages for the Clinic. In addition to the educational enrichment provided by the association, the university has allowed a resident in psychiatry to participate in the Clinic as part of the resident's psychiatric training program. This has allowed the Women's Clinic to grow through the training of new female psychiatrists. In general, the Clinic has been a very popular choice for psychiatric residents who spend from six months to one year of their training at the Clinic.

Conceptually, the clinic is a product of the new psychology of woman, a body of knowledge derived in part from a large body of research conducted in the 1970s (Seiden, 1976a; Seiden, 1976b). The new psychology of woman focuses on sex as an important variable in clinical psychiatry and psychobiological research (Seiden, 1979).

With the emergence of this relatively new body of knowledge has come the realization of the existence of a sexist bias in psychiatry with respect to the treatment of female patients. For example, conditions specific to the lives of women, such as childbirth, sexual abuse or poverty, have traditionally been ignored (Carmen, Notman & Nadelson, 1978, Russo & Miller, 1981). As well, it has become apparent that female psychiatric patients are often overtreated with mind altering drugs, in a manner which tends to reinforce the relative powerlessness of an individual woman's position (Russo, 1985).

Despite the formulation of a body of knowledge loosely defined here as the psychology of woman, and with its growth, a recognition of women as health care consumers of status, the structural changes necessary to formally recognize the latter notion have been slow to develop. To date, limited effort has been made in Canada to relate the new psychology of woman to the investigation and treatment of women's psychiatric disorders in a general hospital setting. The Women's Clinic at the Toronto Western hospital is an attempt to fill this need (Borins & Forsythe, 1985).

OBJECTIVES

The staff at the Women's Clinic includes two part time psychiatrists, a full time psychiatric nursing clinician, a part time social worker and a psychiatric resident. The staffing policy represents a deliberate attempt to respond to requests of patients as consumers to consult professionals of their own sex.

From the outset, the general objectives of the two sections of the Clinic, namely the outpatient and consultative services, have been to study and manage:

1. the traumas of female life, including sexual assault, sexual abuse, physical abuse and incest;
2. the normal and pathological responses to biological events, such as menstruation, pregnancy, childbirth, contraception and menopause; and
3. the psychiatric implications of gynecological and surgical procedures for women, including abortion, hysterectomy, mastectomy and sterilization (Borins & Forsythe, 1985).

The growth of the consultative service section of the Women's Clinic has been influenced by the general directions taken by the Toronto Western Hospital and the particular interests of the medical and surgical disciplines. The consultative service operates within the hospital in the following areas:

a. abortion and sterilization counselling (approximately two thousand induced therapeutic abortions are performed each year at the Toronto Western Hospital)
b. hysterectomy counselling
c. consultations concerning eating disorders, primarily obesity and morbid obesity.

The psychiatric nurse clinician and the psychiatric resident have been particularly involved in the consultation service aspect of the Women's Clinic. As well, students training in the Women's Clinic from the departments of psychology, social work and nursing have participated in the consultation service, especially in the areas of abortion and sterilization counselling.

The outpatient component of the Women's Clinic has primarily developed as a result of four main decisions made by the Clinic's staff collectively when the service was initiated in 1980. They are as follows:

1. Self Referral

The outpatient aspect of the Clinic decided to accept women who are self referred, as well as those who are referred in the more traditional manner of referral by a psychiatric, public health nurse, or social agency. This decision represents an attempt to deal directly with women as health care consumers.

The result has been that approximately 32 percent of the women attending the outpatient service are self referred. A comparison study of the professionally referred and self referred populations has revealed no significant differences between the two groups. As the vast majority of women accepted for treatment in the clinic decides to attend, it would appear that the women using the Clinic's service know what they want in terms of mental health care; that is, they are an educated consumer group (Borins, 1981).

2. Intake Procedure

The second decision involves an intake procedure that constitutes an initial screening for all women applying to the Clinic. This procedure essentially involves each prospective patient completing a lengthy information form.

This procedure has allowed the Clinic to accumulate a large amount of data concerning demographic information, family history, health history and personal data past and present. We have discovered that certain areas, such as physical and sexual abuse, which are difficult to approach informatively by indirect questioning, are best approached directly in the manner of questions in the context of the intake form. A further asset of the intake form is the fact that asking a patient to write down information concerning her own history, such as incidents of trauma and her family background, encourages the patient to address these issues in a manner that aids assessment and therapy.

In summary, in addition to providing the Clinic staff with instructive information concerning a patient's general medical history, the intake form is a source of information about chronic and pervasive conditions as well as areas of acute stress, particular of women's lives. One product of the intake form procedure has been the development of a data bank which aids members of the Clinic in their investigation of specific aspects of women's mental health and allows the development of related research programmes.

3. Expertise

The third decision in forming the outpatient service was that each member of the service would focus on particular areas of interest in women's mental health. Patients with particular difficulties are, therefore, referred to the staff member who works mainly in the area associated with the difficulty in question. This has allowed a gradual development of expertise in particular health care areas and has facilitated the education and development of each staff member.

4. Modality of Treatment

The fourth decision was to focus on a particular modality of treatment which utilized the particular training and ability of each member of the Clinic staff. The treatment specifically employed is insight-oriented, brief psychodynamic therapy (Malan, 1979; Sifneos, 1972).

The patient population has proven to be well suited to this form of therapy. The patient population is comprised primarily of women between 25 and 45 years of age. According to DSM III criteria, the population is socially adaptive, with 89 percent operating in the fair to superior range (Borins & Forsythe, 1981). Seventy-seven (77) percent of the women presenting are under at least moderate stress. Less than one percent of women coming to the Clinic have a psychotic disorder. The modality of treatment chosen reveals that the Clinic is not and does not purport to be a crisis service.

PRELIMINARY OBSERVATIONS

Preliminary observations include the identification in the presenting population of at least three groups of women with a high risk factor for psychiatric illness. They are as follows:

1. a group with a history of trauma, including physical and/or sexual abuse, serious operations and injuries;
2. a group with a history that includes the death of a family member, occurring before the patient reached the age of 18 years; and
3. a group with a family history of chronic illness in a parent, sibling or spouse.

Preliminary observations also include the identification of women seeking treatment primarily for sex specific matters such as abortion, sterilization and gynecological problems.

Clinic members have developed the ability to relate specifically to the needs of the Clinic's patient population. For instance, after completing the intake form, patients who indicate having experienced incidents of trauma complete a more detailed trauma self report inventory. This is followed by clinical interviews with the patient that address, among other issues, the issues of trauma in general and physical and sexual abuse specifically. Clinic members have observed that traumatic incidents occurring early in a woman's life can be expressed later in life in terms of post-traumatic sequelae, both physical and psychological; for example, high stress levels, abortion and sterilization. We have also observed that the early death of a parent or sibling is significantly associated with a request for sterilization.

Data derived from our intake form reveals inter-generational connections between abuses, abortions, stillbirths and other gynecological trauma. Inter-generational repetition of these events is particularly striking.

Finally, a significant proportion of women seen at the Clinic have experienced chronic illnesses personally or in their families. We have observed connections between chronic illness and drug and alcohol related difficulties. We have speculated that sex role expectations and socialization roles of caring for the ill place a particular burden on women in families.

CONCLUSION

The observations noted above suggest that further research based on our preliminary observations will prove worthwhile. In addition to the fact that the Women's Clinic is overwhelmed by applicants for treatment (since the Clinic opened, 1,094 women have applied), a number of other facts suggest that clinically the women's psychiatric treatment center at the Toronto Western Hospital has been a success.

The fact that a large number of the women attending at the Clinic are self referred indicates that the Clinic answers the needs of many female health care consumers. Many women who enter the Clinic have had previous psychiatric care, and many request that the care

a

they receive at the Clinic be provided exclusively by female staff. We, therefore, believe that the guarantee of all-female care has contributed to the overwhelming demand for the Clinic's services. In all probability, our method of treatment, which focuses on psychodynamic therapy, emphasizing greater awareness of conditions specific to an individual woman's life, both in the past and in the present, also contributes to the demand for the Clinic's services.

The psychiatric Women's Clinic located within a general hospital has evolved specific outpatient and consultative areas of expertise. That the Clinic is successful as a treatment center, adaptive to the particular social and economic aspects of Canadian health care delivery is shown by the fact that other university hospitals in Canada have adopted the Clinic as a viable method of delivering health care.

REFERENCES

Borins E. F. M. & Forsythe, P. (1985). Past trauma and present functioning of patients attending a women's psychiatric clinic. *American Journal of Psychiatry, 142*(4), 460-463.

Borins, E. (1981). The women's clinic: At the frontiers of psychiatry. *Canadian Medical Association Journal, 123*, 774-775.

Carmen, E. H., Russo, N. F. & Miller. J. B. (1981). Inequality and women's mental health: An overview. *American Journal of Psychiatry, 138*, 1319-1330.

Ehrenreich, B. & English, D. (1973). *Witches, midwives and nurses*. New York: The Feminist Press.

Kline, S. A., Moldofsky, H. (1986). Fiscal and service analysis in general hospital psychiatry. Unpublished manuscript.

Lipowski, Z. L. (1967). Review of consultation psychiatry and psychosomatic medicine, I: general principles. *Psychosomatic Medicine, 29*, 153-171.

Malan, D. M. (1979). *Individual Psychotherapy and the Science of Psychodynamics*. Toronto: Butterworths.

Notman, M. T. & Nadelson, C. C. (1978). *The Woman Patient, Medical and Psychological Interfaces, Vol. I: Sexual and Reproductive Aspects of Women's Health Care*. New York: Plenum.

Russo, N. F. (1985). Developing a national agenda to address women's mental health needs: a conference report. American Psychological Association.

Seiden, A. M. (1979). General differences in psychobiological illness. In: Gomberg, E. S., Franks, V. (eds.), *Gender and Disordered Behavior: Sex Differences in Psycho-pathology*. New York: Brunner/Mazel.

Seiden, A. M. (1976a). Overview: Research on the psychology of women. In Gender differences and sexual and reproductive life. *American Journal of Psychiatry, 133*, 995-1007.

Seiden, A. M. (1976b). Overview: Research on the psychology of women, II: Women in families, work and psychotherapy. *American Journal of Psychiatry, 133*, 1111-1123.

Sifneos, P. E. (1972). *Short Term Psychotherapy and Emotional Crisis*. Cambridge: Harvard University Press.